Classic Papers in Rheumatology

Classic Papers in Rheumatology

Edited by

Paul Dieppe
Director, MRC Health Services Research Collaboration,
Department of Social Medicine, University of Bristol, Bristol, UK

H Ralph Schumacher, Jr
Professor of Medicine, University of Pennsylvania,
Chief of Rheumatology, VA Medical Center, Philadelphia, USA

Frank A Wollheim
Professor, Lund University Hospital,
Lund, Sweden

First published in the United Kingdom in 2002
by Martin Dunitz Ltd, The Livery House, 7–9 Pratt Street, London NW1 0AE

Tel: +44 (0) 20 74822202
Fax: +44 (0) 20 72670159
E-mail: info@dunitz.co.uk
Website: http://www.dunitz.co.uk

Although every effort has been made to ensure that all owners of copyright material have been acknowledged in this publication, we would be glad to acknowledge in subsequent reprints or editions any omissions brought to our attention.

Although every effort has been made to ensure that drug doses and other information are presented accurately in this publication, the ultimate responsibility rests with the prescribing physician. Neither the publishers nor the authors can be held responsible for errors or for any consequences arising from the use of information contained herein. For detailed prescribing information or instructions on the use of any product or procedure discussed herein, please consult the prescribing information or instructional material issued by the manufacturer.

A CIP record for this book is available from the British Library.

ISBN 1–901865–48–7

Distributed in the USA by
Fulfilment Center
Taylor & Francis
7625 Empire Drive
Florence, KY 41042, USA
Toll Free Tel: +1 800 634 7064
E-mail: cserve@routledge_ny.com

Distributed in Canada by
Taylor & Francis
74 Rolark Drive
Scarborough, Ontario M1R 4G2, Canada
Toll Free Tel: +1 877 226 2237
E-mail: tal_fran@istar.ca

Distributed in the rest of the world by
ITPS Limited
Cheriton House
North Way
Andover, Hampshire SP10 5BE, UK
Tel: +44 (0)1264 332424
E-mail: reception@itps.co.uk

Project management, design and layout: Top Draw Design

Printed and bound in Spain by Grafos SA

Contents

Section 3: Regional and Miscellaneous Disorders

Section 4: Therapy

Contributors

Adewale Adebajo
Consultant Rheumatologist and Honorary Senior Lecturer, Division of Genomic Medicine, The University of Sheffield, Royal Hallamshire Hospital, Sheffield, UK

†Barbara Ansell

Nicholas Bellamy
Professor, Director of CONROD and Chair of Rehabilitation Medicine, Department of Medicine, University of Queensland, Brisbane, Queensland, Australia

Peter M Brooks
Professor, Executive Dean (Health Sciences), University of Queensland, Royal Brisbane Hospital, Herston, Queensland, Australia

W Watson Buchanan
Emeritus Professor of Medicine, Sen. William Osler Health Institute, Hamilton, Ontario, Canada

Jacqui Clinch
Rheumatology Department, Southmead Hospital, Westbury on Trym, Bristol, UK

Cyrus Cooper
Professor of Rheumatology, MRC Environmental Epidemiology Unit (University of Southampton), Southampton General Hospital, Southampton, UK

Paul Dieppe
Professor, Director of MRC Health Services Research Council, University of Bristol, Bristol, UK

Dafna D Gladman
Professor of Medicine, Centre for Prognosis Studies in the Rheumatic Diseases, Toronto Hospital Western Division, Toronto, Ontario, Canada

Brian Hazleman
Rheumatology Research Unit, Addenbrooke's Hospital, Cambridge, UK

Graham RV Hughes
Consultant Rheumatologist and Head of the Lupus Unit, Department of Rheumatology, St Thomas Hospital, London, UK

Michael V Hurley
ARC Research Fellow and Reader in Physiotherapy, Rehabilitation Research Unit, King's College London, Dulwich, London, UK

Malcolm IV Jayson
Professor of Rheumatology, University of Manchester, Manchester, UK

Roland Jonsson
Professor of Medicine (Immunology), Broegelmann Research Laboratory, University of Bergen, Bergen, Norway

Andrew Keat
Consultant Rheumatologist, Arthritis Centre, Northwick Park Hospital, Harrow, Middlesex, UK

Munther Khamashta
Department of Rheumatology, St Thomas Hospital, London, UK

Muhammad Asim Khan
Professor, Metro Health Medical Center, Cleveland, Ohio, USA

E Carwile LeRoy
Professor of Medicine, Department of Microbiology and Immunology, College of Medicine, Medical University of South Carolina, Charleston, South Carolina, USA

Ylva Lindroth
Rheumatology Consultant, Slottsstadens Laekarhus, Malmoe, Sweden

Daniel J McCarty
Will and Cava Ross Professor of Medicine Emeritus, Division of Rheumatology, Department of Medicine, Milwaukee, Wisconsin, USA

Frederick W Miller
Chief, Environmental Autoimmunity Group, Office of Cinical Research, National Institute of Environmental Health Sciences, National Institutes of Health, Bethesda, Maryland, USA

Gabriel S Panayi
Professor of Rheumatology, Arthritis Research Campaign, Department of Rheumatology, Guy's Hospital, London, UK

Paul H Plotz
Arthritis and Rheumatism Branch, National Institute of Health NIAMS, Clinical Center, Bethesda, Maryland, USA

Inga Redlund-Johnell
Department of Radiology, University Hospital MAS, Malmo, Sweden

H Ralph Schumacher, Jr
Professor of Medicine, University of Pennsylvania, Chief of Rheumatology, VA Medical Center, Philadelphia, USA

David GI Scott
Honorary Professor – School of Health Policy and Practice UEA, Department of Rheumatology, Norfolk and Norwich University Hospital, Norwich, UK

Josef Smolen
Professor of Medicine, Department of Rheumatology, University of Vienna, Vienna General Hospital, Vienna, Austria

Hugh Smythe
University Health Network, The Toronto Western Hospital, Toronto, Ontario, Canada

Cathy Speed
Rheumatology Research Unit, Addenbrooke's Hospital, Cambridge, UK

Sophia Steer
ARC Clinical Lecturer, Department of Rheumatology, Guy's Hospital, London, UK

Ralph C Williams, Jr
Master ACR, Santa Fe, New Mexico, USA

Frank A Wollheim
Professor, Department of Rheumatology, Lund University Hospital, Lund, Sweden

Henning K Zeidler
Professor of Internal Medicine and Rheumatology, Medical Highschool Hannover, Division of Rheumatology, Hannover, Germany

Foreword

New paradigms drive out the old. We have had enough of the old history – Hippocrates, Sydenham, Garrods, Pierre Marie and others. This excellent book covers 27 aspects of rheumatology, summarizing what used to be called 'recent advances'. Each of the editorial teams cover up to 14 classic papers each from the 1940s to the present, under the analytic headings 'Summary', 'Key message', 'Why it's important', 'Strengths', 'Weaknesses' and 'Relevance', making them easy to understand. They include a few old classics from 1907, 1912, 1940, and Steinbrocker *et al.* (1949) (see page 8), which have been missed.

Choice is always disputatious, but the contributors here are outstanding and important authorities in their own fields. The theories of 'phlogistom' have perished and, in more recent times, the theories of focal sepsis and the role of physiotherapy versus rehabilitation have undergone drastic criticisms. This book is easy to read, covers the main topics with which rheumatologists (and GPs!) have to deal, and is wholly recommended.

EGL Bywaters
Beaconsfield, UK

Preface

It has been said that we are currently 'drowning in information but thirsting for knowledge'. Through electronic databases we have immediate access to all the recently published literature on any subject we care to think of. But in medicine, in spite of its immediacy, seduction and popularity, current journal literature may not provide us with very much understanding of a subject. An historical perspective and knowledge of the early descriptions of things we now take for granted can add greatly to our understanding and enthusiasm for our subject.

Rheumatology is a relatively young sub-specialty of medicine, which has only come into its own over the last 30 or 40 years. However, we are already drowning in a mass of current literature, with dozens of journals and hundreds of reviews competing for our attention. And we have already forgotten the older literature that set the scene for this present deluge of information. This book attempts to redress the balance by providing readers with access to some of the *classic papers* – the early descriptions of key findings, diseases and phenomena of relevance to clinical rheumatology.

Each chapter starts with a short 'scene-setting' introduction and rationale for the choice of papers that follow, and then each chosen classic paper is presented according to a common template to make it easy to follow and understand. Related references are usually included to help interested readers delve further into the literature.

The contents are split into four sections. In rheumatology, as in any science, technological developments have been of crucial importance to the growth of our subject. In Section 1 we cover the impact of technology on investigative rheumatology; this spans the development of simple clinical measures (metrology) to the impact of modern clinical genetics on our subject. Section 2 covers each of the major disease entities, providing readers access to early descriptive accounts and crucial developmental literature in each area. In Section 3 we address the very common and important regional musculoskeletal disorders, such as back pain, soft tissue disorders and fibromyalgia, as well as miscellaneous disorders. Finally, Section 4 is concerned with the therapy of the rheumatic diseases, and includes key developments in educational and physical interventions, as well as drug therapy.

The authors are all experts in their field, and therefore are well-placed to select the most important papers in their area. Nevertheless, many of them have told us how difficult they found it to make a small selection, and several pleaded with us to allow them to have more papers in their chapter. We were tough, limiting their choices for the sake of space and discipline. We appreciate that others may have made different choices and that some readers may disagree with the choices made. Perhaps we should open a competition for the 'all time top five papers in each category.

We believe that this book should be an important addition to the library of everyone interested in clinical rheumatology. However, it is perhaps of most importance to trainees, as they must surely be expected to develop a greater depth of understanding of their subject while training than can be obtained from modern books and journals. But, of course, we are all trainees. And awareness of history adds good quality to all teaching.

Paul Dieppe
H Ralph Schumacher, Jr
Frank A Wollheim

Dedication

The editors dedicate this book to the late Barbara Ansell (1923–2001).

Section I

Diagnosis

CHAPTER 1

Clinical outcome measurement

Nicholas Bellamy and W Watson Buchanan

Introduction

Validity, reliability and responsiveness are the quintessential requirements of a health status or outcome measure (1). In the last century there has been a steady evolution in the sophistication of measurement techniques. While there remains much to achieve, and accepting that many of the remaining problems are the same problems confronting early pioneers, nevertheless there has been substantial progress in the discipline of musculoskeletal clinical metrology, and there are currently available several advanced high performance techniques with which to quantitate health status in rheumatology. A knowledge of the early work of Taylor, Keele, Steinbrocker and Lansbury, is germane to a comprehensive understanding of the field.

The early pioneers created a foundation for subsequent work in the areas of pain measurement (Keele), functional assessment (Taylor, Steinbrocker), articular index and composite index construction (Lansbury). Their work was without precedent, and unassisted by desk top computers, sophisticated statistical packages and high speed communication. Today, remnants of their early work, can be recognized in the ARA core set measures for rheumatoid arthritis (RA) (9), the ACR response criteria (10), the OARSI core set measures for OA (11) and the OARSI responder criteria (12). The measurement of pain and function remains a challenge but modern instruments, such as the Health Assessment Questionnaire (5), Arthritis Impact Measurement Scales (6, 7), Western Ontario and McMaster Universities Osteoarthritis Index (13) and the Australian/Canadian Osteoarthritis Hand Index (14) are on the leading edge of the development. The problem of weighting and aggregating data from different dimensions, that challenged Lansbury, remains complex, controversial, and without final resolution. Musculoskeletal metrology remains a dynamic and evolving field (1), which owes much to these early pioneers.

References

1. Bellamy N. *Musculoskeletal Metrology.* Lancaster, Kluwer Academic Publishers. 1993: 1–367.
2. Felson DT, Anderson JJ, Boers M, *et al.* The American College of Rheumatology Preliminary Core Set of Disease activity measures for rheumatoid arthritis clinical trials. *Arthritis and Rheumatism* 1993; **36**: 729–740.
3. Felson DT, Anderson JJ, Boers M, *et al.* The American College of Rheumatology Preliminary Definition of Improvement in rheumatoid arthritis. *Arthritis and Rheumatism* 1995; **38**: 727–735.
4. Osteoarthritis Research Society (OARS) Task Force Report: Design and conduct of clinical trials of patients with osteoarthritis: recommendations from a Task Force of the Osteoarthritis Research Society. *Osteoarthritis and Cartilage* 1996; **4**: 217–243.
5. Dougados M, Le Claire P, van der Heijde X, *et al.* Response criteria for clinical trials on osteoarthritis of the knee and hip. *Osteoarthritis and Cartilage* 2000 (In Press).
6. Fries JF, Spitz P, Kraines RG, *et al.* Measurement of patient outcomes in arthritis. *Arthritis and Rheumatism* 1980; **23**: 137–145.
7. Meenan RF, Gurtman PM, Mason JH. Measuring health status in arthritis: The Arthritis Impact Measurement Scales. *Arthritis and Rheumatism* 1980; **23**(2): 146–152.
8. Meenan RF, Jason JH, Anderson JJ, Guccione AA, Kazis LE. AIMS2. The content and properties of a revised and expanded arthritis impact measurement scales health status questionnaire. *Arthritis and Rheumatism* 1992; **35**(1): 1–10.
9. Bellamy N, Buchanan WW, Goldsmith CH, *et al.* Validation study of WOMAC: A health status instrument for measuring clinically important patient relevant outcomes to anti-rheumatic drug therapy in patients with osteoarthritis of the hip or knee. *Journal of Rheumatology* 1988; **15**: 1833–1840.
10. Bellamy N, Campbell J, Haraoui B, *et al.* Development of the Australian/Canadian AUS-CAN Osteoarthritis (OA) Hand Index. *Arthritis and Rheumatism* 1997; **40**(9) (Suppl): S110.
11. Likert R. A technique for the measurement of attitudes. *Archives of Psychology* 1932; **140**: 44–60.
12. Huskisson EC. Measurement of pain. *Lancet* 1974; **2**: 1127–1131.
13. Hochberg MC, Chang RW, Dwosh I, *et al.* The American College of Rheumatology 1991. Revised criteria for the classification of Global Functional Status in rheumatoid arthritis. *Arthritis and Rheumatism* 1992; **35**: 498–502.
14. Lansbury J, Baier HN, McCracken S. Statistical study of variation in systemic and articular indexes. *Arthritis and Rheumatism* 1962; **5**(5): 445–456.

Paper I

A table for the degree of involvement in chronic arthritis

Author

Taylor D

Reference

Canadian Medical Association Journal 1937; June, 608–610

Summary

Taylor reported his recommendations regarding a classification table for chronic arthritis at the Medico-Chirurgical Society of Montreal on 22 January 1937, while Demonstrator in Medicine at McGill University. The Taylor Index was published 5 months later in the *Canadian Medical Association Journal*. Given the relatively limited distribution of the journal at that time, it is not surprising that the paper escaped world attention. In retrospect, Taylor's paper marks the beginning of quantitative measurement in rheumatology. His was the first attempt to rationalize the categorization of musculoskeletal health status. In essence, Taylor described, what he termed four divisions or 'degrees' varying from minimal to advanced stages, in the form of a 'table of degree'. The table was designed for both rheumatoid (atrophic) arthritis and osteoarthritis (hypertrophic), although other applications were envisaged. Indeed Taylor reported two components to the table, one based on x-ray changes, the other based on clinical findings.

The radiographic component provides four gradations within each of which are separate criteria for atrophic and hypertrophic arthritis. The terms commonly used today, such as erosions, osteopenia, bone cysts, joint space narrowing, sclerosis, receive no mention. Each grade is defined by one or more non-exclusive descriptors. The basic radiographic categories are:

Stage I: Soft tissue changes.
Stage II: Joint space is definitely altered.
Stage III: Destruction of joints.
Stage IV: Extreme widespread joint changes.

The clinical component likewise uses combinations of descriptors from the pain stiffness and function domains, creating categorizations that are not mutually exclusive, and which are based on symptom severities across several domains. The basic clinical categories are:

Stage I: Slight symptoms.
Stage II: Moderate symptoms.
Stage III: Severe symptoms.
Stage IV: Extreme symptoms.

The significant feature is the separation of the early or mild cases from those in the advanced stage.

No actual data on reliability, validity or responsiveness are included in the original report. The Taylor Index is important as the first attempt to categorize patients with either RA or OA according to a complex measure based on various radiographic and clinical features.

Key message

The key message was that the severity of musculoskeletal disease could be quantitated, and that quantitative information could play a key role in the evaluation of therapeutic interventions. Taylor noted that detailed clinical and laboratory studies were essential in problem solving and might be facilitated by the use of his table.

Why it's important

Taylor was probably the earliest pioneer, in musculoskeletal clinical metrology. His report not only details the origins of the discipline, but also highlights the challenge of defining a standard, in an era devoid of precedent. Taylor recognized that the rheumatism literature was complex and controversial, and had failed to account adequately for inherent between-patient and within-patient variation. He also recognized the disjunction that can occur between radiographic and clinical findings.

While recognizing the descriptive nature of his table, Taylor also envisaged therapeutic applications. He also recognized that his table would require modification for use in diseases other than RA and OA. The report contains extensive description of the profiles of patients who might fall into the different categories, and in places provides advice as to the preferred method of caring for certain types of patients. It therefore provides a perspective on therapeutic management in the early 1900s.

Taylor recognized the constitutional reaction that can accompany RA, and suggested that it be graded (mild, moderate, severe, extreme). Perhaps most importantly Taylor recognized that through his table, the important observations made on patients differing in disease severity could be more readily communicated to others, and thereby facilitate decision making.

Strengths

1. The first standard method for classifying patients with chronic arthritis according to their radiographic and functional status.
2. Provided a methodology that was easily comprehended and readily applied.
3. Influential in the subsequent development of the Steinbrocker Functional Classification and the ACR Functional Classification.
4. Recognized that radiographic and clinical features should be graded separately.

Weaknesses

1. From a clinimetric perspective, the Taylor Index combines measurements on different clinical domains in the assignment of a single category. The descriptors of pain, stiffness and functional capacity given are not mutually exclusive and therefore may conflict.
2. A lack of data in the original report on validity, reliability and responsiveness is a significant limitation.
3. There are reasons to believe that the Taylor Index may have lacked responsiveness, because of its scale construction. The presence of a restricted number of non-exclusive categories would tend to mitigate against index responsiveness.

Relevance

The Taylor Index is relevant because it was the first of its kind, and formed the foundation of the Steinbrocker Functional Classification and the ACR Functional Classification. In addition Taylor's publication provides insight into concepts and strategies prevalent in the early 1900s.

Paper 2

The pain chart

Author

Keele KD

Reference

Lancet 1948; **255**: 6–8

Summary

Keele described 'a simple method of minimizing errors of description by standardizing terminology, and recording intensity of pain in a pain chart'. His work was inspired by Sir Thomas Lewis and placed priority on the graphic representation of the time intensity of pain by pain charts. Keele described five hierarchical categories of pain: nil, slight, moderate, severe and agony. His seminal paper described temporal variation not only in articular pain, but also in angina pectoris, gastric ulcer, tetany, tuberculous cystitis, Banti's disease and rectal cancer. Patients self-completed the pain charts which were subdivided according to the 24 hours of the day. The descriptors were explained to the patient and were also written on the chart for reinforcement, and reference. Keele's report contains information on the validity and responsiveness of the method but not its reliability. Indication is given regarding potential applications of the method.

Key message

Keele was the first to suggest an adjectival or descriptive Likert scale based on the English adjectives of degree for quantitating changes over time in pain intensity.

Why it's important

Pain is the key symptom in most rheumatic diseases. It is entirely subjective and only appreciable to the sufferer. As such it represents an important but complex metrologic challenge. The classification systems proposed by Taylor and Steinbrocker, encompassed pain but were functionally based measures and of questionable responsiveness. Keele's paper serves as a bridge between the earlier work of Likert in 1932 (reference 11, Introduction) on the measurement of attitude using descriptive terms, and the later work of Huskisson who introduced the visual analogue scale into rheumatology in the 1970s (reference 12, Introduction). To a variable extent, similar descriptors of none, mild, moderate, severe and extreme remain in use today (reference 1, Introduction).

Scaling is a critical element of any health status measure since it is a major determinant of the capacity of a measure to detect change (reference 1, Introduction). Keele had the foresight to recognize the importance of being able to represent pain graphically on a pain chart, in a way that is now commonplace in publications on interventional research in rheumatology.

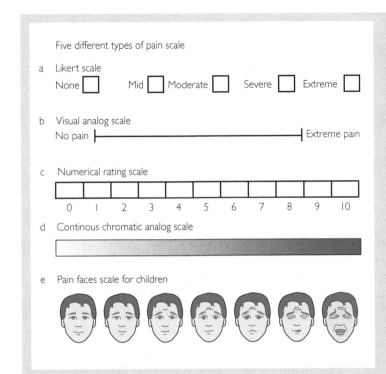

Figure 1.1 Keele described the early use of a Likert scale for the measurement of pain severity in arthritis. The Likert scale is just one of many methods of recording the severity of pain – this illustration shows five of them. (Adapted from Bellamy N, Principles of outcome measurement, in Klippel J, Dieppe P (eds) *Rheumatology*, 2nd edition, 1997, Mosby International, London.

Strengths

1. A simple method for quantitating longitudinal changes in pain intensity.
2. Established a precedent for future pain scales.
3. Emphasized issues of validity and responsiveness.
4. The diagnostic value of the pain chart was exemplified by observations on placebo injections in psychogenic pain.

Weaknesses

1. Report based on only seven selected non-random clinical cases.
2. Statistical methods not employed to establish validity, reliability and responsiveness.
3. Agony might be considered a qualitative aspect of pain rather than a simple measure of intensity.
4. No diagnostic or demographic information were provided for the articular pain case, which is believed to have been RA.

Relevance

The quantitation of pain by a reliable, valid and responsive method facilitates improved diagnostic, prognostic and evaluative activities, and provides a rational basis for developing scaling priorities for unidimensional and multidimensional health status questionnaires in diverse musculoskeletal diseases. Keele established a precedent for standardization in scaling terms and demonstrated its applicability in several different and unrelated conditions.

Paper 3

Therapeutic criteria in rheumatoid arthritis

Authors

Steinbrocker O, Traeger CH, Battereman RC

Reference

Lancet 1949; **140**: 659–662

Summary

Steinbrocker, *et al.* reported criteria for the Committee for Therapeutic Criteria of the New York Rheumatism Association and the Subcommittee for Therapeutic Criteria of the American Rheumatism Association. The report contains a description of three sets of criteria for: (a) Classification of Rheumatoid Progression; (b) Classification of Functional Capacity, and (c) Response of Rheumatoid Activity to Therapy. The criteria for Classification of Functional Capacity are the only ones that remain in use and are generally referred to as the Steinbrocker Functional Classification. Steinbrocker, *et al*'s classification of functional disability in 1949 was similar to that of Taylor, which is not entirely surprising given that Taylor was a member of the aforementioned Committee for Therapeutic Criteria. The Steinbrocker Functional Classification contains four classes defined by whether an individual has complete function, or has function adequate for normal activity, or has limited function, or is incapacitated. The system has been used widely over the last half century, but is acknowledged to lack some sensitivity for use as an outcome measure to detect differential change over time. This problem has been partially addressed by revision of the wording of this simple four point scale by a subcommittee of the American College of Rheumatology (reference 13, Introduction). The Steinbrocker Functional Classification was endorsed by a major international rheumatology association and provided a standard method for classifying functional status in RA. It is of note that the report does not contain any data on the reliability, validity or responsiveness of the classification system.

Key message

The key message is summed up by the authors themselves: the criteria 'provide the common language so sorely needed in the therapeutic investigation of rheumatoid arthritis'.

Why it's important

Prior to 1949, and with the exception of the Taylor Index, there had been no standard system for classifying functional status. While Taylor made the first footsteps on the bare clinimetric landscape, his contribution did not immediately receive endorsement by any major international society. However, Taylor's inclusion in the Criteria Committee of the New York Rheumatism Association and the Criteria Subcommittee of the American Rheumatism Association, is an indication that his earlier contribution had been noted and his opinion sought and respected regarding the exact wording and formulation of the Steinbrocker

Functional Classification. The Steinbrocker Functional Classification allowed patients to be classified as follows:

Class I: Complete. Ability to carry on all usual duties without handicaps.
Class II: Adequate for normal activities, despite handicap of discomfort or limited motion of one or more joints.
Class III: Limited. Able to perform little or none of the duties of usual occupation or self care.
Class IV: Incapacitated, largely or wholly. Bedridden or confined to wheelchair; little or no self care.

While developed for RA patients, the categories appear applicable to many forms of chronic arthritis. The revision recommended by the ACR in a publication by Hochberg, *et al.* (reference 13, Introduction), resulted again in four categories, but using different definitions. The publication on the revised Steinbrocker Functional Classification provided data on validity and reliability, but not on the key requirement for detecting differential change, that of responsiveness (reference 13, Introduction).

Strengths

1. A simple standard method for classifying patients with rheumatoid arthritis according to their functional status.
2. A method endorsed by a major international society and therefore likely to be employed.
3. Established a precedent for future functional scales.

Weaknesses

1. The classification systems proposed by both Taylor and Steinbrocker, are of questionable responsiveness. Individuals categorized in Class IV in 1949 would have been unlikely to improve, while relatively few patients with active RA would have fallen into Class I. This would have effectively restricted the index to a two-point scale for many sufferers.
2. The lack of intermediate gradations between Class II and Class III would have further limited the capacity of the classification index to detect small but important alterations in health status. The more recent availability of superior symptom-modifying and disease-modifying therapies for RA may have altered the situation somewhat, but nevertheless, the principle applies. For RA clinical trials and clinical practice applications, in which sensitivity to change is important, there are better instruments including the Health Assessment Questionnaire (HAQ) (reference 6, Introduction), and the Arthritis Impact Measurement Scales (AIMS, AIMS2) (references 7 and 8, Introduction).
3. The lack of data on the validity, reliability and responsiveness contained in the original report of the Steinbrocker Functional Classification is a significant limitation. The authors noted that the criteria were based entirely on objective information, although none was provided in the report.

Relevance

The ability to classify patients according to standard criteria represented a significant development. In particular the Steinbrocker Functional Classification was a response to the influence of subjective factors in quantitating patient status, the lack of separation between estimates of disease activity and functional status, and the lack of a common language with which to express the results of an assessment. Steinbrocker and colleagues defined a reference standard, which despite its limitations, remains in use today in a modified form.

Paper 4

Quantitation of the activity (manifestations) of rheumatoid arthritis

Author

Lansbury J

References

1. Method for recording its systemic manifestations. *American Journal of the Medical Sciences* 1956; **231**: 616–621
2. Recession of morning stiffness as patients go into remission. *American Journal of the Medical Sciences* 1956; **232**: 8–11
3. The maximum 5-minute Cutler sedimentation rate as an index. *American Journal of the Medical Sciences* 1956; **232**: 12–16
4. Area of joint surfaces as an index to total joint inflammation and deformity. *American Journal of the Medical Sciences* 1956; **232**: 150–155
5. A method for summation of the systemic indices of rheumatoid activity. *American Journal of the Medical Sciences* 1956; **232**: 300–310
6. Correlation of the systemic and joint findings. *American Journal of the Medical Sciences* 1957; **233**: 375–378
7. A numerical method for summing up total deformity. *American Journal of the Medical Sciences* 1958; **235**: 154–156

Summary

Between 1956 and 1958 John Lansbury of Temple University School of Medicine in Philadelphia, published seven of the most important papers in clinical metrology. Because of their extreme value, they will be reviewed as a single entity. Lansbury was professor of clinical medicine when he published methods for the quantitation of the activity of RA. Clearly he was a master of his art, establishing not only a standard in the field, but noting many of the same complexities and conflicts that metrologists still seek to address adequately at the present time. His first paper defined 16 domains for measurement: rest pain, motion pain, morning stiffness, diurnal gelling, fatigue, ASA tablets/day to control pain, 4 pm temperature, basal body weight, grip strength, steps up/down, timed rises from chair, haemoglobin, ESR, serum albumin, serum globulin and CRP. Lansbury also noted the convenience of using a rubber stamp form for recording purposes.

This first paper is conceptual. While it contains no data, it provides the foundation for the remaining papers all of which contain quantitative information. The measurement system was based on the premise that vague impressions conveyed in the general course of a clinical interview were deficient and liable to error. By breaking down the measurement problem into its basic components, and measuring each in relevant units, a multidimensional profile could be constructed, that conveyed the detail in a standardized and structured fashion, and facilitated communication and decision making.

The second paper provides a method for quantitating morning stiffness based on its duration rather than its intensity. Lansbury contended that most patients could distinguish stiffness from pain (an issue that remains controversial to the present day). He noted an association between morning stiffness and Cutler sedimentation rate which he quantitated (construct validity), although he did not express the association using a correlation coefficient.

Lansbury described the dynamic profile of morning stiffness in six patients experiencing a treatment-induced complete remission, and thereby demonstrated the responsiveness of the measure. Interestingly, he regarded morning stiffness as a 'valid index to the total amount of systemic or fibrositic activity of RA in the cases studied'.

The third paper examined the value of the Cutler sedimentation rate as a quantitative measure of rheumatoid activity. No claim was made for superiority over the methods described by Westergren and Wintrobe, and the time-consuming nature of this method, requiring taking readings every 5 minutes, was duly noted. Lansbury described the curvilinear dynamics of the sedimentation rate in 10 patients experiencing a complete remission, and demonstrated the responsiveness of the measure. He observed between-subject variability and described the average sedimentation rate in a further 100 patients.

The fourth paper is extremely important since it describes his development of an articular index, the Lansbury Index. With the collaboration of an anatomist Professor Donald Hart, Lansbury meticulously measured the surface area of the bony surfaces of each individual joint by exactly applying aluminium foil to 'the surface which in life is covered with articulating cartilage'. For each joint the foil was then weighed repeatedly and the average weight (to two decimal places), referred to the weight of a standard square centimeter of the foil used, and the surface area of each joint deduced. It should be noted that all the measurements were conducted on a single skeleton of unknown morphology. Nevertheless, the relative weights would probably be the same or similar in different skeletons. The total joint area in the skeleton studied was 1090.74 cm^2. From the area Lansbury simply rounded to the nearest whole number and in Table 2 of the publication gave values for individual joints. The total amount of inflammation was described by summing the individual values for all affected joints. Using this approach Lansbury created not a direct measure of inflammation, but an index of joint size that could be used to estimate disease activity. In Table 4 of the publication a four point grading system, based on the joint values or weights, is illustrated.

Lansbury divided the total score for each joint into four equal grades: Grade I: Minimal (0–25%), Grade II: Slight (26–50%), Grade III: Moderate (51–75%) and Grade IV: Maximum (76–100%). The value for Grade IV was the actual value or weight for that joint that had been determined by the aluminium foil method. Lesser grades were direct percentages as outlined previously. Lansbury was an astute researcher and cautioned that Grade IV inflammation did not imply four times greater inflammation than Grade I. He also appreciated that while clinicians might agree on what constituted minimal or extreme inflammation, they would be less likely to agree on the intermediate grades.

The fifth paper concerns a method of summating the systemic indices of rheumatoid activity. With humility, Lansbury noted that he was aware that the method had 'been applied to too few cases to permit a conclusive statement to be made as to its ultimate value'. He went on to describe a method of compiling a single composite score based on five subscores (Anaemia, ESR, Grip strength, Fatigability and Aspirin need). Lansbury reasoned that to be acceptable in a composite index, each component must be 'present in the majority of cases and must exhibit statistically significant regularity of trend which correlates with the general trend of the disease'. He proceeded to describe these statistical relationships, the exact methods of ascertainment of the measurements, and highlighted some of the operational difficulties of the methods. Lansbury rationalized that the complete absence of abnormality on any of the indices constituted a clinical remission. The composite score was calculated as follows: The value for the average degree of severity in a series of patients was assigned a value of 100, so that gradations above and below that point could be expressed in percentages. Equivalent percentages for the full range of probable observed data were displayed in a table for ready reference. The status of an individual patient was defined by summing the percentages describing each of the component elements into a so-called Index of Systemic Activity. The exact percentages are shown in Table 2 and a worked example in Table 3 of the original publication. The responsiveness of the index was established in five cases of RA experiencing a remission.

The sixth paper examines the correlation between Articular and Systemic Indices. Based on 80 unselected cases a correlation of 0.78 (p = 0.01) was observed. Lansbury also provided evidence for parallelism, that is synchronous fluctuations, between the Articular Index and Systemic Index scores in a single patient. He recommended that the indices be kept separate and cautioned that parallelism might not be invariable.

The seventh paper concerns a numerical method for summing up total deformity. The so-called Motion Index was based on the Articular Index, and expressed total lost motion as a percentage of total possible lost motion. Lansbury clearly differentiated between this method of quantitating joint motion and functional capacity in the social sense. He acknowledged that the latter depended on other factors such as disease distribution and activity, the patient's courage and type of employment. The Motion Index score was calculated from the sum of all contributing joints. For each joint the difference between the normal and the observed motion (in degrees) was multiplied by the joint size in square centimeters. The values for 28 knuckles, 24 small toe joints and two of all the peripheral movable joints were summed and then divided by 1000. In order to save time, Lansbury accepted that range of movement in small joints might be visually estimated rather than be measured goniometrically. He envisaged that the Motion Index would not be used routinely, but rather be used in long-term studies and rehabilitation environments.

Key message

Lansbury demonstrated that disease activity in RA was amenable to quantitation using standard methods. Although no longer in use, his Articular Index and Systemic Index were conceptually advanced.

Why it's important

Lansbury's seven papers represent a conceptual leap in musculoskeletal clinical metrology. He had a comprehensive understanding of the multidimensional and dynamic nature of the measurement problem in RA. The Articular Index provided a rational basis for weighting and aggregating together unidimensional information from joints of different size, while his Systemic Index attempted to address the complexities of weighting and aggregating together diverse information from different domains, measured on scales differing in length. The weighting and aggregation of multidimensional data remain an on-going challenge.

Strengths

1. The strength of these papers lies in Lansbury's capacity to convey the essence of the metrologic problem succinctly and with balance. He realized the complexity of the problem, was always cautious regarding the generalizability of his observations and acknowledged the necessity for more extensive evaluation. While none of his indices remains in use, they offered partial solutions, and provided a foundation for later developments.
2. Lansbury understood the need to establish the validity and responsiveness of his methods. As a consequence his papers contain more statistical information than others from the same period.

Weaknesses

1. Lansbury's work was constrained by the existent level of understanding regarding the nature of RA.
2. His work preceded the personal computer and the general use of statistical methodology referable to evaluating the clinimetric properties of measuring instruments. Nevertheless, he progressed the field using a combination of refined observational skills and intellectual brilliance.
3. Perhaps the only area of weakness was in his treatment of the pain and function dimensions, which he approached quite superficially by modern standards. While Lansbury's early work was based on complex concepts but simple statistics, his later work showed an increasing sophistication with respect to his use of statistical methodology (reference 14, Introduction).

Relevance

Lansbury's papers are essential reading. For students they provide the necessary background for interpreting progress in the assessment of RA throughout the remainder of the century. For the developers of new measurement techniques they provide reassurance that others have traveled the same path, and in some instances encountered the very same challenges. Finally, they serve as a record of the achievements of an outstanding clinical metrologist and physician.

CHAPTER 2

Imaging

Inga Redlund-Johnell

Introduction

Imaging in medicine began soon after the production of the famous x-ray picture of the normal hand of Roentgen's wife in 1895. The first decades of the 20th century was an epoch when radiology was an issue of concern for every open-minded physician rather than a matter for a few specialized radiologists. At that time the population statistics in western countries showed that there were very few older people compared to the present population demography. For example in the city of Malmö, there were only 5997 people aged over 65 years in 1920 (5% of the population), and 129 (2.1%) of these people had been examined radiologically (according to my survey of the register of the Radiological Department from 1920, Malmö General Hospital). In comparison, in 1995 the corresponding figures were 49 616 persons over 65 years (20% of the population), and 24 057 (48.5%) of them have had skeletal radiological examinations. It is thus not surprising that diseases of older people (such as osteoarthritis (OA)) were not well reported during the first years of radiology. In the patient material of 1920 in Malmö, very few had the diagnosis of arthritis, and in those of 1945, before the introduction of antibiotics, most cases of arthritis were probably of infective origin.

Imaging has an important place in the diagnosis of rheumatic diseases. I have tried to find some of the first published papers that demonstrated the characteristic imaging features of different kinds of arthritis, starting with x-ray papers from the beginning of the 20th century (Papers 1 and 2), and going on to examples of important applications of the newer techniques of computerized tomography (CT) and and magnetic resonance imaging (MRI) (Papers 3 and 4). It has not been easy. The early papers seldom had more than one author and the papers were written in a different style from that of today: the introduction was intermingled with the discussion and case reports were also mixed with discussion points. There were never any presentations of large groups of patients in the early radiological (or in other medical) papers, rather an eagerness to be the first one to present cases with this new diagnostic method. That eagererness was repeated during the 1970s and 1980s when CT and MRI were introduced respectively. One of the differences between these papers, and the early ones on the plain radiograph, is that the number of authors of a paper today are nearly as many as the number of patients studied!

Imaging is also of value in sorting out some of the complications of the rheumatic diseases, and its impact has been particularly important in the recognition of cervical subluxation in rheumatoid arthritis (RA) (Paper 5). Finally, imaging can also help with assessing severity and measuring the progression of the rheumatic diseases, so I have also included the classic papers introducing systems for assessment of the two commonest forms of arthritis, RA (Paper 6) and OA (Paper 7).

Paper 1

The skiagraphy of rheumatoid arthritis

Authors

Bowker GE, Lindsay J

Reference

Edinburgh Medical Journal 1907; **X**:317–320

Summary

Earlier reports on RA have discussed the probability of a specific bacillus responsible for RA. Some infective process may give rise to a general toxaemia and so influence the joint structures that it could produce the features of RA. Many infective processes like gonorrhoea or rectal ulcers may cause acute RA with the same clinical findings, but with the help of x-rays it is possible to differentiate among these cases. In cases of acute RA there has never been any evidence of any change in the configuration of the bony parts of the joints involved but soft tissue swelling may occur. Two case reports, one concerning a man with gonorrhoeal arthritis and one child with acute RA confirm these observations.

In cases of chronicity, the disappearance of cartilage allows a closer approximation of the joints. In further advanced cases the softened joints of the proximal interphalangeal joints are eroded, as are the heads of the metacarpals and the carpal bones. With progression, atrophy of the shafts will appear and the destruction may lead to cupping, and finally a trumpet-shaped appearance may appear as shown in the x-ray illustration. Finally bony ankylosis frequently supervenes.

Related references

(1) Osgood RB. Differential diagnosis of the chronic non-tubercular joint diseases by means of the roentgen ray. *American Quarterly Roentgen* 1906–07; **4**:1. (Summary in R*öfo* 1908; **12**:77).

(2) Reuss E. Über einen fall von knochenatrophie nach gelenkreumatismus (One case of bone atrophy associated with joint rheumatism). *Röfo* 1912–1913; **19**:430–437.

Key message

Joint arthritis can be divided into chronic or RA with x-ray changes (Figure 2.1) and acute (reactive) arthritis without x-ray changes.

Why it's important

This and the related references were amongst the first to show that radiology could discriminate between different kinds of arthritis. It is interesting to note, from the summary, that at this time RA was regarded as likely to be infective in origin. However, the typical x-ray changes of the disease are well described and illustrated, including the erosions.

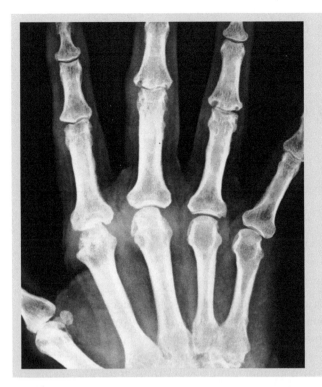

Figure 2.1 A radiograph of the hand in RA showing a characteristic bone erosion at the index finger metacarpophalangeal joint.

Strengths

1. The findings are supported with reproduction of the x-rays.
2. The main features of rheumatoid radiographs, including the characteristic erosions, are well documented.

Weakness

The observations are grounded in only three cases.

Relevance

The typical radiographic features of RA are now well described, but at this time it was not clear that RA was separate from other forms of arthritis. These observations help show contemporary rheumatologists that RA has distinctive features.

Three early descriptions of the radiology of arthritis

Paper 2a

Typical alterations of the bones in gout

Author

Köhler A

Reference

Archives of the Roentgen Ray 1912; **17**:330–333

Summary

According to Huber (1) the bubble-like cavities in the phalanges of the fingers in gout ought to be filled with uric acid salts. These changes would thus not be due to atrophic changes but to the substitution of urates for the natural phosphates of the affected bone. Five cases are presented with x-rays. Typical changes at the articular ends of the phalanges are sharply defined transparent areas. The symmetrical arrangement of the transparent foci seems to point to some connection between the position of the foci and the distribution of the blood vessels. The same destructive lesions may be found in the foot, espcially in the first metatarsal joint. Typical changes have so far not been found in hundreds of x-rays of the larger joints in patients with gout. Along the shafts of the long bones an irritation or stimulus may produce a gouty deposit and erosion of the bone, but the appearance is not diagnostic or typical of gout.

Related reference   (1)   Huber X. Zur verwerthung der röntgen-strahlen im gebiete der inneren medicin. *Deutsche Medizinische Wochenschrift* 1896; **22**:182.

Paper 2b

A case of arthropathia psoriatica

Authors

Ström S

Reference

Acta Radiologica 1920–21; **1**:21–25

Summary

This case-report concerns a 50-year-old man with psoriasis for 30 years in whom treatment with arsenic and chrysarobin had only led to temporary improvement. At the age of 28 years he got thickening of the nails and swelling of the thumbs and big toes, and later on the little fingers and all toes became swollen and shortened without any real pain. He was referred for x-ray with the suspicion of his having syphilis. The x-ray showed a total destruction of several of the affected joints with a tapering towards the ends of the phalanges. The sesamoid bones of the thumbs were three times enlarged with irregular form. Spurs, as in OA, were occasionally found. In some of the toes a total phalangeal destruction was found, resembling that seen in cases with Raynaud's disease. In all the toes there was some bony destruction. Different aetiologies have been proposed in psoriasis, and the findings here support rather the theories of neuropathic origin or that of a disturbance in the internal secretion.

Related reference   **(1)**   Belot X, Chaperon MMJ. Radiographies de lesions et deformations dans le psoriasis arthropathique. *Bulletin Memoires Soc Radiol Med Paris* 1909; **1**:269–271.

Paper 2c

Abnormal calcium deposition inside the knee, a contribution to the question of the primary 'meniscopathy'

Authors

Werwath K

Reference

RÖFO 1928; **37**:169–171

Summary

A 45-year-old, earlier healthy man attended the surgical clinic because of pain and hydrops of the left knee. X-ray revealed calcification of the cartilage and menisci. At operation the diagnosis of calcium deposition was confirmed. A meniscectomy was performed and synovial material was cut out. Microscopy showed spots of calcification of the cartilage as well as scanty cartilage cells and a predominance of fibrous tissue. The findings differed partly from that of OA. The differential diagnosis ought to be a metabolic disturbance or a post-traumatic disorder, but there were neither trauma nor acute arthritis in the anamnesis. The probable diagnosis ought to be a disturbance of the calcium metabolism with secondary deposition in the cartilage.

Related reference **(1)** McCarthy DJ, Haskin ME. The roentgenographic aspects of pseudogout (articular chondrocalcinosis). An analysis of 20 cases. *American Journal of Roentengenology* 1963; **90**:1248–1257.

Key message of the three papers

The key message behind these papers is that different types of rheumatic disease lead to characteristic changes on the plain radiograph (Figure 2.2).

Why they are important

These are early descriptions of the radiological features of gout, psoriatic arthritis (PsA) and chondrocalcinosis respectively. The typical changes found on a plain radiograph in each of these conditons are described and illustrated. The important finding coming from a combination of such studies is that each rheumatic disease results in quite different changes in the bones and spaces of synovial joints, allowing the plain radiograph to be used as a powerful diagnostic tool.

Strengths

1 These papers are amongst the first to describe and illustrate the different radiographic changes of the rheumatic diseases.
2 The descriptions and illustrations are often good, particularly in the gout paper.

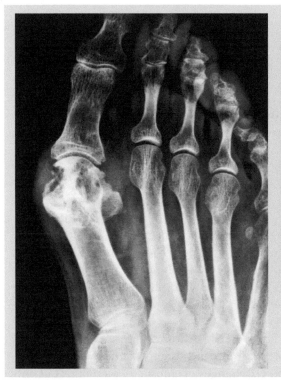

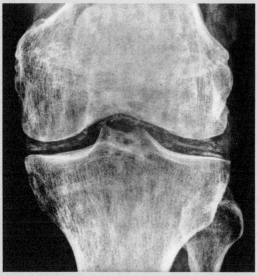

Figure 2.2 Radiographs showing the typical gouty erosion at the first metatarsophalangeal joint (left) and chondrocalcinosis in the knee joint (right).

Weaknesses

1. All papers are of single or a few case reports.
2. The speculation about the nature of the conditons is sometimes misplaced.

Relevance

The authors provide early descriptions of the plain radiographic changes that characterize the different rheumatic diseases.

Paper 3

Computerized tomography of sacroiliitis

Authors

Carrera CT, Foley WD, Kozin F, Ryanand L, Lawson TL

Reference

American Journal of Roentengenology 1981; **136**:41–46

Summary

Sacroiliitis is often difficult to diagnose using conventional radiographs and radionuclide scanning due to low sensitivity and/or specificity for the early diagnosis of sacroiliitis. Computed tomography was used in a study of eight normal volunteers and 20 consecutive patients with a clinical suspicion of sacroiliitis in a double-blind pilot study. The gantry was tilted 30° caudally, and 5mm CT images as well as the plain films were studied for joint narrowing, subchondral sclerosis, erosion and ankylosis.

Three patients did not fulfil clinical criteria of spondyloarthritic syndromes and appeared to be cases with degenerative joint disease, old fracture, and osteitis condensans ilii respectively. Twelve among the other 17 patients had CT changes diagnostic of sacroiliitis but only five had changes at the conventional radiographic examination. Another four patients had equivocal plain film changes and three were normal. The radiation dose was 2.5 times higher with CT but the testicular dose was zero compared to 0.08 rad with plain films. There was no interobserver inconsistency in the interpretation of the CT images but some uncertainty in that of the plain films.

Related references **(1)** Calin A. Abuse of computed tomography. *Arthritis and Rheumatism* 1982; **25**:147–148.

(2) Murphey MD, Wetzel LH, Bramble JM, *et al.* Sacroiliitis: MR imaging findings. *Radiology* 1991; **180**:239–244.

Key message

CT is superior to conventional radiography in diagnosing arthritis of the sacroiliac joints and the gonadal dose is low with the described technique.

Why it's important

The sacroiliac joints are orientated oblique to both the conventional coronal and sagittal planes of the body, and are thus not easy to depict with x-ray. Conventional x-ray tomography with several exposures was formerly a good diagnostic help, but was giving the young patients a high dose of gonadal radiation. This technique with tilting of the gantry is still the best one when examining the sacroiliac joints with CT. MRI is more sensitive, but not more specific.

Strengths

1. This was a double-blind pilot study (the radiologists were not blind but blinded of the possibilities of the new technique).
2. The patient material is compared to a normal material.

Weakness

There were only eight normal controls.

Relevance

This paper shows how to use the new technology with a lower radiation dose to the patient.

Paper 4

Early detection of carpal erosions in patients with rheumatoid arthritis: A pilot study of magnetic resonance imaging

Authors

Gilkeson G, Polisson R, Sinclair H, Voglier J, Rice J, Caldwell D, Spritzer C, Martinez S

Reference

Journal of Rheumatology 1988; **15**:1361–1366

Summary

Standard radiographs taken early in the course of joint arthritis are usually normal or show unspecific changes. This pilot study consisted of 10 patients with classical or definite RA and their radiography and MRI were evaluated by radiologists without knowledge of any connection between the x-ray and MRI films. The MRI appearance of the wrists was also compared with 39 non-rheumatoid patients. MRI was superior in detecting synovial inflammation and erosions in the form of pannus invading carpal marrow. Early erosions were found on the junction between the hamate, capitate and bases of the 3rd and 4th metacarpals. If the expense of MRI was not so great it could be a valuable tool in therapeutic trials.

Related reference   (I)   Ostergaard M, Hansen M, Stoltenberg M, Lorenzen I. Magnetic resonance imaging-determined synovial membrane volume as a marker of disease activity and a predictor of progressive joint destruction in the wrists of patients with rheumatoid arthritis. *Arthritis and Rheumatism* 1999; **42**:918–929.

Key message

MRI is superior to standard radiography in detecting early RA.

Why it's important

The use of MRI in medicine started at the beginning of the 1980s. For the diagnosis of rheumatic diseases it is a sensitive but expensive technique. Even if the time that the patient has to spend in the machine is reduced in the future, film-reading and interpretation will still take a lot longer than with conventional x-rays. However, the cost of MRI is only a fraction of that of some of the new interventions being used to treat RA, so MRI may prove cost-effective in assessing such therapies and monitoring patient progress (1).

In patients with inflammatory arthritis suspected of having RA, it can be very valuable to obtain early evidence of the characteristic anatomical changes, confirming the diagnosis and allowing early use of suppressive therapy. However, it takes several months for changes to appear on a plain radiograph. This paper shows the MRI changes of RA appear earlier in the course of the disease.

Strength

The findings in patients with suspected RA were compared to a normal material.

Weakness

A pilot study with only 10 patients.

Relevance

Early evidence of the potential value of MRI in the early detection of joint damage in RA.

Paper 5

Rheumatoid arthritis with death from medullary compression

Authors

Davis FW Jr, Markley H

Reference

Annals of Internal Medicine 1951; **35**:451–454

Summary

A 58-year old woman with a 25 year history of classical RA and confined to a wheel chair for 6 years was admitted to hospital because of dyspnoea. Three months prior to admission she had been treated for an upper respiratory infection with dysphagia and stridor. A laryngoscopy revealed limitated abduction of the vocal cords. Her neck was unduly short. She gradually deteriorated with increasing stridor, dysphagia and dyspnoea and she died due to what was interpreted as acute bulbar failure. An autopsy revealed an intruding odontoid process through the foramen magnum, impinging on the inferior surface of the medulla. A perforated oesophageal ulcer with subacute osteochondritis of cricoid cartilage and widespread RA deformity were also found.

Related references **(1)** Mikulowski P, Wollheim FA, Rotmil P, Olsen I. Sudden death in rheumatoid arthritis with atlantoaxial dislocation. *Acta Medica Scandinavica* 1975; **198**:445–451.

(2) Redlund-Johnell I. *Dislocations of the cervical spine in rheumatoid arthritis.* Thesis, Lund University, 1984.

Key message

Atlanto-axial and other cervical dislocations are important sources of morbidity in RA and may even be a threat to the life of the patient.

Why it's important

Inflammatory processes such as retropharyngeal abscess as well as odontoid fracture or congenital anomalies of the craniovertebral region were well known causes of fatal medullary compression, but this was the first reported case due to rheumatoid involvement of the craniovertebral region. It was also the first case of laryngeal arthritis to be reported.

Strength

Clear description of cervical disease in RA leading to upward subluxation of the odontoid peg and consequent medullary pressure.

Weaknesses

1. A single case description.
2. The autopsy findings of oesophageal ulcer with cricoarytenoid arthritis were incorrect and were cricoarytenoid arthritis with per continuum spreading into the oesophagus.

Relevance

This paper and the related references led to important changes in radiological examinations in RA, especially in the pre-operative evaluation of the neck, which subsequently included lateral examinations in flexion and extension to demonstrate cervical dislocations.

Paper 6

Radiographic evaluation of rheumatoid arthritis and related conditions by standard reference films

Authors

Larsen A, Dale K, Eek M

Reference

Acta Radiologica (Diagnosis) 1977; **18**:481–491

Summary

A review of radiographic evaluation of RA is given. Standard reference films are introduced for evaluation of RA and related conditions in the extremity joints. In this system numerical evaluation of arthritis is given for individual joints in a patient.

Related references **(1)** Larson A. Radiological grading of rheumatoid arthritis, an interobserver study. *Scandinavian Journal of Rheumatology* 1973; **2**:136.

(2) Larson A, Thoen J. Hand radiography of 200 patients with rheumatoid arthritis after an interval of one year. *Scandinavian Journal of Rheumatology* 1987; **16**:395–401.

(3) Larson A. How to apply the Larson score in evaluating radiographsof rheumatoid arthritis in longterm studies. *Journal of Rheumatology* 1995; **22**:1974–1975.

(4) Kellgren JH, Lawrence JS. Radiological assessment of rheumatoid arthritis. *Annals of Rheumatic Diseases* 1957; **16**:485–493.

(5) Steinbrocker O, Traeger GH, Battermann RC. Therapeutic criteria in rheumatoid arthritis. *Journal of the American Medical Association* 1949; **140**:659–662.

(6) Sharp JT, Lidsky MD, Collins LC, Moreland J. Methods of scoring progression of radiologic changes in rheumatoid arthritis. *Arthritis and Rheumatism* 1971; **14**:706–20.

(7) Van der Heijde DM, van Riel PL, Nuver-Zwart HH. Effects of hydroxychloroquine and sulphasalazine on progression of joint damage in rheumatoid arthritis. *The Lancet* 1989; **1**:1036–1038.

Key message

With the help of standard reference films it is possible to evaluate the severity of joint damage of peripheral joints in RA.

Why it's important

Radiographic evaluation of the severity of RA began in 1949 when Steinbrocker, *et al.* divided the changes into four stages according to occurrence of osteoporosis, cartilage and bone destruction and ankylosis. That method only took consideration of a single joint, not the status of, for example, the whole hand. The present method with standard reference films reflects the severity of the whole hand, foot and other regions. An interobserver analysis demonstrated that nine out of 10 arthritis films were staged uniformly by six observers. The method is not specific for RA and can also be used in psoriatic arthropathy and ankylosing spondylitis. Some problems may occur in cases with OA secondary to arthritis. The method is purely a radiographic evaluation and should not be considered as a general measure of the severity of disease.

The 'Larson method' described in this paper became one of the standard methods for evaluation of joint damage and of radiological progression of RA. This has became very important in the evaluation of new treatments thought to slow disease progression, as well as for studies of the natural history of the disease. Larson has continued to refine and develop the methodology, as outlined in the related references. The main alternative is the Sharp method, and more recently that described by van der Heijde, *et al.* (8).

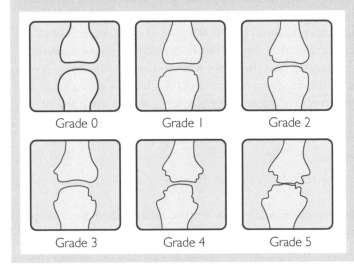

Figure 2.3 Representation of the Larson grades used to assess rheumatois arthritis (as illustrated in Larson (3).

Strengths

1. The method described is simple and easy to learn.
2. The reliability of the method is high.

Weaknesses

1. The most severe form of joint destruction seen in RA (arthritis mutilans), is not included in the Larson grades.
2. Some progression of joint damage can occur without a change in the grade.

Relevance

The described method is still one of the standard techniques used to assess the radiographic progression of RA. Recently, MRI based techniques have been introduced, and they may supercede the Larson technique for the evaluation of new disease-modifying anti-rheumatic drugs.

Paper 7

Radiological assessment of osteo-arthrosis

Authors

Kellgren JH, Lawrence JS

Reference

Annals of Rheumatic Diseases 1957; **16**:494–502

Summary

A series of 510 x-rays from 85 persons in the age group 55–64 years chosen at random from an urban population was graded for osteo-arthrosis by two observers on four occasions to determine the extent of observer difference. Standard films for four grades of osteo-arthrosis for each of eleven joints were chosen. A significant correlation between the two observers was obtained for all joints except the wrist. The stimates of prevalence, however, varied widely because of the cumulative effect of observer bias (+/-31%). It is concluded that comparison of prevalence estimates by different observers could have little value in population studies.

Two readings by the same observer gave only a slightly better correlation on the reading of individual x-rays, but, by excluding observer bias they gave a much closer estimate of prevalence (+/-5%). These two readings however, differed substantially from the mean value for all readings (-8% and -17%). A combined reading by two observers reduced the influence of personal bias and differed little from the mean value (-3%). It is suggested that, where possible, in all population studies the x-rays should be read by either the same observer or preferably by two observers in consultation.

Key message

It is possible to grade x-rays for OA into five categories in a reproducible manner, appropriate for population studies of prevalence.

Related references

(1) Cooper C. Radiographic atlases for the assessment of osteoarthritis. *Osteoarthritis and Cartilage* 1995; **3**(suppl. A):1–2.

(2) Spector T, Cooper C. Radiographic assessment of osteoarthritis in population studies: whither Kellgren and Lawrence? *Osteoarthritis and Cartilage* 1993; **1**:203–6.

(3) Buckland-Wright JC. Quantitative radiography of osteoarthritis. *Annals of Rheumatic Diseases* 1994; **53**:268–275.

Why it's important

The Kellgren and Lawrence system of grading an OA joint into one of five grades has been the 'gold-standard' for reporting and assessing the severity of OA for over 40 years. It is a simple system applicable to population studies and to patient groups, and has been used to assess progression and outcome as well as the presence (or absence) of OA and its severity. There have been however, a number of criticisms of the system, which assumes linear progression between grades and lumps together bone changes such as osteophyte formation with joint space narrowing, which is a surrogate for cartilage loss. These criticisms have led to the development of new atlases which allow individual features to be scored and to the introduction of quantitative methods (see related references). However, in spite of that, most current studies of OA still use or refer to the Kellgren and Lawrence system.

Strengths

1. A simple, plausible system which has four grades of severity and which has an atlas to help reproducibility.
2. Widely used.

Weaknesses

1. The different grades are not well described or clear.
2. There are slightly different descriptions in different publications from the authors.
3. Assumes linearity of progression between grades.
4. Assumes that bone and cartilage changes go together.

Relevance

Introduction of the system which has dominated OA research ever since. However, it could now be overtaken by quantitative MRI.

CHAPTER 3

Serological tests

Josef Smolen

Introduction

It is now difficult to conceive of a time when systemic rheumatic disorders were not thought to have an immunological component. However, prior to the Second World War this was the case. Infections (such as chronic tonsillitis) were thought to be the likely causes of conditions such as rheumatoid arthritis (RA). Furthermore, at that point, there was little or no differentiation made between RA and other systemic rheumatic disorders, and no blood tests available to aid diagnosis. The discovery of a variety of factors (subsequently defined as auto-antibodies) in the serum of patients with rheumatic diseases changed all that. The discovery of these antibodies also led to the development of diagnostic serology, and to a continuing new chapter of research into the etiopathogenesis of rheumatic diseases.

The starting point was the discovery of rheumatoid factor. Waaler's important paper of 1940 (Paper 1) provides the first description of the sheep cell agglutination test for the identification of this anti-immunoglobulin. The test was subsequently developed independently by Rose, and the 'Waaler-Rose test' became the first diagnostic assay for an antibody used in rheumatology. Subsequent technological developments have changed and refined our ways of detecting and measuring rheumatoid factor, but the test remains widely used today.

One of the most active and productive areas of rheumatological research over the last 50 years has centred on the classification and etiopathogenesis of the connective tissue disorders. This all started with Hargreaves' discovery of the 'LE cell' in 1948 (Paper 2). This led to the understanding that in systemic lupus erythematosus (SLE) there were auto-antibodies directed against nuclear antigens. This test was initially also of some value diagnostically, although it has subsequently been overtaken by the more specific and sensitive assays of individual nuclear antigens.

Following these early discoveries, there was then an explosion of serological work in the 1960s, 70s and 80s, leading to the huge spectrum of diagnostic auto-antibody tests available to us today, and stimulating profitable research into the mechanisms of tissue damage in connective tissue disorders. Some of the most important of these discoveries have been picked out. The first non-DNA-non-histone antigen to be identified was the Sm factor found by Tan and colleagues in 1966 (Paper 3). In 1972 Sharp and colleagues described extractable nuclear antigen (ENA) and linked it to a specific phenotype of connective tissue disease expression (mixed connective tissue disease). This was the first disease to be defined serologically (Paper 4). Subsequently a group of other antibodies were discovered which not only aid the diagnosis and classification of connective tissue diseases, but which also provide direct links to tissue damage. These include the Ro and La antibodies found in SLE and Sjögren's syndrome (Paper 5), Scl-70, the first antibody linked to scleroderma (Paper 6) and anti-Jo-1, the first dermatomyositis specific antibody (Paper 7).

Technology has been an important driver of this area of discovery. At the time of writing we are moving into another technologically-derived new era of medicine, the 'post-genome' era, and with this change we are starting to see a shift of interest from the serology to the genome and the production of the proteins that for the antigens and antibodies that are so important in systemic rheumatic diseases.

Paper 1

On the occurrence of a factor in human serum activating the specific agglutination of sheep blood corpuscles

Author

Waaler Erik

Reference

Acta Pathologica Microbiol Scandinavica 1940; **17**:72–188

Summary

Human serum can augment the agglutination of sheep red blood cells (SRBC) coated with anti-SRBC serum and can lead to agglutination of SRBC coated with sub-agglutinating doses of the anti-SRBC serum. The factor, which was independent of natural heteroagglutinins and thus depended on the presence of agglutinins to SRBC, was called agglutination activating factor. Although most human sera contained little or no such factor, some sera were highly active. Both in terms of titre as well as frequency, the most active sera were from rheumatoid arthritis (RA) patients, although 50 of 77 patients did not have the factor and sera from a few patients with non-rheumatic diseases also carried this activity. The activity was not associated with the sedimentation rate nor the presence of anti-streptococcal agglutinins and was thermostable to heating to 60°C for 30 min. The agglutination activating factor was contained in the globulin and not the albumin fraction of serum.

Related reference   (1)   Rose HM, Ragan C, Pearce E, Lipman MO. Differential agglutination of normal and sensitised sheep erythrocytes by sera of patients with rheumatoid arthritis. *Proceedings of the Society for Experimental Biology and Medicine* 1948; **68**:1–6.

Key message

A description of a serum factor (later named rheumatoid factor (RF)) in patient and normal human sera, found most frequently and in highest titres in patients with RA.

Why it's important

Prior to this publication RA was not regarded to be an autoimmune disease and there were no serological tests available to support the differentiation of RA from other rheumatic conditions. Thus, this paper became the starting point for diagnostic tests for RA as well as the search into the immunological etiopathogenesis of the disease. Although the first descriptions of the reported 'agglutination activated activity' was provided by Olsen and by Meyer, Waaler's major contribution was its demonstration in human sera and the observation of its link to RA. Several years later, Rose, *et al.* (without quoting or knowing the paper by Waaler) developed the method for the sheep cell agglutination test widely known and practised until recent years as Waaler–Rose test. In contrast to Waaler, who felt that 'the reaction can not be of any diagnostic value', Rose, *et al.* found a predominance of high titres in patients with RA as well as an association of the magnitude of the reactivity with RA disease activity and suggested that 'the sheep cell differential agglutination test may be of value in determining the activity status of RA' and may 'be helpful as an aid in the differential diagnosis between RA and other diseases with arthritic manifestations'. Singer and Plotz then exchanged SRBC by Latex particles and anti-SRBC serum (from rabbits) with human gamma globulin preparations for reasons of reproducibility and stability (latex fixation test). Although RF is not pathognomonic for RA, it is a helpful diagnostic test and became part of the classification criteria of the American College of Rheumatology. The sheep cell agglutination and the latex fixation test have been now widely replaced by nephelometric techniques.

It has later been shown that the RF activity was an auto-antibody to human IgG (or IgG from other species). The specificity of RF as a diagnostic test is not high, particularly since its frequency in early RA is relatively low. This has prompted several groups to search for other auto-antibodies more specifically associated with RA and has led to interesting and in part diagnostically helpful findings.

Strengths

1. Good example of thorough follow-up of a serendipitous observation with a single serum.
2. Good application of 'classical' serological methods, clear and relevant experimental design.
3. First unequivocal report on anti-protein auto-antibodies in rheumatic diseases.

Weaknesses

1. The nature of the agglutination activating activity as an immunoglobulin was not elucidated, but the methods of those days were relatively poor: electrophoresis had not yet been invented and thus gamma globulin not yet been separated from other globulins, immunoglobulins had not yet been detected and therefore not the immunoglobulin classes either.
2. The conclusion that the RF activity was of no diagnostic value is not easy to follow on the basis of the data presented; it appears to be superficial and partly due to a lack of using statistical analyses and of following patients longitudinally.
3. The diagnostic criteria for RA used in this study are not explained and many patients presumed to have RA may not have had the disease.

Relevance

The discovery of RF led to the search for immunological mechanisms in RA.

Paper 2

Presentation of two bone marrow elements: The 'tart cell' and the 'LE' cell

Authors

Hargraves MM, Richmond H, Morton R

Reference

Mayo Clinic Proceedings 1948; **23**:25–28

Summary

In smears of bone marrow from patients with acute disseminated lupus erythematosus (SLE), a cell type has been found which was called an LE cell and represented a mature neutrophilic polymorphonuclear leukocyte containing chromatin material within a large phagocytic vacuole. The nuclear nature of the material was shown by specific nuclear stain (Feulgen's stain). The LE cell is suggested to be the result of a lytic-phagocytic phenomenon in which neutrophils are chemoattracted by nuclear material released as a consequence of cell destruction and phagocytose this material. Several neutrophils can surround the same mass of material, but once one of the cells has succeeded in ingesting it, the chemotactic action is lost and the other cells move off. The phenomenon has been found only in bone marrow in certain cases of SLE, although the diagnosis may be challenged in some of the more than 25 cases observed with the LE cell phenomenon.

Key message

First description of a reactivity to nuclear material in patients with SLE which has led to a diagnostically valuable test and was the starting point for all subsequent investigations into anti-nuclear antibodies, i.e. auto-antibodies to nucleic acids and nucleic acid binding proteins, as well as the recognition of the autoimmune nature of SLE.

Why it's important

Before the description of the LE cell phenomenon, insight into the pathogenesis of SLE stemmed solely from clinical and histopathological observations. The implication of the description that the LE cell in SLE was somehow associated with a 'lytic-phagocytic' process and that nuclear material in SLE could be modified to become chemoattractive was a first indication of an autoimmune phenomenon (aside from the anti-erythrocyte antibodies). The description of the LE cell phenomenon was followed by the findings that it could be also reproduced in peripheral blood, that the inducing factor ('LE cell factor') was a gamma globulin and that the phenomenon required the presence of nuclear material, the LE cell factor and complement. This laid the grounds for (a) all subsequent laboratory tests in the differential diagnosis of. SLE and other connective tissue diseases, (b) the research in the field of anti-nuclear auto-antibodies, (c) the findings of nuclear antigens as targets of these auto-antibodies, (d) the detection of many nuclear antigens and their biological functions, (e) the recognition of SLE as an immune-mediated and autoimmune disease, and (f) the finding of immune complexes as decisive contributors to the pathology and clinical symptoms of the disease.

The LE cell phenomenon was helpful in the diagnosis of SLE and became one of the classification criteria of the disease. Later, after Coons invented indirect immunofluorescence microscopy, the fluorescent anti-nuclear antibody (FANA) test was described and became a helpful tool in diagnosis and research of connective tissue diseases. ANA patterns soon became discernible and were finally associated with particular diseases.

The nature of the auto-antigen targeted by the LE cell factor had not been unequivocally elucidated until 50 years after the description of the phenomenon, when it could be defined as histone H1 by immunoblotting and various inhibition experiments. The presence of nucleic acids was not necessary to elicit the phenomenon. The LE cell phenomenon and, in particular, the anti-histone H1 auto-antibodies, are associated with more severe courses of the disease. Nevertheless, neither the LE cell phenomenon nor anti-histone H1 antibodies are pathognomonic for SLE.

Strengths

1. Very well observed abnormality in SLE bone marrow and definition of the target moiety as nuclear material.
2. Excellent description of the events governing the phenomenon using only conventional light microscopy and initiating the concept of SLE as characterized by auto-antibodies to nuclear antigens and immune complexes.
3. Diagnostically valuable and stimulating for subsequent research.

Weaknesses

1. The nature of the target antigen remained elusive.
2. Simple observational description without experimental investigations into the basis of the phenomenon.
3. Lack of systematic investigation of different patient cohorts.

Relevance

The discovery of the LE cell began the investigation of anti-nuclear antibodies and autoimmune mechanisms in connective tissue disorders.

Paper 3

Characteristics of a soluble nuclear antigen precipitating with sera of patients with systemic lupus erythematosus

Authors

Tan EM, Kunkel HG

Reference

Journal of Immunology 1966; **96**:464–471

Summary

Precipitating antibodies which reacted with soluble extracts of different human tissues or nuclei including nuclei from calf thymus were found in sera of patients with systemic lupus erythematosus. The antigen was different from DNA and histone, but was associated with protein fractions and insensitive to deoxyribonuclease, ribonuclease and trypsin, but sensitive to periodate treatment. The reactivity was detected by Ouchterlony double-immunodiffusion and by immunoelectrophoresis techniques. The reactive serum factor was shown to migrate in the gamma globulin fraction. The antigen was provisionally termed 'Sm' and the reactivity was described to be found in approximately 75% of SLE patients but only very few patients with other disorders.

Key message

The first description of an auto-antibody reactivity to a non-DNA-non-histone auto-antigen in SLE. This antigenic moiety was termed Sm and the auto-antibodies appeared to be highly specific for SLE.

Why it's important

Prior to this study, only DNA, histones and their complexes had been identified as antigens eliciting auto-antibody reactivities to nuclear antigens in SLE (see chapter on LE cell). The technological advancements of the 1950s and early 1960s, which included the Ouchterlony double-immunodiffusion technique, immunoelectrophoresis and chromatography allowed precipitating antibodies to be distinguished and reactive structures to be better characterized, particularly proteins. The fact that the material extracted from different tissues and nuclei reactive in the precipitation reaction was insensitive to deoxyribonuclease, ribonuclease and trypsin characterized it as clearly different from DNA and histone, but it also gave no line of identity in double-immunodiffusion with the other antigens. In contrast, there were lines of identity when a given serum (from patient Sm) was reacted with soluble extracts from tissues and nuclei of different origin and species. This indicated that the Sm antigen was widely distributed and immunologically identical between species.

Using an anti-Sm positive serum, Steitz and her colleagues were able to identify the antigen as a group of proteins involved in splicing. Thus, the development of auto-antibodies in patients with SLE and the detection of the anti-Sm activity was pivotal for the discovery of hitherto unknown, highly conserved and ubiquitous RNA-binding proteins involved in vital cellular activities. The RNA and protein components of this protein complex (as well as many of their functions) have been well characterized meanwhile, using newer techniques such as immunoblotting and RNA-precipitation, and the characteristic antigenic reactivity was found to reside in the D-antigen. The Sm particle is associated with the 70 kD-U1-RNA particle (see subsequent chapter), and there are certain immunological cross-reactivities between the different components. The antibodies inhibit the splicing process *in vitro*, but their penetration into living cells, although possible, is still debated and does not appear to have major consequences *in vivo*. The proteins are modified during apoptosis.

Strengths

1. Detection of a new reaction with high specificity for SLE.
2. Use of extracts from tissues and nuclei of different organs and different species.
3. Excellent application of existing techniques to define a new auto-antibody, setting the stage for subsequent similar investigations which led to the detection of other auto-antibodies and for investigations into the nature of the nuclear antigens.

Weaknesses

1. The nature of the target antigen remained elusive due to the lack of more sophisticated techniques.
2. Lack of systematic investigation of different patient cohorts (however, this was not the main purpose of the study).
3. Over-estimation of the frequency of anti-Sm antibodies in SLE.

Relevance

The first discovery of an antibody to a non-DNA-non-histone auto-antigen, which was found to be a protein involved in splicing.

Paper 4

Mixed connective tissue disease – an apparent distinct rheumatic disease syndrome associated with a specific antibody to an extractable nuclear antigen (ENA)

Authors

Sharp GC, Irvin WS, Tan EM, Gould RG, Holman HR

Reference

American Journal of Medicine 1972; **52**:148–159

Summary

A nuclear antigen extracted from calf thymus nuclei at low ionic strength, precipitated by acetate and alcohol and solubilized in sodium chloride, containing mainly protein and ribonucleic acid (RNA), was named extractable nuclear antigen (ENA) and used in a haemagglutination test. The antigen was recognized strongly by sera from 25 patients with a mixture of symptoms of SLE, polymyositis and scleroderma (termed mixed connective tissue disease, MCTD) as well as by approximately 50% of SLE patients but not patients with other CTDs. Recognition of the antigen was very sensitive to treatment with RNase, slightly sensitive to trypsin and resistant to DNA. In contrast to SLE, the MCTD sera did not react with Sm and not, or only at low titres, with DNA. The clinical and serological characteristics of MCTD, which included a speckled pattern on indirect immunofluorescence (IIF) and a favourable prognosis, are described.

Related reference **(1)** Mattioli M, Reichlin M. Characterization of a soluble nuclear ribonucleoprotein antigen reactive with SLE sera. *Journal of Immunology* 1971; **107**:1281–1290.

Key message

Demonstration of an anti-nuclear auto-antibody reactivity distinct from Sm but also eliciting a speckled pattern in patients with SLE and an SLE-like syndrome, which led to the description of a new disease entity, mixed connective tissue disease.

Why it's important

The authors described an auto-antibody to an extractable nuclear antigen (ENA) which contained protein and RNA, but in contrast to Sm was RNase sensitive. Their antigen was used in a haemagglutination test and reactivity was found almost exclusively with sera from patients with SLE or SLE-like disease. It was recognized that all 25 patients suffering from a disorder which had features of SLE but also of polymyositis and dermatomyositis, some of whom had also rheumatoid arthritis-like joint involvement, had auto-antibodies to ENA. These patients, in contrast to SLE patients with anti-ENA antibodies, lacked reactivity to Sm and DNA. The reactivity to ENA had been described by the authors previously. A similar antigen named Mo was salt-extracted from thymus nuclei and defined by immunoprecipitation by Mattioli and Reichlin at the same time, but only related to SLE. Sera from patients with MCTD had high titres of both ANA and anti-ENA antibodies. Sera with anti-Sm antibodies had been shown to induce a speckled nuclear fluorescence upon IIF, and so did anti-ENA positive sera. It was later shown that ENA contained mainly 70 kD-U1-RNP and that Sm and U1-RNP were part of the same particle involved in RNA splicing.

MCTD became the first disease which was defined serologically. During the subsequent decades a discussion continued as to the nature of this disease as a clinical entity. However, additional characteristics were found supporting the unique nature of MCTD, such as differences in major histocompatibility antigens when compared to SLE and scleroderma and a highly specific auto-antibody reactivity to a particular epitope of hnRNP-A2, the RA33 antigen. A number of investigators have defined classification criteria for MCTD.

Strengths

1. Description of a new anti-nuclear auto-antibody reactivity.
2. Excellent clinical skills leading to recognition of a new connective tissue disease.
3. First disease defined well by the presence of a particular anti-nuclear auto-antibody.

Weaknesses

1. The nature of the target antigen remained elusive due to the lack of more sophisticated techniques.
2. Antigen only recognized by haemagglutination test.
3. Missed that many patients with SLE also had anti-U1RNP without concomitant anti-Sm and also some scleroderma patients had the antibody.

Relevance

The discovery of MCTD: the first connective tissue disorder to be defined serologically.

Paper 5

Characterization of a soluble cytoplasmic antigen reactive with sera from patients with systemic lupus erythematosus

Authors

Clark G, Reichlin M, Tomasi TB

Reference

Journal of Immunology 1969; **102**:117–122

Summary

A serum of a patient (Ro) with an SLE-like syndrome was shown by complement fixation reaction and double-immunodiffusion technique to react with a cytoplasmic protein contained in several human tissues, but not red blood cells. This protein was distinct from known nuclear antigens such as DNA, histone, nucleohistone, Sm and related extractable antigens. The antigen was found to be an acidic macromolecule containing sulfhydryl groups. Antibodies to this antigen were found in 40% of SLE patients and also in patients with Sjögren's syndrome, but not patients with other connective tissue diseases.

Related references **(1)** Alspaugh M, Tan EM. *Journal of Clinical Investigation* 1975; **55**:1067.

(2) Lerner MR, Boyle JA, Hardin JA, Steitz JA. Two novel classes of small ribonucleoproteins detected by antibodies associated with lupus erythematosus. *Science* 1981; **211**:400–402.

Key message

Description of the reactivity of SLE (and Sjögren's syndrome) sera with a cytoplasmic antigen named Ro. The antigen itself and its cytoplasmic nature made it distinct from the previously recognized nuclear antigens targeted by SLE sera.

Why it's important

While a number of nuclear antigens had been characterized as targets of SLE sera, patient Ro had auto-antibodies directed to a cytoplasmic antigen in her serum. This new reactivity was found in 40% of SLE and in Sjögren's syndrome sera. A similar reactivity was later found primarily in patients with Sjögren's syndrome (and termed SS-A) as a nuclear antigen, but SS-A and Ro were shown to be identical. The riddle's resolution lay in the fact that the antigen shuttled between cytoplasm and nucleus. The Ro antigen turned out to be an RNA-binding protein, but the RNAs that were bound by Ro were hitherto unknown small RNAs, termed Y RNAs. Another antigen which was also recognized by sera from patients with Sjögren's syndrome and SLE and had been termed La or SS-B was associated with yet another group of RNAs, namely 4.5S RNA species which, among other origins, can also be virus associated. Importantly, Ro and La have been found to be associated with each other in a distinct particle. However, the function of the Ro-RNAs as well as the particle have not yet been fully elucidated.

Anti-Ro and anti-La are used in the differential diagnosis of connective tissue diseases, and La is relatively typical (though not pathognomonic) for Sjögren's syndrome. On the other hand, anti-Ro, even though a more promiscuous auto-antibody, has been associated with a series of subtypes of SLE. This includes mild subtypes, such as the so called ANA-negative SLE (which lacked ANA on conventional rat liver sections due to the low concentration of the Ro antigen in rat liver) and subacute cutaneous lupus erythematosus, but also neonatal LE and congenital heart block, both on the basis of transplacentar passage of these (and other) auto-antibodies and their binding to particular organs in the neonate.

Thus, the characterization of the Ro antigen has led to (a) the recognition of the underlying cause of neonatal lupus and congenital heart block, (b) the characterization of particularly mild forms of SLE, (c) the detection of a new ribonucleoprotein particle and (d) the detection of hitherto unknown RNA species.

Strengths

1. Characterization of a new target antigen for auto-antibodies of patients with connective tissue diseases, particularly SLE and Sjögren's syndrome.
2. Demonstrated of the cytoplasmic nature of this antigen as opposed to the nuclear antigens known in those times.
3. Stimulation of further research into cytoplasmic auto-antigens.

Weaknesses

1. Technical limitations of those days precluded better characterization of the antigen.
2. The presence of Ro in a particle was not recognized.
3. Patients were not well characterized clinically.

Relevance

The discovery of Ro antigen which has been found to be associated with a variety of clinical syndromes including neonatal lupus with congenital heart block and mild forms of SLE.

Paper 6

Identification of a nuclear protein (Scl-70) as a unique target of human antinuclear antibodies in scleroderma

Authors

Douvas AS, Achten M, Tan EM

Reference

Journal of Biological Chemistry 1979; **254**: 10514–10522

Summary

Using biochemical and immunological techniques, a 70 kD protein contained in rat liver nuclei was characterized to be reactive with sera from five scleroderma patients. The antigen was termed Scl-70. Absorption experiments revealed that this was the major or only antinuclear reactivity contained in these sera. The preparation of several distinct fractions of nuclear extracts allowed the recognition that the antigen was a basic non-histone nuclear protein associated with the chromatin fraction and localized on the chromosomes of cells in mitosis.

Key message

Characterization of a nuclear, DNA-associated protein as target for sera from several patients with scleroderma. This antigen, Scl-70, is a major, if not sole, target in the sera of these patients.

Why it's important

This is the first nuclear antigen ever characterized as target antigen for patients with systemic sclerosis. Scl-70 was later revealed to be a degradation product of the protein topoisomerase (also named Scl-100 by virtue of its molecular mass). The antigen is found in about 40% of patients with systemic sclerosis and is mainly associated with the diffuse form, while limited systemic sclerosis is associated with auto-antibodies to centromere proteins which typically is present in the CREST syndrome. Other auto-antibody systems also occur in scleroderma. Interestingly, all these auto-antibodies can be localized to the nucleolus, although the exquisite specificity for nucleolar auto-antigens in systemic sclerosis is unresolved.

Anti-Scl-70 auto-antibodies are pathognomonic for scleroderma, but it is uncommon for patients to have more than one scleroderma-typical auto-antibody specificity. The different auto-antibody systems are commonly related to distinct clinical subtypes of the disease and anti-Scl-70 is related to diffuse cutaneous involvement but also pulmonary fibrosis.

The recognition of Scl-70 as a target antigen has significantly advanced the diagnostic armamentarium in the differentiation of the connective tissue diseases and, together with the subsequent detection of other scleroderma-typical auto-antigens, also allowed distinct subsets to be discerned which are characterized by different clinical and particularly prognostic features. All these auto-antibodies are highly characteristic for systemic sclerosis, while other anti-nuclear auto-antibody subsets are virtually never found (with the exception of occasional anti-Ro reactivities).

Strengths

1. Characterization of a new target antigen for auto-antibodies of patients with systemic sclerosis.
2. Use of available techniques to optimize the characterization of the antigen and definition as a non-histone chromosomal protein.
3. Definition of the specificity and selectivity of the immune response in scleroderma patients.

Weaknesses

1. The higher molecular weight parent protein was not detected.
2. Sera from only five scleroderma patients were tested.
3. No description of the patients' clinical features.

Relevance

The discovery of anti-Scl-70, the first of a group of auto-antibodies which are associated with distinct subsets of scleroderma.

Paper 7

Myositis autoantibody inhibits histidyl-tRNA synthetase: a model for autoimmunity

Authors

Mathews MB, Bernstein RM

Reference

Nature 1983; **304**:177–179

Summary

IgG fractions from sera of patients with myositis and anti-Jo-1 antibodies, but not myositis and other auto-antibodies or other autoimmune rheumatic disorders, were used for immunoprecipitation of HeLa cell extracts labelled with 35-S-methionine or 32-P-phosphate. A protein of 50,000 kD molecular mass and an RNA species of tRNA size were detected by polyacrylamide gel electrophoresis. All anti-Jo-1-positive sera induced the same reaction. RNase treatment revealed that the anti-Jo-1[reactivity was retained indicating that the major epitope(s) resided on the protein. Further electrophoretic analyses, including RNA finger-printing, suggested that the RNA species was a tRNA containing the anticodon for histidine. While it had no effect on the stability of the complex between histidine and its cognate tRNA, anti-Jo-1 IgG inhibited 3-H-histidine joining to its tRNA, but not the charging of tRNAs with other amino acids. This inhibition was highly specific for anti-Jo-1-positive sera, since other sera did not inhibit 3-H-histidine-tRNA interaction. Removal of the Jo-1 antigen from the aminoacyl-tRNA synthetase preparation specifically eliminated the capacity to charge tRNA with histidine. It was concluded that the Jo-1 antigen was histidyl-tRNA synthetase or a functional subunit of this enzyme. Importantly, the antigen appeared to be contained only in the cytoplasm. Finally, the authors speculate on the association of autoimmunity to Jo-1 with infections with myotropic viruses capable of carrying a histidine residue attached to its RNA.

Related references   **(1)**   Nishikai M, Reichlin M. Heterogeneity of precipitating antibodies in polymyositis and dermatomyositis – Characterization of the Jo-1 antibody system. *Arthritis and Rheumatism* 1980; **23**:881–888.

(2)   Ross MD, Hendrick JP, Lerner MR, Steitz JA, Reichlin M. *Nucleic Acids Research* 1983; **11**:853–870.

Key message

Characterization of the protein reactive with the most common auto-antibody in sera from patients with poly- and dermatomyositis improve diagnostic approaches and possible search into the etiopathogenesis of myositides.

Why it's important

Poly- and dermatomyositis have been found associated with a large number of precipitating auto-antibodies, anti-Jo-1 being the most common one. While it had been noted at about the same time that anti-Jo-1-positive sera precipitated histidyl-tRNA, the study by Mathews and Bernstein revealed that the reactivity was directed primarily to the enzyme that catalyzes the charging with histidine of the specific tRNA. This finding led to the recognition that a variety of other myositis-specific auto-antibodies were directed to tRNA-synthetases, albeit different species of these enzymes. Although anti-Jo-1 is the most common of these auto-antibodies, the clinical features of patients with auto-antibodies to the different synthetases are similar. One of the features of this 'anti-synthetase syndrome' is involvement of the lung. Thus, the definition of histidyl-tRNA-synthetase as a major auto-antigen in myositis has allowed better diagnostic and prognostic approaches to this disease. Interestingly, the antibodies are not only directed to the proteins but also to the tRNA species themselves. However, completely different auto-antigens are recognized by sera from other patients with myositides, and many of them have other clinical characteristics, frequently with quite aggressive disease.

There are two other important aspects of this study: First, the authors showed that the auto-antibody inhibited the function of the target protein (in this case the charging of histidyl-tRNA with histidine which is catalyzed by the target synthetase); thus, similar to anti-Sm antibodies, the targeted epitope ought to be the functional site of the molecule. Second, this and subsequent investigations also revealed the exquisite specificity of certain auto-antibody systems for particular disorders: anti-Jo-1 and the other anti-synthetases are pathognomonic auto-antibodies, suggesting a common underlying cause for at least one large subset of the myositides. However, despite these highly specific serologic characteristics, the cause(s) of the disease have not yet been elucidated.

Strengths

1. Characterization of the major target antigen for myositis-specific precipitating anti-Jo-1 antibodies.
2. Demonstration of the interference of the auto-antibody with the function of the target enzyme.
3. Demonstration of the cytoplasmic rather than nuclear nature of this auto-antigen.

Weaknesses

1. Other anti-synthetases not described as targets for myositis sera.
2. Target epitope(s) not characterized.
3. Induction of anti-Jo-1 discussed in a speculative way without further data (nor subsequent experimental approach).

Relevance

Anti-Jo-1 was the first specific auto-antibody to be associated with myositis. As outlined in the chapter on polymyositis, the different auto-antibodies found in this family of diseases offer a means of classification.

CHAPTER 4

Other investigations: synovial fluid analysis, arthroscopy and blood biochemistry

Paul Dieppe

Introduction

Rheumatology is a subspeciality of medicine in which diagnoses still depend more on the history and physical examination than on special investigations. Indeed, the relative lack of special diagnostic and therapeutic procedures has been seen as a problem for the discipline. However, the fact that rheumatology is concerned with diseases of joints, particularly synovial joints, means that access to products of the joints, as well as visualization of joint structures have been explored for their diagnostic potential, as well as the insights they provide on disease mechanisms.

The most obvious place to look is in the synovial fluid. The first, definitive studies of human synovial fluid were published as monographs rather than scientific papers. In 1938 Kling published a book describing the synovial membrane and synovial fluid (1), but the most important and 'classic' contribution was that of Marion Ropes and Walter Bauer, published in 1953 (2), a masterful contribution. Hollander was the early proponent of synovial fluid analysis as a diagnostic aid to arthritis, describing it as a 'liquid biopsy' of the synovial joint, and documenting his personal experience of some 100 000 aspirations and injections (Paper 1). The most important development in the diagnostic examination of synovial fluid samples came with Dan McCarty's introduction of polarized light microscopy for the identification of urate (Paper 2) and subsequently pyrophosphate (Paper 3) crystals. Polarized light microscopy is now a routine part of rheumatological practice, and a little known contribution of Ralph Schumacher's group has shown that it is one of the few tests in our armamentarium that actually changes clinical practice (Paper 4). Orthopaedic surgeons, not content with putting small needles into joints to aspirate fluid samples, subsequently introduced arthroscopic examination of joints, allowing direct visualization of structures and biopsy of any structures that appear abnormal (Paper 5). Subsequently mini-arthroscopes have been introduced for office use by rheumatologists, although their value remains disputed.

Joint diseases are characterized by two different pathological processes, first, inflammation of the synovial lining, and second, destruction or altered turnover of structural elements such as the articular cartilage. Both types of process lead to the release of products into the bloodstream, leading to the possibility that simple serum assays might be of diagnostic value. It has long been known that most inflammatory processes in the body (including synovitis) lead to a raised erythrocyte sedimentation rate (ESR). We now know that this is mediated by the release of cytokines from the inflamed tissue, and resulting changes in the synthesis of a range of proteins in the liver. Serum levels of one of these 'acute-phase proteins', C-reactive protein (CRP) are particularly elevated in inflammatory arthritis, and is regularly used to assess disease activity. A particularly important development in this story came with the recognition that CRP levels also had predictive value for subsequent erosive damage to joints in rheumatoid arthritis (RA) (Paper 6) indicating that the measurement of CRP could (and perhaps should) be used to monitor RA and to assess the degree of success of suppressive therapies. More recently, the development of extremely sensitive immunological assays has made it possible to measure serum levels of a variety of products of connective tissue turnover, some of which are relatively specific to joint pathology. Our final selection in this group of papers illustrates the potential value of one of these assays in predicting joint damage in a variety of types of arthritis (Paper 7). Only time will tell what impact the use of these 'biochemical markers' is destined to have on rheumatological practice (3).

References

1. Kling DH. *The synovial membrane and synovial fluid.* Los Angeles Medical Press, 1938.
2. Ropes MW, Bauer W. *Synovial fluid changes in joint disease.* Harvard University Press, 1953.
3. Myers SL. Synovial fluid markers in osteoarthritis. *Rheumatic Diseases Clinics of North America* 1999; **25**:443–449.

Paper 1

Examination of synovial fluid as a diagnostic aid in arthritis

Authors

Hollander JL, Reginato A, Torralba TP

Reference

Medical Clinics of North America 1966; **50**:1281–1293

Summary

From a wide experience with synovianalyses we have concluded that careful examination of joint fluid is the most definitive diagnostic laboratory test for differentiation of the various forms of arthritis. It is also the diagnostic aid least frequently utilized by physicians. Study of the joint fluid is as important in arthritis as urinalysis in renal disease. Synovial fluid is actually a 'liquid biopsy' from the site of inflammation. Many new facts about arthritis are being added to our knowledge each year from studies on the synovial fluid. Some of these advances have been described in this report, together with a detailed description of techniques and findings in various forms of arthritis.

Related references (1) Hollander JL. The most neglected differential diagnostic test in arthritis. *Arthritis and Rheumatism* 1960; **3**:364–367.

(2) Kling DH. *The Synovial membrane and Synovial Fluid.* Los Angeles Medical Press, 1938.

(3) Ropes MW, Bauer W. *Synovial fluid changes in joint disease.* Harvard University Press, 1953.

(4) Hollander JL. In: *Textbook of Rheumatology.*

Key message

Synovial fluid examination is a very important aid to the diagnosis of the different forms of arthritis.

Why it's important

The monograph of Ropes and Bauer (3) is the most important contribution to this field, as it documents synovial fluid findings in health as well as disease, and provides a comprehensive overview of preceding literature as well as the extensive work of the authors. However, it was Hollander, rather than Ropes and Bauer, who championed the routine use of synovial fluid analysis in rheumatological practice. Hollander and colleagues report on their unrivalled experience of synovial fluid analysis in this paper, reporting on findings of gross appearance, mucin clot formation, cell counts, rheumatoid factor levels, culture, and polarized light microscopy. They provide a table of the main findings in different diseases.

Hollander reports on normal synovial fluid, and on total and differential cell counts in inflammatory and non-inflammatory forms of arthritis, findings that have remained largely unchallenged and believed in ever since by subsequent generations of rheumatologists.

Strengths

1. Built on vast experience (Hollander claims that his unit has personal experience of nearly 100 000 joint aspirations and injections).
2. Clear documentation of the main findings of synovial fluid in different forms of arthritis.
3. Comments on all the major available assays of synovial fluids.

Weaknesses

1. No data is presented, just what the authors believe to be the synovial fluid findings in different conditions.
2. It is unclear on what the report of normal synovial fluid findings is based on.
3. This is a review which contains as much propaganda (in favour of aspirating joints) as it does science.

Relevance

Became the established accepted view on synovial fluid findings in different forms of arthritis, and the value of analysis in rheumatological practice.

Paper 2

Identification of urate crystals in gout synovial fluid

Authors

McCarty DJ, Hollander JL

Reference

Annals of Internal Medicine 1961; **54**:452–460

Summary

Urate crystals in synovial fluid and the crystals from a subcutaneous tophus were found to have identical optical properties by polarized light microscopy. They were negatively birefringent with extinction on the long axis. Urate crytals were identified by polarized light microscopy in the aspirated synovial fluid obtained from 15 of 18 patients with clinical gout. The crystals were specifically digested by uricase in all 15 samples and in two instances disappeared in the control specimens as well. Urate crystals were also identified by ordinary light microscopy in 11 of the same 18 synovial fluid samples.

Comparison of the results of ordinary light microscopy with those seen by polariscopic observation revealed that the percentage positive identification was greater when the latter method was used. In two instances, crystals were seen by ordinary light which did not have the characteristics of urate crystals. One of these was from an otherwise typical case of acute gouty arthritis. The concentration of urate in the synovial fluid during the acute attack is probably higher than that found in the serum.

Related reference   (1)   McCarty DJ. The inflammatory reaction to microcrystalline sodium urate. *Arthritis and Rheumatism* 1965; **8**:726–735.

Key message

Polarized light microscopy leads to more accurate identification of urate crystals in the synovial fluid than ordinary light microscopy, which had been used previously. Ordinary light microscopy results in both false negative and false positive results. The highly characteristic properties of urate crystals viewed by polarized light (needle shape and strong negative birefringence) allows easy identification.

Why it's important

Polarized light microscopy of synovial fluid for the identification of urate and pyrophosphate crystals in order to diagnose gout and pseudogout respectively, is now a routine part of our clinical practice. However, prior to the publication of this paper that was not the case. As the authors say in their introduction 'urate crystals have been noted in the synovial fluid from gouty patients in the past, but this finding was believed to be infrequent and of little assistance to the clinician in his attempt to establish a diagnosis'.

With this paper McCarty and Hollander showed that polarized light microscopy allowed the easy identification of urate crystals in synovial fluids, and that they were almost always present in gout. This finding, which has stood the test of time, led to the widespread use of the technique in clinical practice. The paper illustrates the characteristic appearances of urate crystals viewed by polarized light microscopy, as shown in Figure 4.1.

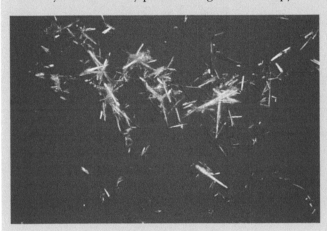

Figure 4.1 Monosodium urate monohydrate crystals from a gouty tophus viewed by compensated polarized light microscopy. Note the needle shaped morphology and strong negative birefringence (resulting in a yellow appearance when the long axis of the crystal is aligned with the axis of the compensator). (Courtesy of Dr Angela Swan.)

Strengths

1. Introduction of a new, reliable technique for the identification of urate crystals.
2. Clear, concise, well illustrated description of the characteristics of the crystals when viewed by polarized light microscopy.
3. Check on the validity of the technique by using uricase to digest crystals.
4. Comparison with the only other method available at the time, i.e. ordinary light microscopy.
5. Discovery of two false positives using ordinary light microscopy pre-empts their discovery of pyrophosphate crystals.

Weaknesses

1. The authors mention, but do not present proper results of the examination of synovial fluids from non-gouty patients. Therefore they were not able to say with certainty that the test was specific for gout.
2. The paper is generally lacking in methodological detail and is rather brief.
3. They do not describe how samples were searched for crystals under either ordinary or polarized light, or how easy or difficult it was to find the particles.
4. Their speculation on urate concentrations in synovial fluid, which reached the summary, has no foundation in data.

Relevance

The paper that led to the introduction of the most important laboratory investigation specific to rheumatology.

Paper 3

The significance of calcium phosphate crystals in the synovial fluid of arthritic patients: the 'pseudogout syndrome'. II. Identification of crystals

Authors

Kohn NN, Hughes RE, McCarty DJ, Faires JS

Reference

Annals of Internal Medicine 1962; **56**:738–745

Summary

In our study of a series of synovial fluids obtained by aspiration from a group of patients with arthritis, we observed seven fluids that contained significant amounts of crystalline material. In five instances, these crystals were shown to be identical crystallgraphically and distinct from apatite and tophaceous material. Physical and chemical studies of these crystals led to the conclusion that they were a form of calcium pyrophosphate. The utilization of x-ray diffraction in obtaining powder pattern photographs proved to be especially useful in this problem. The applicability of this method in the investigation of normal and abnormal biological processes involving the crystalline state is briefly discussed.

Related references

(1) McCarty DJ, Kohn NN, Faires JS. The significance of calcium phosphate crystals in the synovial fluid of arthritic patients: the 'pseudogout syndrome'. I. Clinical aspects. *Annals of Internal Medicine* 1962; **56**:711–736.

(2) McCarty DJ. Calcium pyrophosphate dihydrate deposition disease. *Arthritis and Rheumatism* 1976; **19** (Supplement Volume).

(3) McCarty DJ, Hogan JM, Gatter RA. Studies on pathological calcifications in human cartilage. *Journal of Bone and Joint Surgery* 1966; **48**(A):309.

(4) Dieppe PA, Crocker PR, Huskisson EC, Willoughby DA. Apatite deposition disease, a new arthropathy. *The Lancet* 1976; **1**:266.

(5) Schumacher HR, Sonlyo AP, Tse RL. Arthritis associated with apatite crystals. *Annals of Internal Medicine* 1979; **87**:411.

Key message

Calcium pyrophosphate crystals are found in the synovial fluid of some patients with acute arthritis of the knee joint.

Why it's important

This paper on the 'pseudogout syndrome' should be read alongside the related contribution quoted above (1). The pair make fascinating reading, and represent a major milestone in the development of rheumatology. In the first paper, Dan McCarty and colleagues provide us with the first description of pseudogout. Their paper, as often seems to be the case with original descriptions of diseases, covers all the major features of the condition, including its predilection for the knee and wrist joints of older people, and the presence of radiographic chondrocalcinosis.

The second paper, featured here, is also truly ground breaking, because of the use of complex physical and chemical techniques for the identification of the crystals found in these cases. They did four key, original things: first, they extracted the mineral from the synovial fluids using hyaluronidase digestion (a difficult procedure); second, they synthesized pure crystals of calcium pyrophosphate dihydrate to act as a positive control (an extremely difficult procedure); third, they used the then little known technique of infra-red spectroscopy to compare the extracted mineral with other samples, including their synthetic pyrophosphate crystals, and finally they used x-ray powder diffraction to provide a definitive identification of the crystals. They also compared their 'new crystals' with urates using polarized light microscopy, and describe the weak positive birefringence of pyrophosphate crystals (Figure 4.2). This is painstaking and superb work. They got it right and the work has never been bettered. Some 15 years later other groups used these techniques, along with the new approach of analytical electron microscopy, to identify basic calcium phosphates and other forms of mineral in joint samples, and only then were the findings reported here repeated and confirmed.

The relevance of the finding, as we now know and as was flagged in these papers, is that calcium pyrophosphate dihydrate crystals can cause inflammation and are responsible for the arthritis of pseudogout.

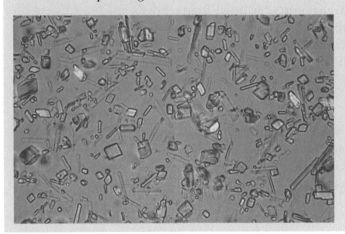

Figure 4.2 Calcium pyrophosphate dihydrate crystals that have been extracted from joint tissues are seen here under compensated polarized light microscopy. Note the varying morphology and weak positive birefringence that help to distinguish them from urate crystals. (Courtesy of Dr Angela Swan.)

Strengths

1. This is a detailed, careful and well presented study using excellent methodology.
2. The use of control samples, including bone apatite and synthetic calcium pyrophosphate crystals (which are very difficult to make).
3. This is one of the first studies in medicine to use physical techniques such as x-ray diffraction.

Weaknesses

1. The numbers of patients studied was small.
2. Only five samples were examined by the physical methods used.

Relevance

The first and definitive, description of pseudogout and of the crystals that cause it.

Paper 4

Usefulness of synovial fluid analysis in the evaluation of joint effusions. Use of threshold analysis and likelihood ratios to assess a diagnostic test

Authors

Eisenberg JM, Schumacher HR, Davidson PK, Kaufmann L

Reference

Archives of Internal Medicine 1984; **144**:715–719

Summary

This study applied threshold analysis and likelihood ratios to determine the usefulness of a diagnostic test. Eleven staff rheumatologists or rheumatology fellows provided probability estimates for the most likely diagnoses both before and after synovial fluid analyses were performed on 180 patients with joint effusions. They also indicated whether the planned therapy was altered by test results. The therapeutic thresholds and log likelihood ratios were derived for the six most frequent diagnoses. Synovial fluid analysis was most useful for patients likely to have gout, pseudogout or infectious arthritis. The derived therapeutic thresholds were consistent with recommended medical practice, for example, with a lower threshold for possible septic arthritis (20%) than for possible gout (65%). This study demonstrates that threshold analyses and likelihood ratios can be used to assess the clinical contribution of diagnostic tests.

Related references	(1)	Pauker X, Kassirer X. The threshold approach to clinical decision making. *New England Journal of Medicine* 1975; **293**:229–235.
	(2)	Schumacher HR. Analyzing synovial fluid: a useful diagnostic aid for practitioners. *Modern Medicine* 1977; **45**:58–63.

Key message

Knowledge of the results of synovial fluid analysis can lead to changes in diagnosis and treatment of arthritis.

Why it's important

This paper was well ahead of its time. In recent years great effort has been put into the analysis of data from clinical trials of interventions, and in finding ways of putting such data to use in routine clinical practice. Similar work is just beginning to appear in relation to diagnostic tests, although very few of the investigations used in arthritis have been subjected to rigorous tests of their validity or value. Yet, as illustrated by this paper, the theoretical basis for such work has been available for a long time, and it is relatively easy to put it into practice.

This paper describes the decisions made by clinicians as to the diagnosis and treatment of arthritis before and after the results of synovial fluid analysis was made available to them. It is one of very few contributions to the rheumatological literature which assesses the value of diagnostic investigations in routine clinical practice. The six most common diagnoses are presented in the paper, and the data show that synovial fluid findings change the diagnosis and treatment in a significant proportion of cases (Table 4.1). Gout was the diagnosis most likely to be changed, and synovial fluid findings were of most value to clinicians in diagnosing septic arthritis and gout. The authors also analysed the data to look at therapeutic thresholds (i.e. the degree of diagnostic certainty required by physicians to institute specific therapy for a condition), and found this was lowest for septic arthritis (20%) and highest for gout (65%).

The paper is important not only because it shows the importance of synovial fluid analysis in clinical practice, but also for the way it applies sound theory and mathematical principles to the analysis of clinical decision-making in rheumatology.

Table 4.1 Data from the paper showing the number of times in which the final diagnosis made by clinicians (after they had access to synovial fluid data) was the same or different from that which they made before aspiration of synovial fluid.

Disease	Same final diagnosis	Different final diagnosis	% changed
Osteoarthritis	31	6	16
Rheumatoid arthritis	24	5	17
Gout	25	9	26
Sepsis	11	3	21
Pseudogout	9	1	10
Traumatic arthritis	7	2	22

Strengths

1. Innovative use of theory and mathematical techniques for decision making and the value of diagnostic tests in rheumatology.
2. Analysis of a relatively large number of clinical cases (180).
3. Comprehensive reporting of the data.

Weaknesses

1. This is a difficult paper to read, which does not explain the theoretical background of the approach very well.
2. Clinicans taking part were asked to list their four most likely diagnoses and to suggest a therapy, which made it difficult to understand what they thought they were treating or why.
3. It was not possible to assess the importance of other types of information, such as serum uric acid levels, in clinical decision making.

Relevance

One of the few papers in the rheumatology literature which show that an investigation can alter clinical practice.

Paper 5

Arthroscopy of the knee in rheumatic diseases

Authors

Jayson MIV, Dixon ASTJ

Reference

Annals of Rheumatic Diseases 1968; **27**:503–511

Summary

Arthroscopy offers a safe and simple method of examining the morphology of the synovial membrane of the knee joint and of obtaining biopsies under direct vision. The technique is described in detail and typical results are presented.

Related references

(1) Burman MS, Finkelstein H, Mayer L. Arthroscopy of the knee joint. *Journal of Bone and Joint Surgery* 1934; **16**:255.

(2) Johnson LL. *Comprehensive arthroscopic examinantion of the knee*. Mosby: St Louis. 1977.

(3) Halbrecht JL, Jackson DW. Office arthroscopy: a diagnostic alternative. *Arthroscopy* 1992; **8**:320–326.

(4) Ike RW, O'Rouke KS. Detection of intra-articular abnormalities in osteoarthritis of the knee: a pilot study comparing needle arthroscopy with standard arthroscopy. *Arthritis and Rheumatism* 1993; **36**:1353–1363.

Key message

Biopsies taken under direct vision via an arthroscope, so that areas of abnormality are sampled, are more likely to provide a diagnosis than a blind biopsy.

Why it's important

The authors describe the technique of arthroscopy done under local anaesthetic (as a day case procedure) in detail. They then describe and illustrate the results of a series of 23 cases performed by themselves. They pay particular attention to their findings on examination and biopsy of the synovium, pointing out that the changes in early inflammatory arthritis are very patchy (Figure 4.3). They show that using this technique they are able to visualize and biopsy abnormal areas, whereas a blind biospy might easily result in areas of normal synovium being sampled. They also describe cartilage changes, point out that it is difficult to see the menisci using this technique, and record the fact that the attending irrigation of the joint seemed to result in a clinical improvement in the joint in many cases.

This paper was the first one to describe the use of arthroscopy as a part of rheumatological practice, rather than by orthopaedic surgeons (who had been using arthroscopy for some years). It pre-empted the extensive use of the technique over the following two decades, after which the office mini-arthroscopy approach was introduced. They were also amongst the first people to describe the improvement in joints that can result from lavage.

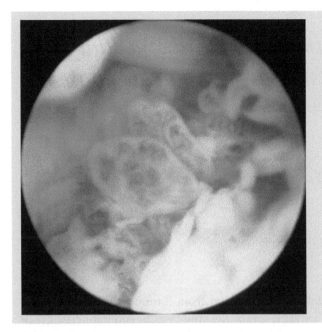

Figure 4.3 Typical appearance of inflamed synovium seen through an arthroscope. While this area of synovium show extensive hypertrophy and inflammation other areas in the same joint looked relatively normal.

Strengths

1. It was highly innovative to introduce arthroscopy under local anaesthetic into rheumatological practice.
2. The illustrations of the synovial and cartilage changes that can be seen using this technique are extensive, in colour and of a high quality.
3. The technique is described in sufficient detail for others to be able to reproduce it.

Weaknesses

1. They only describe 23 cases.
2. Most of the cases described had RA, so the range of changes and uses for arthroscopy that subsequently became apparent (such as its value in picking up pigmented vilonodular synovitis) were not apparent.
3. They do not discuss the extent to which the findings changed their diagnosis or treatment of these 23 cases.
4. There was no formal assessment of outcome resulting from lavage.

Relevance

The introduction of arthroscopy into rheumatological practice.

Paper 6

The assessment of rheumatoid arthritis: a study based on measurements of the serum acute-phase reactants

Authors

McConkey B, Crockson RA, Crockson AP

Reference

Quartely Journal of Medicine 1972; **41**:115–125

Summary

We have studied 187 patients with RA for periods ranging from 3 months to 6 years; 55 of them were observed for more than 3 years. The aim of the study was to compare changes in clinical state with changes in measurements of the blood levels of two acute-phase proteins (CRP and haptogolobin).

The results showed that measurements of the serum acute-phase reactants reflected exacerbation or remission of arthritis when such changes occurred over short periods of time, for example a few months. The serum acute-phase reactants also reflected the course of RA over longer periods of time; in patients studied for more than 3 years there was a close correlation between the course of the disease and the levels of the acute-phase reactants. We suggest that measurements of the serum acute-phase reactants provide an accurate and objective way of assessing the progress of RA and of its response to treatment.

Related references (1) Lansbury J. Report of a three-year study on the systemic and articular indexes in rheumatoid arthritis. *Arthritis and Rheumatism* 1958; **1**:505–522.

(2) Crockson RA. A gel diffusion precipitin method for the estimation of c-reactive protein. *Journal of Clinical Pathology* 1963; **16**:287–289.

Key message

C-reactive protein levels in the serum reflect disease activity in RA; sustained elevation of CRP levels is a poor prognostic factor. In the long-term therapy of RA one should aim to reduce CRP levels to as near normal as possible.

Why it's important

The authors of this paper note that in 1958 Lansbury had pointed out that what was needed in RA was a test which tells us how well the disease is controlled (1). Before the pioneering work of this group on CRP the ESR had been the standard blood test used to assess disease activity. In addition, clinical assessments, such as the 'Lansbury Index' were used.

Crockson showed that CRP was a good acute-phase reactant and developed an accurate measurement of serum levels. He then teamed up with McConkey to apply his assay to the assessment of RA. This paper summarizes their work, which clearly shows that CRP measurements are superior to ESR assays in both short-term and long-term assessments of RA. Although there was a strong statistical association between ESR and CRP in the whole group, in many individual instances the ESR did not correlate with the CRP, and in these cases it was the CRP which correlated with clinical activity and progression and not the ESR.

In addition, they showed that serial measurements have a great advantage over single point measurements, and that there were correlations between long-term disease progression and the general levels of CRP in the serum. This led them to conclude that regular measurement of CRP levels should provide the test that Lansbury wanted. Now, most rheumatologists do use serial assays of CRP to help them monitor the activity and response to therapy of their patients with RA. Thus this paper represents the initial evidence base for one of the currently accepted approaches to the management of this disease.

Strengths

1. The authors applied their extensive experience of the measurement of acute-phase proteins to a large number of patients with RA studied over many years.
2. The hypothesis is clear and well-founded.
3. Clear presentation of a lot of data.

Weaknesses

1. The clinical assessments against which the CRP was correlated are very poor, relying largely on physician and patient assessments of change (better, same or worse).
2. They say that they also measured x-ray progression, but do not present data relating CRP to x-ray changes.
3. The patients are a highly selected group from one hospital base, and may not be representative of RA as a whole.

Relevance

Led to the introduction of CRP as the key serum assay for the assessment of disease activity and responses to treatment in RA.

Paper 7

Cartilage oligomeric matrix protein: a novel marker of cartilage turnover detectable in synovial fluid and blood

Authors

Saxne T, Heinegard D

Reference

British Journal of Rheumatology 1992; **31**:583–591

Summary

Cartilage oligomeric matrix protein (COMP) is a tissue-specific non-collagenous protein. We have developed an enzyme-linked immunosorbent assay for the detection of this protein in the synovial fluid and serum. The protein has been quantified in these fluids in patients with RA, reactive arthritis (ReA), juvenile chronic arthritis, osteoarthritis (OA) and in sera of control subjects. The protein was detectable in all fluids and the synovial fluid levels were always higher than in serum in paired samples. The highest knee joint synovial fluid levels were found in ReA and the lowest in RA patients with advanced destruction of the knee joint. However, the relative synovial fluid content of COMP was higher in these RA patients than in patients with advanced OA. In patients with long-standing reactive synovitis the concentrations were decreased. This decrease, however, was less marked than for proteoglycan concentrations. The serum concentrations were low in patients with juvenile chronic arthritis and in patients with RA with advanced cartilage destruction of the studied knee joint. In the other groups serum levels did not differ between groups or from controls.

Related references

(1) Saxne T, Heinegard D, Wolheim FA, Pettersson H. Differences in cartilage proteoglycan level in synovial fluid in early rehumatoid arthritis and reactive arthritis. *The Lancet* 1985; **8447**:127–128.

(2) Petersson IF, Boegard T, Svensson B, Heinegard D, Saxne T. Changes in cartilage and bone metabolism identified by serum markers in early osteoarthritis of the knee joint. *British Journal of Rheumatology* 1998; **37**:46–50.

(3) Lohmander LS, Saxne T, Heinegard DK. Release of COMP into joint fluid after knee injury and in osteoarthritis. *Annals of Rheumatic Diseases* 1994; **53**:8–13.

(4) Sharif M, Saxne T, Shepstone L, Kirwan J, Elson C, Heinegard D, Dieppe P. Relationship between serum COMP levels and disease progression in osteoarthritis of the knee joint. *British Journal of Rheumatology* 1995; **34**;306–310.

Key message

That serum and synovial fluid levels of a cartilage-specific protein reflect both normal turnover and different pathological processes occurring in different forms of joint disease.

Why it's important

Prior to this work there had been other attempts to use the measurement of cartilage macro-molecules released into the synovial fluid and blood as potential markers of disease process and progression. Most of these had concentrated on proteoglycans or their glycosaminogly-can side chains, such as keratan sulphate, and the results had, in general, been disappointing. In this paper Saxne and Heinegard describe the application of an assay of a different cartilage macromolecule, COMP, which at that time was thought specific to articular cartilage. They describe a careful set of experiments which first of all provide the characteristics and validation of the COMP assay, and then apply it to relatively large groups of patients with a variety of different joint diseases, whose disease status had been carefully documented both clinically and radiographically.

What they found was that synovial concentrations of COMP showed similar differences to those seen when proteoglycans are assayed, suggesting that release is due to changes in the articular cartilage. They also found that COMP was readily detectable in the serum of normal controls, suggesting that there is normal turnover of the protein. They also found marked differences in the levels found in different disease states, suggesting that turnover and release differs in the different types of joint pathology. In a thoughtful discussion, the authors consider the difficulties in interpretation of data of this sort, dependent as it is on synthesis as well as release of COMP, and, in the case of serum assays, on what is happening in multiple joints.

This paper is important, not only because of the high standard of the work, but also as it is the original description of this group's work on COMP, which has proved to be one of the more promising 'biochemical markers' of joint disease. Subsequent work (cited in the related references) showed that COMP levels were predictive of joint damage.

Strengths

1. Careful characterization of the COMP assay.
2. Application to large numbers of well characterized patients.
3. Inclusion of normal control subjects.
4. An excellent discussion on the difficulties of interpreting marker assays.

Weaknesses

1. The data are cross-sectional and not prospective.
2. No normal synovial fluid data are included.

Relevance

COMP is one of the few biochemical markers that is both joint-specific and showing signs of being of value in the prediction of outcome in arthritis, as well as indicative of different pathological processes.

CHAPTER 5

Clinical genetics

Sophia Steer and Gabriel S Panayi

Introduction

In the last two decades the field of human genetics has advanced and expanded perhaps more than any other in human biology. The realization that the presence of genetic markers and the study of their transmission through disease pedigrees could localize chromosomal regions linked with disease (from where positional cloning could be used to identify the precise disease gene) drove the initial attempts to establish a genetic map. The recognition of DNA polymorphisms as genetic markers allowed this to start in earnest in the 1980s. The first generation of markers were restriction fragment length polymorphisms, the typing of which was laborious. These were superceded by microsatellites which are amenable to typing by polymerase chain reaction (PCR), and these in turn are being replaced by single nucleotide polymorphisms. The application of this reverse genetics philosophy (i.e. isolating a disease-causing gene without knowing its function) coupled with the advance of recombinant DNA technology has resulted in the identification of genes responsible for many Mendelian diseases. This progress has been relevant to the field of rheumatology with disease loci located for Marfan's syndrome, Ehlers–Danlos syndrome and osteogenesis imperfecta, but we have chosen to focus the papers in this chapter on the more common inflammatory rheumatic diseases which remain a substantial challenge in terms of gene localization.

The application of similar techniques to these diseases has been less rewarding than initially hoped. Their pattern of familial clustering suggests that they are polygenic or oligogenic in origin with each contributing susceptibility locus potentially having only a small effect. Approaches to localizing such disease genes include the candidate gene approach, where a suitable gene is tested for association with disease, usually on the basis of a putative pathogenic role, and the use of linkage analysis in family studies.

The first two papers in this chapter are examples of the candidate gene approach. They both look for the association of an human leucocyte antigen (HLA) gene with disease in a cohort of unrelated cases and compare the prevalence of the allele with that in a control population. Both are very successful studies demonstrating a strong association that has in each case been replicated on many occasions. Before the 1980s the direct analysis of candidate genes was the only approach available and the major histocompatibility complex (MHC) antigens were one of the few genetic determinants known. These studies demonstrate the power of this approach when there is a good *a priori* hypothesis for the gene in question and when cases and controls are well characterized and matched.

Recently candidate gene studies have fallen out of favour largely because findings in one disease cohort have often failed to be replicated in others. This has been attributed to population stratification occurring as a result of inadequate matching of cases and controls. However candidate gene studies offer huge advantages in terms of power and case ascertainment and are likely to be the future for gene localization studies.

The use of multicase pedigrees for classical linkage analysis is difficult in polygenic multi-factorial diseases where the precise mode of inheritance is not known. A best fit model of transmission of disease is used in the analysis. Errors in this model can lead to false linkage assignment. Family studies do however have the advantage of internal genetic homogeneity thus avoiding the potential for false conclusions being drawn due to inadequately matched case and control populations. Methods that do not rely on models of disease transmission (nonparametric methods) have been developed to take advantage of this, and the transmission disequilibrium test described in the fourth paper in this chapter is an example of one of these. These methods are being applied more widely with promising results but are less powerful than candidate gene studies in case-control populations, and have the inherent difficulties of family finding which can be particularly difficult in late- onset diseases. Methods using siblings rather than parents in the transmission disequilibrium test have been developed to make this less of a problem.

The final two papers of the chapter illustrate how the molecular structure of disease susceptibility genes can both lend support to existing hypotheses of disease causation and provoke further discussion of pathological mechanisms. One of the most persuasive reasons for investing so much in discovering the genes determining susceptibility and severity in rheumatic diseases is the elucidation of their underlying aetiology and pathogenesis. This of course requires not only gene localization but much more in the form of functional *in vitro* and *in vivo* studies.

The third paper in this chapter introduces the field of pharmacogenetics. The ultimate aim is the development of specific targeted therapy that cures disease (assuming that disease cannot be averted) without adverse effect in each and every affected individual. The sequencing of the the entire human genome, combined with the development of genome wide single nucleotide polymorphism maps and chip-based technologies, will allow the scale of current approaches to increase by several orders of magnitude. Parallel advances in statistical techniques and approaches that allow case-control studies to emerge as robust and powerful, combined with functional studies, may allow us to reach this goal.

Paper I

HLA-Dw4 in adult and juvenile rheumatoid arthritis

Authors

Stastny P, Fink CW

Reference

Transplantation Proceedings 1977; **9**(4):1863–1866

Summary

HLA-D typing of patients with adult onset erosive seropositive rheumatoid arthritis (RA) was performed using the mixed lymphocyte reaction between the patients' cells and homozygous stimulating cells for several HLA-D loci. HLA-Dw4 was present in 16% of normal white controls and in 59% of the white RA patients. This difference was highly significant (p<0.001) and suggested that HLA-Dw4 conferred a relative risk of 7.5 times that of other HLA-D antigens. The frequency of HLA-Dw4 in black Dallas residents with RA was 14% and in patients of Mexican origin it was 10%, but there were no non-white control groups for comparison.

Related references **(1)** Stastny P. Association of the B-cell alloantigen DRw4 with rheumatoid arthritis. *New England Journal of Medicine* 1978; **298**(16):869–871.

(2) Panayi GS, Wooley P, Batchelor JR. Genetic basis of rheumatoid disease: HLA antigens, disease manifestations, and toxic reactions to drugs. *British Medical Journal* 1978; **2**(6148):1326–1328.

Key message

The frequency of HLA-Dw4, later reclassified within HLA-DR4, in white patients with adult-onset RA was significantly increased at 59% compared to a rate of 16% in a white control population. This increase was not apparent in non-white adults with the disease.

Why it's important

By the early 1970s there was some evidence implicating the immune system in RA, such as rheumatoid factor production and the development of lymphoid nodules in the synovial membrane of affected joints. An association of the disease with the HLA antigens seemed likely but previous studies looking at class I antigens using serological methods had been negative. The poor response of peripheral blood lymphocytes from patients with RA in mixed lymphocyte culture (MLC) against cells from other RA patients led Stastny to investigate their lymphocyte defined (LD) histocompatibility determinants, subsequently known as HLA-D. He demonstrated that the low MLC reactions were due to the sharing of an LD determinant among RA patients and defined this further as LD-104 which subsequently became HLA-Dw4.

This paper set out to confirm the preliminary work outlined above and was the first case-control study of a candidate gene in RA to show a positive association. It demonstrates the importance of ethnicity in population-based case-control studies as with a less homogeneous group of patients the result would have been much less significant. Panayi, *et al.* (2) replicated these findings using serological methods for detecting HLA-DR antigens and as did Stastny in the same year (1).

The location of this gene close to the HLA region, a region known to be analogous to the immune response gene in mice and monkeys, allowed further speculation as to the role of the immune system in RA. Thus this finding lent support to the rationale for the extensive immunologically-based research that followed.

Strengths

1. The first example of an association study in RA, a technique that continues to play a major role in the analysis of complex genetic disease.
2. It placed the genetic basis for RA on a firm footing.

Weakness

None.

Relevance

The association of RA with DR4 remains the strongest genetic association for this disease and has been pivotal to our understanding of its pathogenesis and the involvement of T cells in particular.

Paper 2

Ankylosing spondylitis and HL-A27

Authors

Brewerton DA, Hart FD, Nicholls A, Caffrey M, James DC, Sturrock RD

Reference

The Lancet 1 (7809) 1973; 904–907

Summary

Sixty-five caucasian men and 10 caucasian women attending hospital rheumatology clinics with undoubted classical ankylosing spondylitis (AS) underwent HL-A typing using a lymphocytotoxicity method. The HL-A27 antigen was identified in 72 out of 75 patients (96%) and in 3 out of 75 controls (4%). To investigate the possibility that this high frequency might result from the disease or its treatment 60 first degree relatives were also HL-A typed. Thirty-one of the 60 (52%) possessed the HL-A27 antigen.

Related references **(1)** Schlosstein L, Terasaki PI, Bluestone R, Pearson CM. High association of an HL-A antigen, W27, with ankylosing spondylitis. *New England Journal of Medicine* 1973; **288**(14):704–706.

  (2) Rubin LA, Amos CI, Wade JA, Martin JR, Bale SJ, Little AH, *et al.* Investigating the genetic basis for ankylosing spondylitis. Linkage studies with the major histocompatibility complex region. *Arthritis and Rheumatism* 1994; **37**(8):1212–1220.

  (3) Taurog JD, Richardson JA, Croft JT, Simmons WA, Zhou M, Fernandez-Sueiro JL, *et al.* The germfree state prevents development of gut and joint inflammatory disease in HLA-B27 transgenic rats. *Journal of Experimental Medicine* 1994; **180**(6):2359–2364.

Key message

HL-A27, later reclassified as HLA-B27, is present in 96% of caucasian patients with AS and in 52% of their first degree relatives versus a control population frequency of 4%.

Why it's important

The suggestion of a genetic contribution to AS was first made in the 1950s following reports of multicase families and increased disease concordance in monozygotic twins. These provided the rationale for examining the association of genetic determinants with AS. This paper reports a highly significant result which was replicated at the same time by Schlosstein, *et al.* (1). Claims that this association would lead to discovery of the pathogenic mechanisms underlying disease and the rational design of treatment were made then but have yet to be realized.

Despite the strong association of AS with B27 only a small proportion of B27 positive individuals develop disease and the explanation for this remains elusive. It seems unlikely to be due to a rare environmental trigger as the disease is geographically widespread and variations in prevalence seem to reflect variations in B27 gene frequency. Furthermore, twin concordance studies suggest the disease is strongly genetic with a heritability of 90%. The contribution of B27 to the genetic susceptibility of AS is estimated to be 20–50% of the total (2), with the remaining components coming from a number of weaker susceptibility loci. This is supported by B27 transgenic rat models of disease where the background strain of the rat influences the expression of disease. The location of the non-MHC genetic contributions to disease susceptibility are not known. The first genome wide screen in AS was in 105 affected sibling pair families and demonstrated several regions of linkage in addition to that at the MHC locus.

However the absence of disease in transgenic HLA B27 positive rats raised in a germ free environment (3) emphasizes the importance of interplay between genes and the environment. Disease causation hypotheses building on the normal role of B27 in its presentation of antigenic peptide to cytotoxic T cells and natural killer (NK) cells are numerous and include molecular mimicry and arthritogenic peptide theories, but the pathogenesis of this disease remains unknown more than 25 years on from this important paper.

Strengths

1. Clear significant result.
2. Well designed with respect to cases and controls.

Weakness

None.

Relevance

This robust association has provided the stimulus for further family and genetic studies of AS. These are likely to suggest additional candidate genes and improve our understanding of the disease pathogenesis.

Paper 3

HLA-DR antigens and toxic reactions to sodium aurothiomalate and D-penicillamine in patients with rheumatoid arthritis

Authors

Wooley PH, Griffin J, Panayi GS, Batchelor MD, Welsh KI, Gibson TJ

Reference

New England Journal of Medicine 1980; **303**(6):300–302

Summary

Ninety-one consecutive patients selected because they had classic or definite RA (according to the American Rheumatism Association criteria) which was severe enough to warrant treatment with sodium aurothiomalate or D-penicillamine, were HLA typed. Their notes were reviewed for evidence of drug toxicity, classified as rashes, proteinuria or haematological problems (eosinophilia, thrombocytopenia). Seventy-one patients had toxic reactions to either or both drugs; the total number of toxic episodes was 95. The remaining 20 patients took one of the drugs for at least 6 months without toxicity. Nineteen of 24 patients in whom proteinuria developed were positive for HLA-B8 and HLA-DRw3; 14 of 15 episodes of aurothiomalate-induced proteinuria and 9 of 13 episodes of penicillamine-induced proteinuria occurred in patients with these antigens. The relative risk of proteinuria during aurothiomalate therapy was increased 32 times in patients with the DRw3 antigen but there was no statistically significant association between HLA-DRw3 and proteinuria during penicillamine therapy. No significant associations were found between any HLA antigen and the development of skin rashes or haematological complications.

Related references   **(1)**   Panayi, GS, Wooley P, Batchelor JR. Genetic basis of rheumatoid disease: HLA antigens, disease manifestations, and toxic reactions to drugs. *British Medical Journal* 1978; **2**(6148):1326–1328.

           (2)   Sinigaglia F, Scheidegger D, Garotta G, Scheper R, Pletscher M, Lanzavecchia A. Isolation and characterization of Ni-specific T cell clones from patients with Ni-contact dermatitis. *Journal of Immunology* 1985; **135**(6):3929–3932.

           (3)   Romagnoli P, Spinas GA, Sinigaglia F. Gold-specific T cells in rheumatoid arthritis patients treated with gold. *Journal of Clinical Investigation* 1992; **89**(1):254–258.

Key message

Toxicity during aurothiomalate or penicillamine treatment for RA may be under genetic control.

Why it's important

A previous study (1) had found a significant association between HLA-DRw2 and DRw3 and toxic effects of therapy with these two drugs. This study was undertaken to confirm or refute that association. In confirming an association with HLA-DRw3 the principle that susceptibility to drug toxicity may be genetically determined was established for rheumatic disease. This study also implied that mechanisms of toxicity may be under the control of the major histocompatibility system and this has since been confirmed in work by Sinigaglia, *et al.* and others (2, 3). They have demonstrated the important role of HLA class II molecules in the stimulation and proliferation of nickel and gold specific T cell clones.

The first clinical observations of inherited differences in drug effects such as haemolysis after antimalarial therapy and inherited levels of glucose 6-phosphate dehydrogenase activity, and peripheral neuropathy with isoniazid and inherited differences in the acetylation of the drug were reported in the 1950s. The molecular basis for these began to be elucidated in the 1980s with the discovery of a polymorphic locus encoding the enzyme CYP2D6 and since then many such pharmacogenetic traits have been discovered. For drugs that have a narrow therapeutic index and are metabolized by a polymorphic enzyme, for example azathioprine metabolized by thiopurine methyltransferase, or warfarin metabolized by cytochrome P450, the influence of such a monogenic trait can be profound in terms of toxicity. The importance of this was highlighted recently by the high incidence of serious and fatal adverse drug reactions reported in US hospitals.

Genetic polymorphisms have now been identified in more than 20 drug-metabolizing enzymes and exist for almost every gene involved in drug metabolism and disposition as well as for many drug receptors, transporters and cell signalling pathways. The overall effect of a drug is therefore not a monogenic trait but determined by the interplay between several genes. The rapidly expanding knowledge of the genetic sequence of target genes combined with the development of single nucleotide polymorphism (SNP) maps and automated screening for SNPs will allow the identification of functionally important polymorphisms. This approach should lead to the development of individual pharmacogenetic profiles and prescription advice based on genotype. In the longer term it may lead to the development of new drug regimes specifically for genetically identifiable subgroups of the population with the aim of improving outcome.

Strength

Established the role of genetics in drug toxicity in rheumatic disease.

Weaknesses

1. Skin rashes not precisely delineated which may explain lack of association with HLA.
2. Relatively small number of cases.

Relevance

The first report of a genetic association with drug toxicity in RA, which has been pivotal in the development of thinking about tailoring therapies to the genetic backgrounds of individual patients.

Paper 4

Transmission disequilibrium as a test of linkage and association between HLA alleles and pauciarticular-onset juvenile rheumatoid arthritis

Authors

Moroldo MB, Donnelly P, Saunders J, Glass DN, Giannini EH

Reference

Arthritis and Rheumatism 1998; **41**(9);1620–1624

Summary

This study aimed to establish whether HLA class I and II alleles previously found to be associated with pauciarticular-onset juvenile rheumatoid arthritis (POJRA) in population association studies are transmitted from heterozygous parents to affected offspring to an extent different from the expected 50%. One hundred and one white North American families that had been serologically HLA typed during earlier studies were used in the analysis. Each family had a single child with POJRA and serological HLA data were available for both parents, the proband, and unaffected siblings in 95% of families. HLA-A2, B27 and B35 were the class I alleles that showed a significant increased frequency of transmission to affected offspring, as did the class II alleles HLA-DR5 and DR8. HLA-DR4 was transmitted to affected subjects significantly less frequently than expected. When the data were stratified by age and sex, HLA-A2, HLA-B35, DR5 and DR8 were all transmitted at higher than expected rates to female patients, particularly among those with a young age at disease onset. HLA-B27 showed strong transmission disequilibrium among male patients with disease onset after the age of 8 years. HLA-DR4 was transmitted less frequently than expected to females younger than 8 years at disease onset.

Related references **(1)**   Stastny P, Fink CW. Different HLA-D associations in adult and juvenile rheumatoid arthritis. *Journal of Clinical Investigation* 1979; **63**(1):124–130.

(2)   Glass D, Litvin D, Wallace K, Chylack L, Garovoy M, Carpenter CB, *et al.* Early-onset pauciarticular juvenile rheumatoid arthritis associated with human leukocyte antigen-DRw5, iritis, and antinuclear antibody. *Journal of Clinical Investigation* 1980; **66**(3):426–429.

Key message

HLA alleles A2, B27, B35, DR5 and DR8 are transmitted from heterozygous parents to affected offspring significantly more frequently than expected, establishing linkage and association between the MHC and POJRA.

Why it's important

In the Western world POJRA is the most common of the group of phenotypically heterogeneous childhood arthritides previously classified as juvenile chronic arthritis (JCA) in Europe and juvenile rheumatoid arthritis (JRA) in the US, now classified as juvenile idiopathic arthritis (JIA). Although the observed familial occurrence of JIA is low and no large twin study has been performed for any subgroup, the evidence in support of a genetic basis came from the observation that first degree relatives can present with the same phenotypic features of JIA.

The HLA system and the POJRA subgroup have been researched the most intensively. The first association study in JCA was reported by Stastny and Fink in 1979 (1) and showed a positive association with HLA-DR8. This was followed shortly by Glass, *et al.*'s report of association of POJRA with HLA-DR5 (2). Subsequently associations with HLA-DR6, HLA-DPw2, HLA-A2, and a specific HLA-DP beta allele were reported in POJRA. All these studies were population-based association case-control studies which may give false positive results as they are vulnerable to population stratification, particularly in outbred populations, which may in theory have genetically heterogeneous cases and controls.

By using the transmission disequilibrium test this problem is avoided as the controls are within family and therefore genetically homogeneous. The disadvantages apart from the obvious difficulties in recruiting families, include the loss of power due to overmatching of controls and the test's ability to detect linkage between a marker locus and a disease locus only if association due to linkage disequilibrium is present. It is a particularly valid way of designing a replication study, which is how it has been used here, as it provides definite confirmation of the previous findings in a way that another population association study could not.

The strong evidence of linkage and association between multiple HLA alleles and POJRA from this study leads one to question why this should be. It is not explained by linkage disequilibrium either between different HLA alleles or with other closely related genes. There is some evidence to suggest that these alleles share a consensus amino acid motif and could thereby influence disease pathogenesis possibly by affecting the development of the T cell repertoire, or by binding specific 'arthritogenic' peptides. Another explanation would be that within the subgroup of POJRA there is in fact further clinical heterogeneity and this has been supported by studies looking at outcomes of this group.

Strengths

1. Excellent study design.
2. Confirms and clarifies the previous population-based association data.

Weakness

Relatively small number of families which may result in real effects being missed.

Relevance

This paper demonstrates the genetic heterogeneity that exists amongst POJRA which raises questions regarding the clinical homogeneity of the disease. The confirmation of linkage and association with the MHC region suggests that immune mechanisms are important for the pathogenesis of POJRA; the involvement of T cells seems likely given the association with specific HLA-DR molecules.

Paper 5

The shared epitope hypothesis. An approach to understanding the molecular genetics of susceptibility to rheumatoid arthritis

Authors

Gregersen PK, Silver J, Winchester RJ

Reference

Arthritis and Rheumatism 1987; **30**(11);1205–1213

Summary

Much work investigating the inheritance of RA has focussed on the associations between HLA class II serological specificities and disease. This has demonstrated association with different DR4 serological subtypes in some populations, lack of association with DR4 in others and association with certain other DR alleles, particularly DR1 in DR4 negative patients. Analysis at DNA sequence level revealed that the DR4 serological subtypes differed only in the DRB1 gene and that these differences were restricted to the codons surrounding position 70 of the N-terminal domain of the molecule, the region corresponding to the third hypervariable region of the DRB1 molecule. The differences in sequence lead to amino acid substitutions with substantial implication in terms of charge and therefore protein binding. The substitutions in the DR4 subtypes associated with RA (Dw4, Dw14, Dw15) and in DR1 are of similarly charged amino acids, whereas those not associated (Dw10) differ markedly. These regions of shared sequence therefore have a similar conformation when expressed as protein, with similar properties in terms of antigen binding, presentation and immune regulation. The protein epitope is thereby shared by serologically distinct HLA haplotypes.

Related references **(1)** Wordsworth BP, Lanchbury JS, Sakkas LI, Welsh KI, Panayi GS, Bell JI. HLA-DR4 subtype frequencies in rheumatoid arthritis indicate that DRB1 is the major susceptibility locus within the HLA class II region. *Proceedings of the National Academy of Sciences USA* 1989; **86**(24):10049–10053.

(2) Nepom GT, Seyfried CE, Holbeck SL, Wilske KR, Nepom BS. Identification of HLA-Dw14 genes in DR4+ rheumatoid arthritis. *The Lancet* 1986; **2**(8514):1002–1005.

(3) Cairns JS, Curtsinger JM, Dahl CA, Freeman S, Alter BJ, Bach FH. Sequence polymorphism of HLA DR beta 1 alleles relating to T-cell-recognized determinants. *Nature* 1985; **317**(6033):166–168.

(4) Brown JH, Jardetzky TS, Gorga JC, Stern LJ, Urban RG, Strominger JL, *et al.* Three-dimensional structure of the human class II histocompatibility antigen HLA-DR1 (see comments). *Nature* 1993; **364**(6432):33–39.

Key message

The seemingly conflicting serological data on HLA class II disease associations in RA can be explained by analysis of RA populations at the sequence level; the lack of association with the Dw10 subtype of DR4 and the positive association with DR1 are both accounted for by this hypothesis.

Why it's important

This hypothesis is based on the immune response being dependent on antigenic peptide presented in the groove of the class II MHC molecule to the T cell receptor. This concept suggests that one specific HLA molecule or protein conformation should be associated with a disease and did not fit easily with the multiple reports of different HLA-DR4 subtypes being associated with RA in various populations. Previous work involving alloreactive T cell clones had provided evidence of shared T cell recognition sites amongst class II molecules from DR4 positive and DR4 negative patients with RA (3), but it was the sequencing of the different HLA-DR4 subtypes (1) that finally demonstrated that they shared a common antigen binding structure.

Further support for the relationship between structure and immune response has since been derived from experiments involving site directed mutagenesis of the DRB1 gene, and by the confirmation of the HLA class II molecule crystal structure which has localized the shared sequence motif in the antigen binding groove (4). Furthermore, since the publication of this hypothesis the results of studies testing it in patients of different ethnic backgrounds have lent it additional support (2).

The mechanism through which the shared epitope might determine the immune response has been debated at length and may be through presentation of arthritogenic peptide to T cells. However there are variations in sequence between DR4 subtypes outside the shared sequence that may also influence antigen binding which would not be taken into account by this model. Alternatively the shared epitope may play a role in the selection of the T cell repertoire via thymic education.

Strength

Explains the majority of the population association data in RA.

Weakness

Does not provide an explanation for DR4/DR1 negative RA.

Relevance

This hypothesis provides an explanation for the majority of population association data in RA, lends great support to a central component of immunology and provides a framework for further analysis of class II association data in other immunological diseases.

Paper 6

HLA heterozygosity contributes to susceptibility to rheumatoid arthritis

Authors

Wordsworth P, Pile KD, Buckely JD, Lanchbury JS, Ollier B, Lathrop M, Bell JI

Reference

American Journal of Human Genetics 1992; **51**:585–591

Summary

The HLA-DR genotypes of 184 patients with severe RA and of 46 patients with Felty's syndrome were analysed with the aim of establishing the relative contribution of the RA associated subtypes of DR4 (Dw4, Dw14, Dw15). The relative risks for RA associated with particular genotypes were calculated using the observed frequencies of these genotypes in patients and controls; they were calculated relative to DRX/DRX where DRX is any antigen except DR4 or DR1. There was an excess of DR4 homozygotes, particularly Dw4/Dw14 compound heterozygotes. The risk associated with the Dw4 subtype of DR4 depended on which other allele was present. It was highest for the Dw4/Dw14 genotype (RR 49) and also high for the Dw4/DR1 genotype (RR 21). Dw4/Dw4 homozygotes were at intermediate risk (RR 15) while Dw4 combined with a non-DR4, non-DR1 allele was associated with the lowest RR of 6. Four cases of the rare Dw4/Dw15 genotype were found (expected <0.5).

The results were compared with the genotypes of 63 patients with RA who were ascertained on the basis of being known DR4 homozygotes without reference to disease severity. The excess of Dw4/Dw14 in this group was less apparent and not statistically significant (RR1.4), suggesting that this genotype may be associated with severe disease.

Related references

(1) Nepom BS, Nepom GT, Mickelson E, Schaller JG, Antonelli P, Hansen JA. Specific HLA-DR4-associated histocompatibility molecules characterize patients with seropositive juvenile rheumatoid arthritis. *Journal of Clinical Investigation* 1984; **74**(1):287–291.

(2) Nepom GT, Seyfried CE, Holbeck SL, Wilske KR, Nepom BS. Identification of HLA-Dw14 genes in DR4+ rheumatoid arthritis. *The Lancet* 1986; **2**(8514):1002–1005.

(3) Weyand CM, Hicok KC, Conn DL, Goronzy JJ. The influence of HLA-DRB1 genes on disease severity in rheumatoid arthritis (see comments). *Annals of Internal Medicine* 1992; **117**(10):801–806.

(4) Weyand CM, Xie C, Goronzy JJ. Homozygosity for the HLA-DRB1 allele selects for extraarticular manifestations in rheumatoid arthritis. *Journal of Clinical Investigation* 1992; **89**(6):2033–2039.

Key message

Combinations of the alleles Dw4, Dw14, Dw15 and DR1 predispose to severe RA.

Why it's important

Prior to this study HLA-D heterozygous genotypes had been identified in seven out of 12 patients with JRA (1) and in six out of seven adult patients with RA who were DR4 homozygotes (2). However, neither the high prevalence of compound heterozygotes amongst DR4 homozygotes nor the significance of the effect of heterozygosity on disease severity were well established. Much of the previous work addressing HLA association with disease had used differences in allele frequencies between populations rather than analysis of individual genotypes. However, shortly after this publication work by Weyand, *et al.* emphasized the importance of this approach. They demonstrated that clinical subsets with different disease manifestations could be characterized through HLA-DRB1 genotyping. Extra-articular disease was strongly associated with Dw4 homozygosity (4).

This paper and the work by Weyand *et al.* (3,4) demonstrate that both HLA haplotypes contribute to the phenotypic expression of the disease and to the genetic risk of RA. The mechanism is not clear but some revision of the shared epitope hypothesis is obviously necessary to take account of these findings. It is probably not explained by the concentration of HLA class II antigens on the cell surface as there was only a limited increase in Dw4/Dw4 and Dw14/Dw14 homozygotes in this study.

The increase in all of Dw4/DR1 and Dw4/Dw15 and Dw4/Dw14 genotypes where Dw14, Dw15 and DR1 all share identical amino acid sequences differing from Dw4 by a single amino acid substitution, strongly suggests a role for synergy in mediating the heterozygote effect. Dw4 and Dw14 haplotypes may act synergistically possibly by enabling more efficient binding of arthritogenic peptides. The above work suggests that whatever the underlying mechanism it does not function only at the initiation of disease but also in its progression. Perhaps by playing a role in T cell selection in the thymus the HLA molecules determine an increased repertoire capable of recognizing a specific antigen and regulate the overall composition and diversity of the T cell compartment. An understanding of this mechanism may shed more light on the pathogenesis of RA.

Strengths

1. Demonstrates the importance of analysing clinical subsets of disease to obtain clear evidence of a genetic effect.
2. Unequivocally confirms the importance of HLA heterozygosity.

Weakness

None.

Relevance

This paper demonstrates how advances in molecular methods can provoke further questioning of central immunological mechanisms and challenge prevailing views of disease pathogenesis.

Section 2

Diseases

CHAPTER 6

Rheumatoid arthritis

Frank A Wollheim

Introduction

In several countries Rheumatology was in the past very much focussed on rheumatoid arthritis (RA), which was the major cause of disability. Although the picture has changed RA remains a major problem for many sufferers amounting to 0.5% to 1% of the adult population in most populations. Expanded knowledge of the pathophysiology of joint inflammation and destruction, as well as therapeutic advances occur at a fast pace. It is possible to control disease activity and help patients to a better or even normal life. However, we are still ignorant regarding aetiology and no cure is in sight.

The selection of 'the' most important papers in the vast field encompassed under the title of RA is an impossible task. I have tried to select papers dealing with both fundamental issues, such as the nature of RA, when does it start, and what makes it chronic, as well as the more practical issues regarding classification, clinical assessment and outcome measures. Each of these topics could easily be dealt with in one whole chapter. Several important papers regarding genetics, rheumatoid factors (RFs), imaging and pharmacotherapy will be covered in other chapters. I hope the reader will forgive my biases and find some interest in the selections.

The selected papers range from very pragmatic ones, like the American Rheumatism Association (ARA) criteria from 1958 and the Health Assessment Questionnaire (HAQ) from 1980, to important clinical discoveries exemplified by the description of low complement levels in synovial fluid made in 1964 and the description of the nailfold vasculitis in 1956. More basic classics constitute the discovery of the GM system in 1956 and that of microchimerism in RA in the 1990s. Classics in drug therapy is covered in another chapter, but one therapy paper dealing with joint surgery is included.

I would like to dedicate this chapter to two of the great scholars and inspirators, who helped to make rheumatology academically strong by training generations of young rheumatologists from several countries, Eric GL Bywaters (1) and Morris Ziff (2). The cited papers bear witness of their stringent and to the point style from which we can still learn.

References

1. Bywaters EGL. Historical aspects of the aetiology of rheumatoid arthritis. *British Journal of Rheumatology* 1988; **27**(suppl. 2):110–5.
2. Ziff M. Rheumatoid arthritis – Its present and future. *Journal of Rheumatology* 1990; **17**:127–133.

Paper 1

1958 revision of diagnostic criteria for rheumatoid arthritis

Authors

Ropes MW, Bennet GA, Cobb S, Jacox R, Jessar RA

Reference

Annals of Rheumatic Diseases 1957; **16**:118–25

Abstract

A committee chaired by Marion Ropes was appointed by the ARA to define criteria best suited to define RA. A number of physicians 'particularly interested in rheumatic diseases in various sections of the United States and Canada' were asked to each contribute data from their clinics of the five most recent patients with definite RA, five recent patients with probable RA and five patients with no evidence of RA. In all 332 patients were analysed for presence of 11 criteria that had been selected on the basis of clinical experience by the authors. Sensitivity and specificity was calculated for presence of five or more criteria (definite disease), 3–4 criteria (probable disease), and less than 3 of the 11 criteria (no disease). In order to avoid inclusion of false positives, 19 exclusions were also listed.

Summary

The 11 selected criteria vary individually with regard to specificity and sensitivity (Table 6.1), but the combination gave a sensitivity of 0.70 and specificity of 0.91 for greater than five criteria for definite RA, and a sensitivity of 0.88 and a specificity of 0.77 for probable RA. It is not clear from the publication how much was added when applying the 19 exclusions. It was pointed out that one of the exclusions, antinuclear antibodies, would remove 3–5% of RA patients. It was stressed that objective joint changes such as swelling, tenderness and nodules, had to be verified by a physician.

Table 6.1 Selected criteria to define RA.

1. Morning sickness
2. Pain on motion or tenderness in at least one joint
3. Swelling of one joint, representing soft tissue or fluid
4. Swelling of at least one other joint
5. Symmetrical joint swelling
6. Subcutaneous nodules
7. Typical radiological arthritic changes
8. Positive test for rheumatoid factor in serum
9. Poor mucin precipitate from synovial fluid
10. Characteristic histological changes in synovial membrane
11. Characteristic histopathology of rheumatoid nodules

Related references (1) Ropes MW, Bennet GA, Cobb S, Jacox R, Jessar RA. 1958 revision of diagnostic criteria for rheumatoid arthritis. *Bulletin of Rheumatic Diseases* 1958; **9**:175–176.

(2) Arnett FA, Edworthy SM, Bloch DA, *et al.* The American Rheumatism Association 1987 revised criteria for the classification of rheumatoid arthritis. *Arthritis and Rheumatism* 1988; **31**:305–314.

Key message

RA can be defined with the help of standardized criteria and further subdivided into categories of certainty.

Why it's important

Proper classification of a condition is an absolute requirement for prognostic and therapeutic studies. Pathogenetic as well as aetiological research must be based on precise clinical diagnosis. This was a simple instrument allowing stringent classification of a disease of unknown cause and variable expression. This was a prerequisite for epidemiological investigations and geographical comparisons between different populations.

Strengths

1. The simple nature of the instrument facilitated universal testing and use.
2. The instrument could be used even if not all criteria were available.
3. The list of criteria was didactically useful in teaching students what RA is about.

Weaknesses

1. The long list of exclusions require extensive work up.
2. The exclusions could falsely exclude patients with features of overlap symptoms.
3. The criteria are not really diagnostic in the clinical setting.
4. The category of possible RA included a substantial number of patients who never developed established disease.

Relevance

The 1958 revision (1) actually only added one additional exclusion, agammaglobulinaemia. This revised form was then in universal use for three decades and must be one of the most cited papers in rheumatological literature. It was replaced in 1988 (2) by what is now called the 1987 ACR criteria, which are actually only moderately better, although simpler to use. Many investigators have questioned whether RA is one disease or a designation for a mixed bag of different conditions. A further signum of relevance was accumulating evidence, that the number of positive criteria correlated to disease severity and indeed to mortality. The robust nature of the criteria tell the message, that RA is until proven wrong, indeed one condition.

Paper 2

Prevalence of rheumatoid arthritis

Author

Lawrence JS

Reference

Annals of Rheumatic Diseases 1961; **20**:11–17

Summary

A random sample of 751 males and 814 females in the town of Leigh in Lancashire and an area sample of 485 males and 540 females in Wensleydale in Yorkshire, UK, have been investigated clinically, radiologically, and serologically to determine the prevalence of RA. The examination was completed in 86% of the Leigh sample and in 87% of the Wensleydale sample.Using the ARA criteria, the minimal prevalence of 'definite' disease was 0.4% in males, and 1.4% in females, and that of 'probable' disease was 1.7% in males and 3.8% in females. Radiological evidence of erosive arthritis was present in 8% of all those x-rayed, both in males and females, but the disease was more severe in females. Changes were most frequently encountered in the cervical spine. A positive sheep cell agglutination test was found in 4% of males and in 5% of females.

It is estimated that, in Great Britain in 1959, approximately 377 000 males and 1 034 000 females had 'probable' or 'definite' RA.

Related references

(1) Silman AJ. Has the incidence of rheumatoid arthritis decline in the United Kingdom? *British Journal of Rheumatology* 1988; **27**:77–79.

(2) Gabriel SE, Crowson CS, O'Fallon WM. The epidemiology of rheumatoid arthritis in Rochester, Minnesota. *Arthritis and Rheumatism* 1999; **42**:415–420.

(3) Wiles N, Symmons DP, Harrison B, *et al.* Estimating the incidence of rheumatoid arthritis: trying to hit a moving target? *Arthritis and Rheumatism* 1999; **42**:1339–1346.

Key message

RA is a common disease. Its prevalence is 2–3 times higher in women, and the prevalence increases with age, in particular in women (Figure 6.1). RA is more severe in women.

Why it's important

This was probably the first population-based application of the ARA criteria of 1958. It also compared a rural and an urban population. Although it involved clinical examination of some 2500 individuals, it was the work of one author, showing firstly this man's assiduity and second, giving proof that the method was practicable. The author states in all modesty, that his data might be of use to other UK investigators who would like 'a standard to compare their own findings'. In fact, solid data on prevalence in a defined population and point in time, are universally useful.

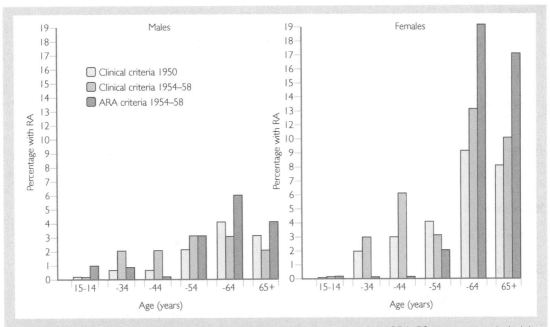

Figure 6.1 RA diagnosed clinically in the 1950 complaints survey and the 1954–58 x-ray servey in Leigh, and by the ARA criteria in the latter; this figure is based on unpublished material. The Wensleydale data have been excluded.

Strengths

1. Application of new methodology to population-based samples.
2. High response rate strengthens reliability of the observations.
3. Same observer compares different populations.

Weaknesses

1. The radiological data are incomplete and confusing. Probably they do not distinguish RA from osteoarthritis lesions.
2. The prevalence of individual criteria is not presented.
3. No data on disease duration or functional status are provided.
4. No incidence data are provided.

Relevance

This study, simple as it may seem, has withstood the test of time. Many more recent studies have confirmed much of the Lawrence data. It is not possible to summarize all important progress in a few sentences that followed this early study. One area of controversy is whether or not RA is becoming less severe or less prevalent (1). Only solid population-based prospective studies are helpful to address this problem (2, 3). Several recent prevalence studies indicate lower than 1% prevalence and higher age of onset in the adult population, but it has not been convincingly shown that the disease is actually diminishing in defined populations.

Paper 3

The ameliorating effect of pregnancy on chronic atrophic (infectious rheumatoid) arthritis, fibrositis, and intermittent hydrarthrosis

Author

Hench PS

Reference

Proceedings of the Staff Meetings of the Mayo Clinic 1938; **13**:161-167

Summary

'Rheumatic women have long been devotees of the sun; perhaps it is important for them to invoke also the kindly and regular auspices of the moon. At least many physicians during the last century have believed that a normal regular menstrual cycle is good insurance against rheumatism, and have listed menstrual irregularities among the common predisposing caus-es of the disease. Some still hold that (1) chronic arthritis is etiologically related to defective catamenia or other uterine disorders, the menopause, too rapid child-bearing or prolonged lactation and that (2) pregnancy is dangerous for arthritic women because the joints are apt to flare up after parturition. I have studied the effect of thirty-seven pregnancies on twenty-two women with chronic articular disease, and have concluded that, regardless of its after-math, pregnancy (like jaundice) involves a physiologic state which is decidedly antagonistic to the continuation of symptoms of certain articular disease, especially chronic atrophic (infectious rheumatoid) arthritis.'

Key message

The author cites a large number of authorities who have pointed out the dangers of female reproduction to the joints, including Charcot, AR and AE Garrod, Bannantyne, Kersley and van Breemen. In contrast only few authors had observed beneficial effects of pregnancy, and these were mostly related to intermittent hydrathrosis. Although some authors had hinted at beneficial effects even in 'atrophic' arthritis, Hench was impressed by the absence of real observations and set out to produce just this. 20 of the 22 patients experienced relief, usually during every pregnancy, and most often within the first month. He also noticed that relapse was the rule, usually within one or a few months post-partum. Furthermore it was stated that the two women who did not improve during pregnancies, also had failed to improve during unrelated episodes of jaundice.

Why it is important

Like so many landmark observations, this one went counter to current dogma, although in retrospect, there were several hints around pointing to the benefit of pregnancy. The documentation that symptoms of RA could be influenced in a predictable way created, as Dr Hench points out a possibility to investigate pathogenesis and search for therapies. On another note, as also recognized by the author, it was important to be able to inform patients with RA what a pregnancy could mean to them, and such information did not exist. Furthermore RA was then and even much later, considered as a relentlessly progressive condition, 'chronic progressive polyarthritis', and this paper indicated that this perhaps was not entirely true.

Strengths

1. This is patientside research asking a distinct question and arriving at a clear-cut result.
2. The paper is based on an original hypothesis and follows a logic from a previous study of jaundice.
3. The author proves that he is both an independent thinker and has a balanced knowledge of previous work in the field.
4. The author realises the importance of the observation.

Weakness

1. No predefined definitions of improvement or relapse.
2. The observations seem to be gathered both prospectively and retrospectively, and the mix could have introduced bias.
3. The results are presented in a verbal and subjective way, without attempt to quantify results or present objective measures.
4. The follow up period is not standardized, one pregnancy was still ongoing.

Relevance

The implication of this paper are far reaching. The author makes the interesting statement that it would seem likely, that the agent responsible for improvement would be similar in jaundice and pregnancy, and that therefore neither bile salts or female sex hormones would be a likely cause. This, in fact, was the seed for the later discovery of the effect of cortisone on RA. The relevance of the paper can best be appreciated by considering the 1000 or so hits relating to pregnancy and RA in Pub Med since 1965, 50 of which were published in the last year.

Paper 4

Participation of monocyte-macrophages and lymphocytes in the production of a factor that stimulates collagenase and prostaglandin release by rheumatoid synovial cells

Authors

Dayer JM, Breard J, Chess L, Krane SM

Reference

Journal of Clinical Investigation 1979; **64**:1386–92

Summary

Cultured mononuclear cells from human peripheral blood produce a soluble factor (MCF) that stimulates collagenase and prostaglandin E2 (PGE2) release by cultured rheumatoid synovial cells up to several hundred-fold. These target rheumatoid synovial cells lack conventional macrophage markers. To determine which mononuclear cells are the source of MCF, purified populations of monocyte-macrophages, thymus-derived (T) lymphocytes, and bone marrow-derived (B) lymphocytes were prepared. The monocyte-macrophages alone produced levels of MCF that were proportional to cell density but unaffected by phytohaemagglutinin or pokeweed mitogen. No detectable collagenase activity was produced by the cultured monocyte-macrophages or lymphocytes. Purified T lymphocytes produced levels of MCF approximately equal to 1–3% those of purified monocyte-macrophages in the presence or absence of the above lectins. Purified T lymphocytes modulated the production of MCF by the monocyte-macrophages, however, in a manner dependent upon relative cell densities and the presence of lectins. For example, at optimal ratios of T lymphocytes : monocyte-macrophages, MCF production was markedly stimulated by pokeweed mitogen. Thus, interactions of T lymphocytes and monocyte-macrophages could be important in determining levels of MCF, which regulate collagenase and PGE2 production by target synovial cells in inflammatory arthritis.

Related references (1)   Dayer JM, Robinson DR, Krane SM. Prostaglandin production by synovial cells: stimulation by a factor from human mononuclear cells. *Journal of Experimental Medicine* 1977; **145**:1399–1404.

(2)   Mizel SB, Dayer JM, Krane SM, Mergenhagen SE. Stimulation of rheumatoid synovial cell collagenase and prostaglandin production by partially purified lymphocyte-activating factor (interleukin 1). *Proceedings of the National Academy of Sciences USA* 1981; **78**:2474–2477.

(3)   Burger D, Rezzonico R, Li JM, *et al.* Imbalance between interstitial collagenase and tissue inhibitor of metalloproteinases 1 in synoviocytes and fibroblasts upon direct contact with stimulated T lymphocytes: involvement of membrane-associated cytokines. *Arthritis and Rheumatism* 1998; **41**:1748–1759.

Key message

Macrophages interact with synovial fibroblasts and stimulate them to produce mediators of inflammation. This effect is due to a soluble factor, later called IL-1beta and it can also be effectuated through direct cell-cell interaction.

Why it's important

This report clearly demonstrated a key interaction between macrophages and synovial cells, where IL-1 is involved, and which can be modulated by T lymphocytes, and which results in chronic destructive synovitis. Understanding more about this process could be expected to identify possible targets for therapeutic intervention.

Strengths

1. The highly original approach to study cell interactions in an *ex vivo* system.
2. The combination of experimental and analytical skills with biological fantasy.

Weakness

Molecular biology was not yet available to the author in the 1970s. It would have allowed the author to characterize the factor or indeed factors involved in signalling. This work was left to other laboratories, and is still not complete.

Relevance

The relevance of this early observations has become increasingly obvious with the evolving explosion in cytokine research. One need only mention the IL-1 family of cytokines and their receptors and natural inhibitors, among them IL-1Ra as well as IL-18 and IL-18 binding protein. The demonstration of stimulation of PGE2 secretion by a factor of 200 antedated the discovery of cyclooxygenase 2 by a decade. Dr. Dayer was involved in the discovery of IL-1Ra and of the natural tumour necrosis factor inhibitors, which now are transforming rheumatological therapy.

Paper 5

Appearance of anti-HLA-DR reactive cells in normal and rheumatoid synovium

Authors

Klareskog L, Forsum U, Malmnäs Tjernlund UK, Kabelitz D, Wigren A

Reference

Scandinavian Journal of Immunology 1981; **14**:183–192

Summary

The reactivity of rabbit anti-HLA-DR antigen antibodies with cells in normal and rheumatoid synovial tissue was investigated by indirect immunofluorescence on frozen sections of tissue. The antibodies reacted with a significant portion of the synovial lining cells of both normal and rheumatoid synovial tissue, with endothelial cells, and with a number of, most probably, migratory cells. After dispersion of cells from rheumatoid synovial tissue by digestion with collagenase and DNase, adherent cells of both a macrophage-like and a dendritic appearance reacted with the HLA-DR antigen antibodies. The adherent cells were also found to be potent stimulators in the allogeneic MLR. In addition, it was found that a high proportion of T lymphocytes from both peripheral blood and synovial tissue from rheumatoid patients bound anti-HLA-DR antibodies. The present data suggest a role for synovial lining cells in HLA-D-locus-dependent events of importance in the pathogenesis of RA and other joint diseases, and point to the need for further investigations on T lymphocytes derived from the site of inflammation in the study of RA.

Related references
(1) Janossy G, Panayi G, Duke O, *et al.* Rheumatoid arthritis: a disease of T-lymphocyte/macrophage immunoregulation. *The Lancet* 1981 Oct 17; **2**(8251):839–844.

(2) Klareskog L, Forsum U, Scheynius A, *et al.* Evidence in support of a self-perpetuating HLA-DR-dependent delayed-type cell reaction in rheumatoid arthritis. *Proceedings of the National Academy of Sciences USA* 1982; **79**:3632–3636.

(3) Kingsley GH, Panayi GS, Lanchbury O. Immunotherapy of rheumatic diseases – practice and prospects. *Immunology Today* 1991; **12**:177–179.

(4) Burmester GR, Yu DT, Irani AM, Kunkel HG, Winchester RJ. Ia+ T cells in synovial fluid and tissues of patients with rheumatoid arthritis. *Arthritis and Rheumatism* 1981; **24**:1370–1376.

Key message

Macrophage/monocytes arriving in the joint of RA patients can activate T lymphocytes by means of their cell surface HLA-DR expression.

Why it's important

This report in conjunction with *The Lancet* publication (1), which appeared a few months later focussed interest on the involvement of antigen presenting cells (APC, Figure 6.2) interacting with resident lymphocytes as a central pathogenetic event in RA. The nature of this interaction, and ways to influence the interaction or its consequences, are still hot items after two decades in basic and applied RA related research. The activated T cell presence had been reported earlier (4).

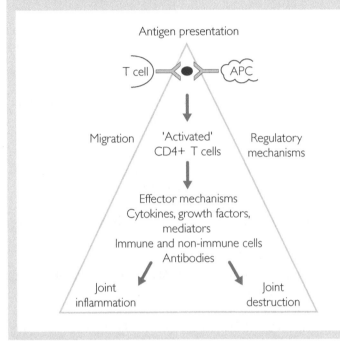

Figure 6.2 Pathogenesis of RA (from Related reference 3).

Strengths

1. These investigators built the bridge between established bench technology and the operating room.
2. They asked the right question – which cells are involved in RA synovitis?
3. They used the right reagents to identify them.

Weaknesses

1. The patients' clinical data are largely absent.
2. The definition of 'normal' tissue can be questioned.

Relevance

This observation stimulated scientists world wide in attempts to identify the antigen. This has proved frustrating, perhaps because there is not *one* antigen but several. It has furthermore motivated therapeutic efforts targeting T lymphocytes, which have been unsuccessful. Nevertheless, it has given rise to the paradigm which is still useful 20 years later (3). However, therapies targeting macrophage function are now in the forefront of RA therapy. Both the Swedish and the British groups of investigators extended observations from other fields of pathology to RA. It shows how important interfaces and bridges are for progress in science.

Paper 6

Measurement of patient outcome in arthritis

Authors

Fries JF, Spitz P,Kraines RG, Holman HR

Reference

Arthritis and Rheumatism 1980; **23**:137–145

Summary

A structure for representation of outcome is presented, together with a method for outcome measurement and validation of the technique in RA. The paradigm represents outcome by five separate dimensions: death, discomfort, disability, drug (therapeutic) toxicity, and dollar cost. Each dimension represents an outcome directly related to patient welfare. Quantitation of these outcome dimensions may be performed at interview or by patient questionnaire. With standardized, validated questions, similar scores are achieved by both methods. The questionnaire technique is preferred since it is inexpensive and does not involve interobserver validation. These techniques appear extremely useful for evaluation of long-term outcome of patients with rheumatic diseases.

Related references   **(1)**   Meenan RF, Gertman PM, Mason JH. Measuring health status in arthritis. The arthritis impact measuring scales. *Arthritis and Rheumatism* 1980; **23**:145–152.

            (2)   Steinbrocker O, Traeger CH, Batterman RC. Therapeutic criteria in rheumatoid arthritis. *Journal of the American Medical Association* 1949; **140**:659–662.

            (3)   Fries JF. Toward an understanding of patient outcome measurement. *Arthritis and Rheumatism* 1983; **26**:697–704.

Key message

A simple self administered patient questionnaire was proven to give robust, relevant and reproducible quantitative information concerning physical health in patients suffering from established RA.

Why it's important

The HAQ proved for the first time that patients could respond to the right questions in a reproducible fashion, that the test could be repeated over time and could be used to measure changes. Furthermore the scale was more continuous than the classical functional classes of Steinbrocker (2). The HAQ index allows characterization of the severity of disability in individual patients and comparisons between patient groups. In contrast to laboratory measures such as CRP, which relate to the process rather than to the outcome, and surrogate measures, such as grip strength, which may or may not be critical for function. HAQ is a direct measure of functional qualities with high patient relevance (3).

Strengths

1. Limited number of questions.
2. Simple standard for answers.
3. Concerns functions of obvious relevance to most patients and may alert health care providers to important disabilities.
4. Minimal cost to administer.

Weaknesses

1. Patient's mood may influence answers.
2. Requires translation and validation in different settings.
3. Measures only physical consequences of RA.

Relevance

Every rheumatologist treating RA patients may benefit from the routine use of the HAQ in daily practice. It is in wide use in therapeutic trials and modifications are developed for other diseases. HAQ impairment measured in early disease has been shown to predict mortality. It should be said that the AIMS instrument (1), which was published in the same issue of *Arthritis and Rheumatism* as the HAQ, is more comprehensive and measures social performance, pain, anxiety and depression as well. This more complex approach is no doubt an advantage in several situations, but also explains the more limited use.

Paper 7

When does rheumatoid arthritis start?

Authors

Aho K, Palosuo T, Raunio V, Puska P, Aromaa A, Salonen JT

Reference

Arthritis and Rheumatism 1985; **28**:485–489

Summary

Some 10 000 sera had been collected and stored in connection with a community-based population survey in eastern Finland in 1972 and 1977. Tests for RF were performed on a representative sample amounting to 1500 sera. Thirty of these patients had developed RA as diagnosed by specialist physicians between a few months and 9 years after sampling. Nine of these pre-onset sera were Waaler-Rose positive and 16 latex test positive. The proportion of positive sera was higher the closer to onset of RA the sera had been drawn.

Related references **(1)** Hench PS, Rosenberg EF. Palindromic rheumatism: a 'new' oft recurring disease of the joints (arthritis, periarthritis, para-arthritis) apparently producing no articular residues: report of 34 cases; its relation to 'angioneural arthrosis', 'allergic rheumatism', and rheumatoid arthritis. *Archives of Internal Medicine* 1944; **73**:293–321.

(2) Williams MH, Sheldon PJDS,Torrigiani G, *et al*. Palindromic rheumatism. *Annals of Rheumatic Diseases* 1971; **30**:375–380.

(3) Schumacher HR, Kritridou RC. Synovitis of recent onset. A clinico-pathologic study during the first month of disease. *Arthritis and Rheumatism* 1972; **15**:465–485.

(4) Schumacher RH. Palindromic onset of rheumatoid arthritis. Clinical, synovial fluid, and biopsy studies. *Arthritis and Rheumatism* 1982; **25**:361–369.

(5) Gonzales-Lopez L, Gamez-Nava JI, Jhangri G, *et al*. Decreased progression to rheumatoid arthritis or other connective tissue diseases in patients with palindromic rheumatism treated with antimalarials. *Journal of Rheumatology* 2000; **27**:41–46.

(6) Gran JT, Husby G, Thorsby E. HLA antigens in palindromic rheumatism, nonerosive rheumatoid arthritis and classical rheumatoid arthritis. *Journal of Rheumatology* 1984; **11**(2):136–140.

(7) Aho K, Heliövaara M, Knekt P, *et al*. Serum immunoglobulins and the risk of rheumatoid arthritis. *Annals of Rheumatic Diseases* 1997; **56**:351–356.

(8) Masi AT. Sex hormones and rheumatoid arthritis: cause or effect relationships in a complex pathophysiology. *Clinical and Experimental Rheumatology* 1995; **13**:227–240.

Key message

Rheumatoid factor positivity is a common finding in asymptomatic patients who later develop RA. In a later extended report increased serum immunoglobulin (Ig) G and IgA levels were found predictive of RA (7).

Why it's important

Hench first described a dramatic episodic arthritis termed palindromic rheumatism in the 1940s (1), and later it was shown sometimes to develop into RA (2). Although no definite evidence of RA was identified on careful histological examination in patients with very recent onset of synovitis (3) or palindromic rheumatism later developing RA (4), therapy with anti-malarials had recently been shown to delay or prevent development of RA in palindromic rheumatism (5). Decreased levels of male hormone had also been found in stored pre-disease onset sera (8), pointing to early abnormalities in body fluids which may influence disease susceptibility. The unique Finnish studies present convincing evidence of ongoing pathology sometimes preceding RA, even in apparently asymptomatic individuals. These observations open the possibility to explore pre-clinical events that may pertain to the aetiology of RA. The identification of individuals like those in Finland could clearly help to identify triggering events in the environment.

Strength

The utilization of a unique serum collection to study pre-clinical serology of RA.

Weaknesses

1. Clinical data regarding disease evolution or severity are not presented.
2. It was not clear whether any of the patients had suffered from palindromic rheumatism before disease onset.

Relevance

The material from the so-called Mini-Finland study has shown that serologic events precede clinical disease in many patients. This study opens important approaches. It was later shown, using samples from 124 RA patients from the same material, that hyper IgG and IgA was also common before disease onset. It is not known whether tissue types were predictive in these patients. It could be of interest to study the samples of these patients with regard to evidence of microbial infections or other environmental events. Perhaps one study could try an interventional approach in line with that in reference (4). It has been established in a Norwegian study, that HLA-DR 4 is common in patients with palindromic rheumatism developing RA (6).

Paper 8

Agglutination of erythrocytes coated with 'incomplete' anti-RH by certain rheumatoid arthritic sera and some other sera

Author

Grubb R

Reference

Acta Pathol Microbiol Scand 1956; **39**:195–197

Summary

Some pathological sera, notably certain RA sera, agglutinate Rh-positive cells coated with 'incomplete' anti-Rh despite dilution. Human serum can be grouped with the aid of some rheumatoid sera.

Related references **(1)** Grubb R, Laurell A-B. Hereditary serological human serum groups. *Acta Pathologica et Microbiologica Scandinavica* 1956; **39**:390–398.

(2) Eberhardt K, Grubb R, Johnson U, Pettersson H. HLA-DR antigens, Gm allotypes and antiallotypes in early rheumatoid arthritis – their relation to disease progression. *Journal of Rheumatology* 1993; **20**:1825–1829.

(3) Grubb R, Grubb A, Kjellén L, *et al.* Rheumatoid arthritis – a gene transfer disease. *Experimental and Clinical Immunogenetics* 1999; **16**:1–7.

(4) Bjarnadottir M, Nathansson C, Balbin M, *et al.* Nucleotide sequences specific for nonnominal immunoglobulin allotypes in rheumatoid arthritis patients and in normal individuals and their expression in synovial tissue of rheumatoid arthritis patients. *Experimental and Clinical Immunogenetics* 1999; **16**:8–16.

(5) Nelson JL. Maternal-fetal immunology and autoimmune disease: is some autoimmune disease auto-alloimmune or allo-autoimmune? *Arthritis and Rheumatism* 1996; **39**:191–194.

Key message

Sera of patients with RA have potency to agglutinate sheep erythrocytes coated with sub-agglutinating doses of human gamma globulin depending on genetic variations of the employed source. Thus is was possible for the first time to show genetic polymorphism among human gamma globulins, the Gm (Gamma gobulin marker) system was discovered.

Why it's important

The observation that immunoglobulin allotypes in man display mendelian inheritance changed the fundamental understanding of immunoglobulin control. The Gm system became a powerful instrument in population genetics. The significance of anti-Gm antibody formation in RA is yet to be fully understood. The intriguing observation of the presence of 'forbidden' or nonnominal allotypes in RA, made using homozygous RA patients blood and PCR amplification (4), is still a puzzle which Professor Grubb was trying to elucidate at the time of his untimely death in 1998. He interpreted the results as indicating transfer of genetic material by means of viral infection, called transduction. Accordingly he proposed the hypothesis that RA is a gene transfer disease (3).

Strengths

1. An unexpected observation of antibody activity in RA sera opened a new field of genetics.
2. It has given a handle for exploration into the aetiology of RA.

Weakness

Understanding the full implication of the observation requires a good amount of basic knowledge. Or as Professor Grubb liked to phrase it: 'He who is not confused is not informed'.

Relevance

The Gm system was the first genetic gammaglobulin allotypic variation, several other have followed. Gm antibodies and the Gm allotypes offer opportunities to test the gene transfer hypothesis of RA. This involves a virus vector which incorporates foreign antigenic material into a susceptible recipient, who under the right conditions develops RA. Support for the hypothesis has been published recently (5). The observation of microchimerism among patients with RA is another supporting observation. Although no direct toxic effect has been linked to Gm antibodies in RA, occurrence of anti-G1m(a) antibodies in early disease was highly predictive of small joint erosions (2).

Paper 9

Identification of immunoglobulins and complement in rheumatoid articular collagenous tissues

Authors

Cooke TD, Hurd ER, Jasin HE , Bienenstock J, Ziff M

Reference

Arthritis and Rheumatism 1975; **18**:541–551

Summary

Ninety-three patients with a variety of joint diseases were studied for evidence of immune complexes in articular collagenous tissue. Frozen sections of freshly obtained biopsies of hyaline articular cartilage and menisci were stained with fluoresceinated monospecific antisera for evidence of human Igs (IgG, IgM,IgA) and the beta1c component of complement. The criterion for the presence of complexes was the staining of two or more Igs and beta1c in an identical location of sequentially-cut sections. Of the 42 patients with RA 83% were positive by this criterion. In those with classic RA the incidence was 92%. Sixteen patients with fresh joint trauma or non-arthritic disease had negative findings. Among 26 patients with non-inflammatory disease, four of eight with polyarthritis whose features suggested primary degeneration, one of 11 patients with secondary degenerative arthritis, and a single case of synovial osteochondromatosis also had positive findings. Among nine patients with miscellaneous inflammatory arthritides, all of three with psoriatic arthritis were negative; however two of six with other inflammatory arthritides were positive. The findings in classic RA suggest that immune complexes are deposited in the articular collagenous tissues. The persistence of these complexes may play a significant role in the chronicity of the synovitis.

Related references **(1)** Cooke TD, Hurd ER, Ziff M, Jasin HE. The pathogenesis of chronic inflammation in experimental antigen-induced arthritis II. Preferential localization of antigen-antibody complexes to collagenous tissue. *Journal of Experimental Medicine* 1972; **135**(2):323–338.

(2) Smiley JD, Sachs C, Ziff M. *In vitro* synthesis of immunoglobulin by rheumatoid synovial membrane. *Journal of Clinical Investigations* 1968; **47**:624–632.

(3) Ishikawa H, Smiley JD, Ziff M. Electron microscopic demonstration of immunoglobulin deposition in rheumatoid cartilage. *Arthritis and Rheumatism* 1975; **18**:563–576.

Key message

The paper establishes the presence of immune complexes in articular cartilage from patients with inflammatory joint disease. The presence of immunoglobulin in RA cartilage was also confirmed using electron microscopy (3). This indicates that this tissue may be an important reservoir of disease perpetuating material.

Why it's important

This paper brings convincing proof of penetration of immune complexes as defined by Ig plus complement in identical location. The authors had previously shown such deposits in the antigen-induced model of monarthritis (1). If large proteins like these can penetrate cartilage, this tissue could also harbour other macromolecules and these could contribute to chronic inflammation by immunological mechanisms. An early important paper from Dr. Ziff's laboratory (2) had shown that synovial tissue has the same capacity to produce Ig as lymph nodes.

Strengths

1. Large and well characterized clinical material.
2. Patient application of careful previous animal experiments.

Weaknesses

1. No identification of the putative antigen. However this has still to be found 25 years later.
2. The 'control' group is not clearly defined. It included post-traumatic joint problems, but also 'other conditions'.

Relevance

These observations clearly implicated cartilage as a possible reservoir of substances attracting what appeared to be complement-binding immune complexes, and gave rise to an attractive hypothesis of persisting antigen as a driving force for chronicity in RA. This was before the cytokine era, and today one would probably implicate cytokines and proteases to have done the ground work, opening the entrance for the gamma globulin and complement. However the electron microscopic deposits (3) speak for themselves, and it should not be ruled out that gamma globulin and complement interact with pro-inflammatory mediators to support inflammatory tissue damage.

Paper 10

Prognosis of rheumatoid arthritis. A prospective survey over 11 years

Authors

Jacoby RK, Cosh JA, Jayson MI

Reference

British Medical Journal 1973; **2**(858):96–100

Summary

One hundred patients with 'definite' or 'classical' RA were followed in a hospital clinic from within 1 year of the onset of the arthritis. The average interval between onset and first attendance was 3.7 months. Onset was commoner in the winter, transient prodromal symptoms being noted in 23 patients, with possible precipitating factors in 14. The serum RF test was positive at some time in 88 patients.

The patients were reassessed between 8 and 14 years later. Seventeen died during this period, five possibly as a result of the disease or its treatment. The remaining patients had improved as a whole in terms of the blood sedimentation rate, haemoglobin, titre of RF test, and status of the disease, but there was an overall deterioration in functional capacity. Both the RF titre and the functional capacity at an earlier review could be directly correlated with the outcome, but other factors were not found to influence the ultimate prognosis.

Related references **(1)** Reilly PA, Cosh JA, Maddison PJ, *et al.* Mortality and survival in rheumatoid arthritis: a 25 year prospective study of 100 patients. *Annals of Rheumatic Diseases* 1990; **49**:363–369.

(2) Corbett M, Dalton S, Young A, *et al.* Factors predicting death, survival and functional outcome in a prospective study of early rheumatoid disease over fifteen years. *British Journal of Rheumatology* 1993; **32**:717–723.

(3) Fex E, Jonsson K, Johnson U, Eberhardt KB. Development of radiographic damage during the first 5–6 years of rheumatoid arthritis. A prospective follow-up study of a Swedish cohort. *British Journal of Rheumatology* 1996; **35**:1106–1115.

Key message

RA is a heterogeneous disease with modestly increased mortality. Survivors have a reduced inflammatory activity contrasting to progressive joint damage.

Why it's important

This was one of the first long-term cohort studies of RA, which together with its follow-up report (1) contains a number of important observations. The patients were all seen by Dr. Cosh within 1 year from onset, and all could be traced for decades or until death. It gives the causes of death for the 17 patients, four of which were directly related to disease manifestations: vasculitis, renal amyloidosis, constrictive pericarditis and 'rheumatic' heart disease. The authors also try to identify precipitating events, such as trauma or infection. This Bath/Bristol cohort, together with a similar one from London (2) form the background to which later cohort studies can be compared if one wants to address questions related to change in disease pattern or severity.

Strengths

1. 'He has the best view who has seen the thing from its start' (Aristoteles).
2. The comprehensive inclusion of relevant variables.
3. The complete tracing of the patients.

Weaknesses

1. The selection of classical and definite RA only selected for severe disease.
2. No attempt was made to separate natural course from influence of therapy.

Relevance

The two British studies are evidence against some claims of the association between more benign nature and later age of onset of RA. The radiological data, although qualitative, are of interest in assessing the more recent detailed quantitation of progression rate (3). Of particular interest are the mortality data. It is possible, that some of the cardiovascular mortality may be related to a chronic inflammatory state. With the advent of early aggressive intervention with potent therapeutic agents in RA, it needs to be remembered what the disease evolution would be without these measures. Such evidence is never easy to identify. We should perhaps not forget, that many RA patients even before the methotrexate era fared rather well.

Paper II

Studies on the depressed hemolytic complement activity of synovial fluid in adult rheumatoid arthritis

Author

Hedberg H

Reference

Acta Rheumatologica Scandinavica 1963; **9**:165–193

Summary

Synovial fluid from the knee joints and serum of 68 patients with various joint diseases were analysed by measuring the concentration of haemolytic complement (CH50). Decreased synovial fluid levels were found in patients with SLE and active RA. Lower levels in RA correlated with disease activity and presence of subcutaneous nodules and rheumatoid factor. The low levels were found in both fresh and stored fluids. The findings were also consistent in sequential samples. Fluids from patients with seronegative RA had intermediate CH50 levels and those from osteoarthritis patients were not depressed. Serum CH50 levels were normal in RA but low in SLE.

Related references **(1)** Pekin JT, Zvaifler NJ. Hemolytic complement in synovial fluid. *Journal of Clinical Investigations* 1994; **43**:1372–1382.

(2) Hedberg H. Studies on synovial fluid in arthritis. I. The total complement activity. *Acta Medica Scandinavica* 1997; **479**(suppl.):1–137.

(3) Franco AE, Schur PH. Hypocomplementemia in rheumatoid arthritis. *Arthritis and Rheumatism* 1971; **14**:231–238.

(4) Winchester RJ, Agnello V, Kunkel HG. The joint fluid gammaG-globulin complexes and their relationship to intraarticular complement diminution. *Annals of the New York Academy of Sciences* 1969; **168**:195–203.

Key message

Synovial fluids collected from patients with RF positive RA are characterized by a diminished concentration of haemolytic complement in contrast to fluids from patients with OA.

Why it's important

The observation of unexpectedly low total complement levels in the synovial fluid was made independently in another laboratory (1). It pointed at local complement consumption in the joint and thus was an important clue to pathogenesis of seropositive RA. Serum complement levels have been studied by a number of investigators and often considered unaffected. However, this is not the case. If one considers that two dominating components of complement, C3 and C4, are regulated as acute phase components, one would expect elevated rather than normal or low levels, as are often observed (2, 3). Thus it seems evident that complement consumption is a feature of active RA. A direct correlation of low synovial fluid levels of complement and amount of immune complexes supports a role for immune complexes in the pathogenesis of RA.

Strengths

1. A sound methodology approach allowing comparison between individuals.
2. Looks at the site of pathology rather than just in the blood.
3. Realization of the importance of the observation.

Weakness

Paper has a dull lay out and was not published in a high impact journal.

Relevance

Initial hopes that testing for synovial fluid complement levels would become a diagnostic tool to distinguish different forms of arthritis have not held up. Complement is important in the normal immune defence, and genetic deficiency is often correlated to lupus-like syndromes or susceptibility to infection. The precise role of low complement in RA has not been fully worked out. Figure 6.3 clearly documents selective local complement consumption.

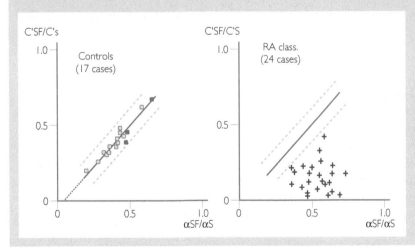

Figure 6.3 Ratio of synovial fluid/serum concentrations of CH50 and alpha-globulin in controls and RA patients (from Heberg [1963]).

Paper 12

Orthopedic surgery in rheumatoid arthritis

Authors

Laine V, Vainio K

Reference

Bulletin of Rheumatic Diseases 1964; **15**:360–361

Summary

Since 1952, when close cooperation was established between the rheumatologist and orthopaedic surgeon, more than 6500 operations have been performed on patients with RA at the Rheumatism Foundation Hospital (317 beds) in Heinola, Finland. In summary our experience shows that patients with RA tolerate orthopaedic surgery very well and with few complications. The results are best when surgery is performed early in the disease before severe deformities are produced. However, much can be offered to the severely deformed patient by surgical procedures.

Related references **(1)** Vainio K. History of surgery of rheumatoid arthritis in Europe. *Scandinavian Journal of Rheumatology* 1983; **12**:65–68.

(2) Laine K. General discussion. In: *Early Synovectomy in Rheumatoid Arthritis,* W Hijmans, WD Paul (eds.). Amsterdam: Excerpata Medica Foundation, 1969:214–215.

Key message

Patients with active RA tolerate joint surgery and benefit in the short-term from so-called 'early synovectomy'.

Why it's important

As Vainio points out (1) the history of orthopaedic surgery in general was rather short and surgery was mostly used as a last resource in rehabilitation of the patient with advanced 'burn out' disease. This was to a large extent due to fears that the surgical procedure could somehow activate the rheumatoid process. It took some courage to challenge this view, but starting in the early 1960s, rheumatologists and orthopaedic surgeons in large numbers visited Heinola and exported the message. This led to the establishment of several centres modelled after the Heinola experience in Europe and overseas. In particular great hopes were put on early synovectomy as a means to halt the disease process or at least ameliorate its consequences. Dr. Laine (2) realized the difficulties relating to controlled trials of the outcome of surgical interventions. Time has shown that early synovectomy is effective to relieve pain but does not halt progression of destruction. Nevertheless, the Heinola experiences formed a foundation upon which later surgical rehabilitation was built, largely consisting of total joint replacement.

Strengths

1. The establishment of interdisciplinary cooperation around the RA patient.
2. The appreciation of difficulties of standardizing surgical technique.
3. The coining of stages of joint damage where 'early' and 'late' refer to severity rather than to duration of the disease.

Weaknesses

1. No controlled trials emerged from Heinola regarding effects of surgery.
2. Failure to promote the idea that outcome assessment should be performed by the rheumatologist or some other neutral assessors, rather than by the orthopaedic surgeon responsible for the procedure.

Relevance

The introduction of joint surgery as a routine therapy in management of RA (Figure 6.4) was an immense step forward. Although synovectomies did not stop progression, which was the initial hope, it provided some years of relief to a large number of patients. It also stimulated widespread interest in the development of better procedures for joint replacement, which continues to be a mainstay of successful rehabilitation in RA. It has a long history.

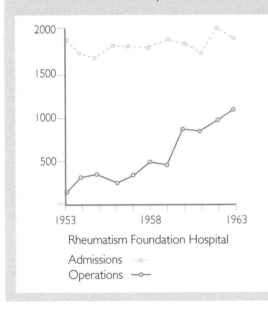

Figure 6.4 Number of admissions and number of operations (from Laine and Vainio [1964]).

Paper 13

Peripheral vascular obstruction in rheumatoid arthritis and its relation to other vascular leisons

Author

Bywaters EGL

Reference

Annals of Rheumatic Diseases 1957; **16**:84–103

Summary

Ten cases of RA have been described, which showed vessel obliteration associated with symptoms ranging from small infarcts, presenting as brown lesions of the nailfold, nailedge, or digital pulp, to gangrene of all four limbs with visceral lesions. This is not thought to represent polyartheritis nodusa or Buerger's disease, but to resemble more closely the arterial changes seen in scleroderma and SLE, and perhaps also the changes described as 'remittent necrotizing acrocyanosis' (1) or 'non-specific obliterative angiitis' (2). None showed the ordinary symptoms of Buerger's disease, although all except one were ambulant. It is not felt that cortisone played any important part, since only three of the 10 had had such preceding treatment.

Related references **(1)** Edvards EA. *Journal of the American Medical Association* 1956; **161**:1530.

(2) Pennoch LL, Primas DH. *Angiology* 1956; **7**:32.

Key message

Occluding vascular lesions causing nailfold infarcts or major gangrene occur in rare cases of RA and can be distinguished from polyangiitis nodusa.

Why it's important

The realization that RA is a systemic disease was based on careful clinical and pathological examinations and only individuals with expertise in both fields could see relevant connections. Professor Bywaters was both pathologist and clinician and had the insight to distinguish the novel type of nailfold necrotic pathology now called 'Bywater's lesion' (Figure 6.5). Classification of conditions with vascular occlusion was never easy and this paper does not pretend to give a final answer. However it points to a new type of pathology easily recognized based on the careful description and illustration in this article. The observation that cortisone therapy was not a likely cause is also important, and has been amply supported by numerous later observations.

Strengths

1. The stringent clinical description, relevant pathology, and the realization that nailfold necrosis and pulp lesions were related.
2. A large number of very fine illustrations.
3. The balanced discussion of published and unpublished observations.
4. The realization that the real knowledge of the nature of the lesions was not at hand.
5. The realization of the existence of rare cases of 'malignant' RA.

Weaknesses

1. Perhaps giant cell artheritis (GCA) should have been discussed as a differential diagnosis. Some of the arterial lesions bear similarities to GCA.
2. The statement that the lesions were not specific for RA.

Relevance

The observations have since been included in medical student teaching, and it appears that Bywater's lesions are indeed specific for RA. The observation that rheumatoid nodules were present in all cases indicated the possibility that vascular changes could have pathogenetic importance for the formation of rheumatoid nodules.

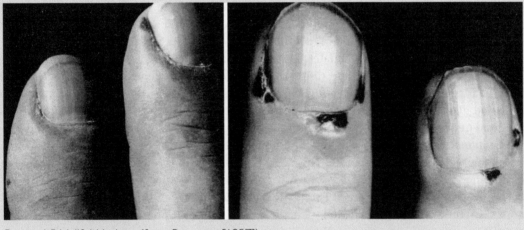

Figures 6.5 Nailfold lesions (from Bywaters [1957]).

CHAPTER 7

Chronic arthritis in children

Jacqui Clinch and †Barbara Ansell

Introduction

Juvenile idiopathic arthritis is the most common rheumatic condition of childhood, with an annual incidence of 1.4 cases per 10 000 under the age of 16 years and a prevalence of 1.0 per 1000. It was in 1897 that George Frederic Still described a series of 22 cases of polyarthritis in childhood. Twelve cases had fever and florid lymphadenopathy; with these cases he brought together almost all the distinctive features of systemic-onset childhood arthritis except for the rash which was subsequently investigated by Isdale and Bywaters. At the end of the Second World War, the Canadian government presented the hospital at Taplow, England, to the people of Britain to serve as a memorial to the work of the Canadian Red Cross Society in this country during the War. It was established as a special unit for juvenile rheumatism under the directorship of Professor Eric Bywaters. Initially most children were admitted with rheumatic fever, in later years chronic arthritis became more prevalent.

Still considered that there were different entities of childhood arthritis and this view has been confirmed and many different classification systems have ensued. The terms 'juvenile rheumatoid arthritis' (JRA) and 'juvenile chronic arthritis' (JCA), both major sources of disagreement in the past, were discarded. In 1997 Petty and Southwood proposed the International League of Associations for Rheumatologists (ILAR) classification for juvenile idiopathic arthritis (JIA) (Paper 2). This was adopted as an umbrella term to indicate disease of childhood-onset, characterized primarily by arthritis persisting for at least 6 weeks, and currently having no known cause. The ILAR classification divides the disease into seven categories; systemic-onset, oligoarthritis (persistent or extending), polyarthritis (rheumatoid factor (RF) negative), polyarthritis (RF positive), psoriatic arthritis, enthesitis-related arthritis and 'other arthritis'.

The aetiology of JIA remains elusive. Many factors have been implemented but none proven. Possible causes include infection, autoimmunity, trauma and stress, with genetic predisposition having an important role. There is mounting evidence that viral and bacterial infections are associated with both acute and chronic childhood arthritis. In 1985 Chantler and co-workers described the finding of persistent rubella infection in children with JIA. More recently streptococcal infections have become the target of much research. The association between JIA and iridocyclitis was noted in the 19th century where children with seemingly low-grade arthritis developing ocular inflammation that led to irreversible visual impairment. Smiley and co-workers described a large cohort of children with Still's disease in Taplow (Paper 3) who underwent opthalmological investigations regularly over a set time period.

Treatment up until recent years concentrated on first-line anti-inflammatory medications such as non-steroidal anti-inflammatory drugs (NSAIDS) and corticosteroids. Approximately one-third of all patients with JIA achieve adequate control of their disease with NSAIDS. However, these medications do need to be monitored particularly with regard to gastric irritation and, in the higher doses, renal impairment. Corticosteroids allow rapid reduction in inflammation while second-line agents have time to reach therapeutic levels. The side-effects of steroids in children (including the marked reduction in growth velocity) render their long-term use undesirable. More recently the treatment of difficult JIA has been revolution-ized by the anti-metabolite methotrexate. In 1992 a large multicentred trial concluded that methotrexate given weekly in low doses was extremely effective for children with resistant JIA (Paper 1). Later in that year Wallace and Sherry reported their encouraging experience with higher doses of methotrexate, particularly in the oligo- and polyarticular subtypes. Over the past 2 years much research has been published in the adult literature regarding Cox-2 inhibitors, tumour necrosis factor (TNF)-alpha receptor inhibitors and other biological ther-apies. Long-term outlook with these therapies in children is currently unknown.

In three of the papers reviewed the new ILAR classification was not in existence. Hence the terms JRA, JCA and Still's disease are used. These terminologies are now combined under the umbrella term JIA.

Paper 1

Methotrexate in resistant juvenile rheumatoid arthritis: Results of the USA–USSR double-blind, placebo-controlled trial

Authors

Giannini EH, Brewer EJ, Kuzmina N, Shaikov A, Maximov A, Vorontsov I, Fink C, Newman A, Cassidy J, Zemel L

Reference

New England Journal of Medicine 1992; **326**:1043–1049

Summary

One hundred and fourteen children were entered into a multicentre, randomized, double-blind clinical trial designed to evaluate the effectiveness and safety of orally administered methotrexate in JRA. The children, with a mean duration of disease of 5.1 years, were randomized to receive 10 mg/m^2 methotrexate, 5mg/m^2 methotrexate, or placebo weekly for 6 months. Two NSAIDs and prednisolone less than 10 mg daily were allowed. The authors showed that the higher dose of methotrexate was extremely effective in the treatment of resistant JRA. Only three children had the drug discontinued because of mild side-effects.

Key message

First large randomized trial showing that low-dose methotrexate has anti-inflammatory activity and clinical effectiveness in resistant JRA.

Why it's important

Prior to methotrexate the choice of second-line agents in children with resistant JRA was limited both by clinical effectiveness of the medications and some severe toxic side-effects. Cyclophosphamide, cyclosporin, penicillamine and sulphasalazine are all used in resistant cases but many are discontinued due to side-effects or no perceived benefit. High-dose steroids, previously used as long-term treatments, have proved disastrous to many children and young adults who have markedly delayed growth velocity, severe osteoporosis and changes in body appearance that affect morale and social integration.

Methotrexate has distinct advantages over other second-line agents, including its oral or subcutaneous route, once weekly dosage and lack of known long-term side-effects (such as oncogenicity and fertility). This trial also illustrated a trend towards a dose-response relation with the higher dose proving more effective. Methotrexate is now the standard second-line treatment of pauci- and polyarticular JRA that is not controlled by NSAIDs alone. Subsequent papers have gone on to show increased effectiveness in higher doses than used here and also benefit from the subcutaneous route of administration.

Strengths

1. Large randomized controlled trial.
2. Wide range of outcome measures.
3. Clearly shows the benefit of methotrexate in children with resistant disease.

Weakness

No long-term data on clinical effectiveness and toxicity.

Relevance

The treatment of resistant JIA has always involved weighing the risks of second-line treatments against benefits they may provide. Methotrexate has provided physicians with an effective, apparently safer option in these difficult cases.

Paper 2

Revision of the proposed classification criteria for juvenile idiopathic arthritis: Durban 1997

Authors

Petty RE, Southwood T, Baum J, Bhettay E, Glass D, Manners P, Maldonado-Cocco J, Suarez-Almazor M, Orozco-Alcala J, Prier A-M

Reference

The Journal of Rheumatology 1998; **25**:10 1991–1994

Summary

For many years a united international classification for chronic childhood arthritis has been absent. The lack of consensus has led to difficulties in trial structure and data interpretation. The authors put forward the new ILAR classification in which the term JIA replaces JRA and JCA. The classification is based on clinical characteristics during the first 6 months of disease and divided into seven distinct categories. The ILAR classification aspires to define categories of arthritis that are clinically homogenous such that to a degree this may predict response to therapy and outcome. A detailed account of the new classification and possible pitfalls is given.

Key message

The ILAR classification arguably provides an international classification system for chronic childhood arthritis that allows professional unity and a structured approach to ongoing and future trials.

Why it's important

The classifications of childhood arthritis represent attempts of many generations of physicians to introduce order in what is often viewed as heterogeneity of chronic inflammatory joint disease. Previously there have been two different classifications (North American (ACR) and European (EULAR)) which have made comparability of clinical trials difficult and interpretation of serological, epidemiological and genetic data almost impossible.

Using an international assembly of paediatric rheumatologists unambiguous terminology was developed to describe seven separate categories of childhood arthritis. These categories are based on clinical description in the hope that clinical clarity may contribute to understanding of the disease processes. The ILAR classification highlighted psoriatic arthritis as a separate entity, whereas previously this heterogeneous form of childhood arthritis was included in the spondyloarthropathy category and felt to be a 'contaminant'.

Oligoarticular diseases also received attention. Many paediatric rheumatologists have reported initial oligoarticular arthritis extending into a more difficult polyarticular form that is RF negative. By reclassifying this as an extending oligarticular JIA alternate, more aggressive therapies can be introduced earlier and multidisciplinary input 'stepped up'.

Strengths

1. Provides a clear, primarily clinical classification of chronic childhood arthritis.
2. Devised by international working party thus enables comparability of outcome data and further research progress.

Weakness

There remains an 'other' category that serves as a potentially confusing area for collections of symptoms that do not fit elsewhere. A caveat to this however is that, with careful evaluation, these children could enable other categories to be developed or existing ones broadened.

Relevance

Paediatric rheumatology is an expanding speciality with increasing numbers of paediatricians and rheumatologists becoming involved in the care of children with complex forms of arthritis. It is important that all physicians involved use the same classification internationally so that we can work together to further our understanding of chronic childhood arthritis.

Paper 3

Iridocyclitis in Still's disease: its complictions and treatment

Authors

Smiley WK, May E, Bywaters EGL

Reference

Annals of Rheumatic Diseases 1957; **16**:371

Summary

This paper is one of the original, comprehensive descriptions of iridocyclitis associated with JIA (referred to here as Still's disease). The authors looked at their own population in Taplow and also comprehensively reviewed the literature. One hundred and eighty-three children with Still's disease were examined regularly over a range of 1–9 years after the first appointment for ocular abnormalities. Ten cases were found. The clinical characteristics and complications of iridocyclitis are described. The insidious nature of iridocyclitis is stressed, particularly as this often leads to progressive impairment of vision unless treated. Band keratopathy, secondary glaucoma, cataracts and eventual blindness were all described in their cohort. Treatment with mydriatics, steroids (topically and systemically) and surgery are described.

Key message

There is a strong association between Still's disease and iridocyclitis. The onset of this ocular inflammation may be silent and, unless recognized and treated early, leads to permanent visual disability.

Why it's important

This paper is the first large study of children with chronic arthritis that particularly investigates ocular inflammation. Previous to this study there had been many reports of associated eye disease but no prospective data on larger numbers. Smiley and co-workers concentrate on the complications of iridocyclitis in Still's disease and the importance of diagnosing and treating as early as possible. Many of the complications they describe have not previously been associated with Still's disease, in particular band keratopathy, a condition not associated with iridocyclitis in adults.

Iridocyclitis has been the subject of much research in paediatric rheumatology since these reports from Taplow and other institutions. We now know that chronic anterior uveitis (iridocyclitis) is strongly associated with oligoarticular disease, anti-nuclear antibodies and the female sex (approximately 20% incidence in this group). It is less common in polyarticular disease and very rarely seen in the systemic disease. The importance of early investigations has been further supported in subsequent studies. In almost half of patients, iridocyclitis is present at the time the arthritis is diagnosed. The risk of developing ocular inflammation continues for at least 5 years even if the joint disease is quiescent.

Strengths

1. Original paper looking prospectively at a large cohort of children with arthritis and their risk of developing iridocyclitis.
2. Detailed descriptions of iridocyclitis and its many complications seen in children with chronic arthritis.
3. Comprehensive review of other literature published in this period.

Weaknesses

1. The importance of long-term ocular follow-up in chronic arthritis was not stressed at this time. The incidence of 5.5% quoted is low compared to current figures and probably represents shorter follow-up and the heterogeneity of the group they observed.
2. The accounts of their cases are occasionally repetitive.

Relevance

Chronic anterior uveitis continues to cause significant morbidity in children who often suffer very mild episodes of joint inflammation. These children may present late to specialist centres with advanced eye disease that proves resistant to the treatment that earlier would have restored normal vision.

Paper 4

Prognosis in juvenile chronic polyarthritis

Authors

Ansell BA, Wood PH

Reference

Clinics in Rheumatic Diseases 1976; **2**:397–412

Summary

This paper documents the clinical characteristics and outcome of 243 children who fulfilled the criteria for Still's disease (then relating to a juvenile chronic polyarthritis) when first seen. The children were reviewed regularly during a 15 year period. The authors divide the children into five main clinical disease categories; JRA (RF +ve), monoarticular disease, systemic disease, juvenile ankylosing spondylitis, and chronic iridocyclitis Still's disease (in this last group the authors recognize the association of iridocyclitis in young females with monoarticular disease).

There is a thorough review of outcomes looking at disability, mortality and behaviour. Much of the data presented highlights the improved outcome of many forms of childhood arthritis when compared to adult disease. Overall mortality was 7%; disability measures showed that 40% recovered with no limitation and 30% with slight limitation, those that presented later in their disease had a less favourable outcome. Quality of life in these children at the end of their paediatric follow-up is discussed.

Key message

Childhood arthritis, when diagnosed and treated early, has an encouraging prognosis in many children.

Why it's important

This series (collected between 1947 and 1958) enabled the comprehensive study of the characteristics and outcome of childhood chronic arthritis. Previous reports from orthopaedic centres painted a depressing picture; in contrast the experience at Taplow showed the outcomes of these diseases to be improved (particularly when compared to adult disease). Prognosis can only be assessed when different outcome measures are known for each 'set' of characteristics. The authors here were able to describe prospectively the identity of variants in childhood polyarthritis as the disease progressed and group them accordingly. From this data they were able to look at outcome measures for each group and thus develop prognostic indicators. The delay in time-to-diagnosis and treatment in its relation to ultimate outcome is highlighted; particularly recognizing the 'reversibility' of many forms of juvenile arthritis when dealt with in the early stages.

From this series Ansell and Wood are able to describe five main syndromes. Of particular interest are the specific characteristics they found with JRA, iridocyclitis and systemic disease. They show the association between clinical differences in different groups and correlation with the differences in ultimate outcome. Their mortality and long-term disability figures provided early evidence that juvenile chronic arthritis had a better overall outcome (without subdividing into disease categories) than adult disease.

Strengths

1. Original paper prospectively studying a large series of children over a long period (15 years).
2. Detailed clinical descriptions of clinical variants within this initially homogenous group.
3. Relates outcome measures to presentation, clinical developments of the disease and environment.
4. Comprehensive literature review.

Weaknesses

1. Series of children and their long-term outlook in period of time when therapeutic possibilities more limited.
2. Unable to assign a significant minority of children to a diagnostic group at this time (not able to study human leucocyte antigen (HLA) or anti-nuclear antibody (ANA) status), thus degree of difficulty in assessing their outcomes.

Relevance

Many forms of childhood arthritis are now recognized to have a favourable outlook, particularly when diagnosed and treated early. In a majority of cases we are able to demonstrate clinical signs and symptoms that fit a category in which we are able to advise the child and parents on ultimate outcome of the disease. This early work of Ansell and Wood is of utmost importance in developing the diagnostic and outcome measures we have today.

CHAPTER 8

Ankylosing spondylitis

Muhammad Asim Khan

Introduction

Ankylosing spondylitis (AS) has a long and interesting history. There is evidence favouring antiquity, although there can be some difficulty differentiating AS from DISH (diffuse idiopathic skeletal hyperostosis) when examining paleopathological specimens (1). The skeletal radiograph of the famous Egyptian Pharoah Rameses II (1290–1221 BC) shows evidence of the disease (2). However, recognition of AS as a clinical entity came in the 19th century; Brodie (1841) is sometimes credited with the definitive description, although the disease has eponyms that come from the later work of Strümpell (1897), Marie (1898), and von Bechterew (1893) (3).

Developments in the 20th century started with the application of clinical radiography, allowing the detection of the characteristic sacroiliitis and spondylitis. In the imaging chapter an early example (Fraenkel, 1907) is reviewed (chapter 2), a later more comprehensive description of the imaging changes came from Buckley in 1931 (4). However, in spite of these early descriptions, it was not until the second half of the century that AS became clearly differentiated from rheumatoid arthritis (RA), and as recently as 1960 Graham was having to argue that the term 'rheumatoid spondylitis' was unhelpful (5).

Our selection of papers spans the second half of the 20th century, which has seen major developments in our understanding of AS, and are confined to key clinical developments. Paper 1 is the definitive description of the major characteristic pathological feature of the condition, i.e.enthesitis, and the next two papers (Papers 2a and b) are the definitive clinical descriptions, both of AS and of the family of disorders known as the 'spondyloarthritides', more often called 'spondyloarthropathies'. The ground breaking work relating AS to the HLA-B27 gene was published in 1973, and is described in the clinical genetics chapter of this book (chapter 5). This was a great stimulus to research on AS, which had been relatively neglected up to that point. It has led to major recent developments in our understanding through highly sophisticated work on the structure and function of HLA-B27, and with transgenic mice (6). The third selection (Paper 3) describes the more clinically orientated work that led to an association being made between the 'HLA-B27 positive spondyloarthropathies' and gastrointestinal inflammation, even if there were no signs or symptoms of inflammatory bowel disease (although it transpires that the gut inflammation is not directly associated with HLA-B27). This type of work has fuelled the continuing debate that gut infections and inflammation are critical in the pathogenesis of AS and related disorders. In this context it is of interest that sulphasalazine can be of therapeutic value in AS, but only for peripheral arthritis, and not the axial disease.

The final selections are concerned with the very important issues of classification and assessment. There have been a variety of systems used as potential diagnostic or classification criteria, but the two best appear to be those of the European Spondyloarthropathy Study Group (ESSG) and of Bernard Amor, as described in Papers 4a and 4b. The assessment of disease activity and progression has been a major obstacle to clinical research in AS. However, recent work, described in Papers 5a and 5b have led to the development of useful assessment instruments, now called the WHO/ILAR core sets and remission criteria that have been found to be very helpful in fully assessing the dramatic efficacy of the TNF-alpha blocking therapy in AS (7).

References

1. Rogers J, Watt I, Dieppe P. Paleopathology of spinal osteophytosis, vertebral ankylosis, ankylosing spondylitis and vertebral hyperostosis. *Annals of Rheumatic Diseases* 1985; **44**:113–120.

2. Dastugue J. Les maladies de nos ancestres. *La Recherche* 1982;**13**:980–988.

3. O'Connell D. Ankylosing spondylitis. The literature up to the close of the 19th century. *Annals of Rheumatic Diseases* 1956; **15**:119–123.

4. Buckley CW. Spondylitis deformans. *British Medical Journal* 1931; **1**:1108-12.

5. Graham W. Is rheumatoid arthritis a separate entity? *Arthritis and Rheumatism* 1960; **3**: 88–90.

6. Taurog JD, Maika SD, Satumtira N, *et al.* Inflammatory disease in HLA-B27 transgenic rats. *Immunological Reviews* 1999; **169**:209–213.

7. Brant J, Haibel H, Cornely D, *et al.* Successful treatment of active ankylosing spondylitis with the anti-tumor necrosis factor alpha monoclonal antibody infliximab. *Arthritis and Rheumatism* 2000; **43**:1346–1352.

Paper 1

Enthesopathy of rheumatoid and ankylosing spondylitis

Author

Ball J

Reference

Annals of Rheumatic Diseases 1971; **30**:213–223

Summary

This paper, which is the Heberden Oration in 1970, for the first time clearly demonstrated the differential pathology of AS and RA. It is a histological description of autopsies and biopsy data, and represents changes observed in relatively advanced AS. The involved sites in AS show multiple focal inflammatory lesions, primarily localized to the ligamentous attachments with active erosive lesions, and also lesions in various stages of healing, that may culminate in new bone formation and progressive ankylosis of the axial skeleton.

Ball emphasized a striking and characteristic inflammatory enthesopathy (enthesitis) in AS, and pointed out that the natural history or course of this enthesitis could explain some of the clinical and pathological features of this disease. He demonstrated that the enthesitis observed in the extraspinal sites was also present in the axial skeleton of AS patients, involving the sacroiliac and apophyseal joints, and the intervertebral discs. The enthesis is the point of bony attachment of the tendon, ligament, joint capsule, or fascia to bone. It is a metabolically active site, especially during the growth phase, and it is of interest that AS oftens begins in adolescence and young adults. Enthesopathy is seen in many arthropathies, but inflammatory enthesopathy is the cardinal feature and possible unifying inflammatory lesion of AS and related spondyloarthropathies (SpA). This enthesitis often leads to new bone formation but the underlying mechanism is not yet understood.

Related references (1) Braun J, Bollow M, Neure L, Seipelt E, Seyrekbasan F, Herbst H, Eggens U, Distler A, Sieper J. Use of immunohistologic and *in situ* hybridization techniques in the examination of sacroiliac joint biopsy specimens from patients with ankylosing spondylitis. *Arthritis and Rheumatism* 1995; **38**:499–505.

(2) McGonagle D, Khan MA, Marzo-Ortega H, O'Connor P, Gibbon W, Emery P. Enthesitis in spondyloarthropathy. *Current Opinion in Rheumatology* 1999; **11**:244–250.

Key message

There is a striking and characteristic inflammatory enthesopathy (enthesitis) in AS, and the natural history or evolution of this enthesitis can explain many of the clinical and pathological features of this disease. The enthesitis observed in the extraspinal sites also involves the axial skeleton, including the sacroiliac and apophyseal joints, and the intervertebral discs.

Why it's important

Enthesitis is now considered a characteristic feature of AS and related SpA, but because of the relative inaccessibility of the enthesis, the inflammatory, microbiological, and immunological events at that site have not as yet been well defined. Recent magnetic resonance imaging studies have drawn attention to the ubiquitous nature of enthesitis in AS and associated SpAs, especially adjacent to synovial joints, and have delineated the early changes, including the oedematous bone marrow spaces in the immediate vicinity of the enthesitis that Ball described in his seminal paper.

This paper also popularized the use of the term enthesopathy/enthesitis in the English language. The word enthesopathy came into use to signify traumatic changes to tendon insertions, e.g. tennis elbow, because the word enthesis means 'insertion or implantation'. Czech physician Niepel and his colleagues first used the term in the 1960s to describe the inflammatory symptoms at insertional sites that are an important feature of AS and related SpA. Although the term enthesopathy or inflammatory enthesopathy was initially used, the term enthesitis was subsequently preferred. Enthesopathy is seen in many arthropathies, but inflammatory enthesopathy (enthesitis) is the cardinal feature and possible unifying inflammatory lesion of AS and related SpA. Clinically, the concept of enthesitis had gained sufficient recognition to be included as one of the classification criteria for SpA and for subsets of juvenile chronic arthritis.

Needle biopsies of the sacroiliac (SI) joints in five AS patients with active disease have now been performed by Braun, *et al.* for immunohistological studies. Dense cellular infiltrates of T cells and macrophages were found in the synovial portion of the SI joints of all patients. In these infiltrates a high amount of tumor necrosis factor alpha (TNF-alpha) messenger RNA (mRNA) was detected by *in situ* hybridization, and near the site of new bone formation, a lower amount of transforming growth factor beta (TGF-ß) mRNA were detected, while no message for interleukin-1 was found in the three patients examined by this technique. Further investigation of such biopsy specimens showed the absence of DNA of reactive arthritis-associated bacteria. The authors suggested that their finding of abundant TNF-alpha message in the SI joints could have implications regarding potential immunotherapeutic approaches to this disease. In fact they have now reported in an open label pilot study a dramatic improvement in more than 90% of active AS patients treated with anti-TNF-alpha antibody infliximab (Remicade) (reference 7, Introduction).

Strength

Demonstrates clearly for the first time that the natural history or course of enthesitis could explain many of the clinical and pathological features of AS. The other two papers have taken the next steps to understand the mechanism of enthesitis and its more effective therapy.

Weaknesses

1. A histological description of autopsies and biopsy specimens.
2. Represents changes observed in relatively advanced disease.

Relevance

The involved sites in AS show multiple focal inflammatory lesions, primarily localized to the ligamentous attachments, with active erosive lesions, and also lesions in various stages of healing, that may culminate in new bone formation and progressive ankylosis of the axial skeleton. Understanding the mechanism of enthesitis will lead to its more effective therapy. The mechanisms responsible for the increased bone formation in AS is not yet fully understood.

Paper 2a

Ankylosing spondylitis

Authors

Hart FD, Robinson KC, Allchin FM, Maclagan NF

Reference

Quarterly Journal of Medicine 1949; **18**: 217–238

Paper 2b

Associations between ankylosing spondylitis, psoriatic arthritis, Reiter's disease, the intestinal arthropathies, and Behçet's syndrome

Authors

Moll JM, Haslock I, Macrae IF, Wright V

Reference

Medicine 1974; **53**:343–364

Summary

Hart, *et al.* provided the first complete and most accurate clinical description of AS, and defended the name AS rather than rheumatoid spondylitis. Describing the early lumbo-sacral backache they noted many patients complained of pain in the buttock or buttocks, while in some the first complaint was mid-lumbar ache, or mid-thoracic or cervical pain. They pointed out that 'at the onset such aches and pains were usually trivial and often ignored by the patient's medical officer, or resulted in the patient being treated as a case of "fibrositis", "rheumatism", or occasionally "psychoneurosis".' Many of their patients had wrongly been given psychiatric treatment, and many had been suspected of malingering. The most effective treatment those days was deep x-ray therapy.

The term 'spondylarthritides' was proposed by Moll, *et al.* for the group of related inflammatory joint diseases, the centre piece of which is AS, and they clarified the shared characteristic clinical features that they emphasized so well in their paper. Clinical and radiological involvement of the SI joint is an outstanding feature of the SpA, especially AS. Patients with Reiter's syndrome/reactive arthritis, psoriasis, ulcerative colitis and Crohn's disease can often develop AS. The reverse has also been known, that is, AS patients are more often found to have Crohn's disease, ulcerative colitis or psoriasis. Reiter's syndrome/reactive arthritis can sometimes be difficult to differentiate from psoriatic arthritis.

Related references **(1)** Hersch AH, Stecher RM, Solomon WM, Wolpow R, Hauser H. Heredity in ankylosing spondylitis. A clinical description of fifty families. *American Journal of Human Genetics* 1950; **2**:391–408.

(2) McEwen C, DiTata D, Lingg C, Porini A, Good A, Rankin T. Ankylosing spondylitis and spondylitis accompanying ulcerative colitis, regional enteritis, psoriasis and Reiter's disease. A comparative study. *Arthritis and Rheumatism* 1971; **14**:291–318.

Key message

These two papers provide the basic foundation for the more accurate and detailed clinical description of AS and the diseases that are grouped with it under the term 'spondyloarthritides'.

Why it's important

The clinical features of AS that should provide the earliest diagnostic clues were emphasized by Hart, *et al.*: AS should not be diagnosed if SI joints were radiologically normal, unless other evidence was strong, and they described one of the two such patients they had diagnosed when their SI joints were as yet normal. They also pointed out that the disease was very often not diagnosed until it was relatively far advanced, and that it 'can be diagnosed with greater ease than most conditions in medicine'.

The concept of SpAs was put forward by Moll, *et al.*, in which AS formed the centre piece of this group of diseases that share clinical features and genetic predisposing factors; the remarkable association with the major histocompatibility complex class I molecule HLA-B27 that was discovered while their paper was in press, confirmed the validity of their proposal. Five subgroups can be now differentiated: AS, reactive arthritis (ReA) that encompasses Reiter's syndrome, psoriatic arthritis, arthritis associated with inflammatory bowel disease, and undifferentiated SpA (including enthesitis related arthritis).

Moll *et al.* also emphasized that extra-articular organ systems may also be involved in these diseases, especially the gastrointestinal tract. Mielants, *et al.* (see Related reference (1), Paper 3) were subsequently able to demonstrate on ileocolonoscopic studies 11 years later the presence of inflammatory gut lesions in all the diseases in the SpA group, even in the absence of gastrointestinal symptoms. Bowel inflammation is present in a large number of patients with SpA who had no intestinal symptoms or overt inflammatory bowel disease (IBD). Enteropathic arthritis develops in up to 20% of patients with chronic IBD, and most of these patients have peripheral synovitis that correlates with flare up of bowel disease, but one-fourth have axial disease which does not fluctuate with bowel disease activity.

Strengths

1. Hart, *et al.* provided one of the first accurate and comprehensive clinical description of the early stages of AS, and emphasized the clinical features that should provide the earliest diagnostic clues.
2. Moll, *et al.* proposed the term 'spondylarthritides' for the group of related inflammatory joint diseases, the centre piece of which is AS, and they clarified the shared characteristic clinical features of this group of diseases.

Weaknesses

1. The paper by Hart, *et al.* did not contain any pathological findings but it was because none of their patients had come to autopsy.
2. The paper by Moll, *et al.* included Behçet's syndrome in the spondyloarthritides group but it is not generally considered to belong to this group of diseases.

Relevance

Hart, *et al.* emphasized more than 50 years ago the clinical features of AS that should lead to early diagnosis. It took more than 40 years for these clinical features to be incorporated in the classification criteria. Moll, *et al.* emphasized the shared characteristic clinical features of this group of diseases, and this concept was further reinforced by the discovery of the genetic marker, HLA-B27, that shows a remarkable association with this group of diseases.

Paper 3

HLA-B27 related arthritis and bowel inflammation. Part 2 Ileocolonoscopy and bowel histology in patients with HLA-B27 related arthritis

Authors

Mielants H, Veys EM, Cuvelier C, De Vos M, Botelberghe L

Reference

Journal of Rheumatology 1985; **12**:294–298

Summary

The concept of SpAs put forward by Moll, *et al.* gathers together a group of chronic rheumatological diseases, where extra-articular organ systems may also be involved, especially the gastrointestinal tract. Mielants, *et al.* (1, 2) were the first to demonstrate on ileocolonoscopic studies the presence of inflammatory gut lesions in all the diseases in the SpA group, in the absence of gastrointestinal symptoms. The prevalence of these inflammatory gut lesions varied between 20% and 70% in the different diseases. Their recent data are based on performance of biopsies of the terminal ileum and proximal colon in 108 patients with SpA (55 had ReA and 53 had AS), and 56 controls (47 patients with other rheumatic diseases, and 19 patients with chronic constipation, colonic polyps or adenocarcinoma). There was histological evidence of IBD with features either of acute enterocolitis, or early Crohn's disease in 30 of 53 (56.6%) AS patients, 37 of 55 (67%) patients with ReA, and in only one of 56 controls (2%). These lesions were histologically 'acute' in approximately 25% and 'chronic' in 30%. Only 18 of the 67 (27%) patients with histological gut inflammation, however, had intestinal symptoms.

Related references **(1)** Mielants H, Veys EM, Cuvelier C, De Vos M. Ileocolonoscopic findings in seronegative spondylarthropathies. *British Journal of Rheumatology* 1988; **27**:95–105.

(2) Mielants H, Veys EM, Cuvelier C, De Vos M, Goemaere S, De Clercq L, Schatteman L, Elewaut D. The evolution of spondylarthropathies in relation to gut histology. *Journal of Rheumatology* 1995; **22**:2266–2284. (This work is in 3 parts: Part I covers clinical aspects (pp. 2262–2272). Part II covers histological aspects (pp. 2273–2278). Part III covers the relationship between gut and joint (pp. 2279–2284).)

Key message

Subclinical inflammatory lesions in the gut have been observed on ileocolonoscopic mucosal biopsy in SpA patients without gastrointestinal symptoms, or clinically obvious IBD or psoriasis. Persistent subclinical gut inflammation was observed in active joint disease.

Why it's important

They have hypothesized that subclinical inflammatory bowel disease is present in some patients with SpA, in which the joint inflammation can be the only clinical manifestation. Their studies support the aetiopathogenetic role of the gut in SpA. The link between gut inflammation and arthropathy has also been demonstrated in the HLA-B27 transgenic rats, that make a nice animal model for SpA. The development of gut inflammation precedes the development of SpA, and if these animals are born and raised in a germ-free environment they do not develop gut inflammation or SpA, although they may develop psoriasiform skin and nail lesions. Thus presence of gut flora are needed for the SpA, except the psoriasiform skin and nail lesions.

Presence of chronic (Crohn-like) gut inflammation and mild complaints of diarrhoea implies a high risk of evolution to AS and IBD. The presence of these gut lesions is not associated with HLA-B27, and the data support the existence of a B27-independent common pathogenic link between gut inflammation and SpA. SpA patients with acute or chronic inflammatory gut lesions seem to respond better to sulphasalazine treatment than those with normal gut histology, suggesting that sulphasalazine may have a beneficial effect on the patients with SpA by healing their gut inflammation. Sulphasalazine has a beneficial effect on articular activity by controlling gut inflammation, but it does not prevent evolution to IBD.

Mielants, *et al.* have also studied long-term evolution of gut inflammation in patients with SpA (1, 2). Evolution to IBD was observed in 7% of these patients. Follow-up studies of SpA patients with the subset with chronic inflammatory gut lesions suggest that anywhere between 15–25 % of them will develop clinically obvious Crohn's disease, suggesting that these patients had initially a subclinical form of IBD. The presence of these Crohn-like gut lesions is not associated with HLA-B27. Persistent gut inflammation was observed in active joint disease. Presence of chronic gut inflammation and mild complaints of diarrhoea implies a high risk of evolution to AS and IBD.

Strengths

1. Their studies suggest the aetiopathogenetic role of the gut in SpA.
2. The link between gut inflammation and arthropathy has been further supported by the HLA-B27 transgenic rat model for SpA (reference 6, Introduction).

Weakness

Unable to pinpoint the precise bacterial trigger for AS, if there is one.

Relevance

These authors have identified a group of SpA patients with inflammatory chronic, or relapsing acute arthritis who have histological evidence of ileocolitis, even in the absence of any gastrointestinal symptoms. The presence of these gut lesions is not associated with HLA-B27. Evolution to IBD can occur in some of these patients on follow-up. Sulphasalazine has a beneficial effect on articular activity (peripheral arthritis) by controlling gut inflammation, but it does not prevent evolution to IBD and does not benefit axial disease.

Paper 4a

A wider spectrum of spondyloarthropathies

Authors

Khan MA, van der Linden SM

Reference

Seminars in Arthritis and Rheumatism 1990; **20**:107–113

Paper 4b

The European Spondyloarthropathy Study Group preliminary criteria for the classification of spondyloarthropathies

Authors

Dougados M, van der Linden S, Juhlin R, *et al.*

Reference

Arthritis and Rheumatism 1991; **34**:1218–27

Summary

The clinical spectrum of these diseases is now understood to be much wider and no longer implies necessarily the presence of sacroiliitis or spondylitis. For example, the disease may start with features such as enthesitis (inflammation of the sites of attachment of ligaments and tendons to bone), dactylitis, or oligoarthritis that in some cases may progress to sacroiliitis and spondylitis, with or without any extra-articular features such as acute anterior uveitis or muco-cutaneous lesions. The various forms of SpA show a strong association with the histocompatibility antigen HLA-B27; however, the strength of this association varies markedly not only between the various SpA but also among racial and ethnic groups. Khan and van der Linden, primarily based on their earlier studies, pointed out that features typical of SpA may occur in different combinations so that the existing criteria for disease classification and diagnosis were inappropriate or too restricted, and that these criteria do not recognize the existence of a much wider disease spectrum.

The disease spectrum of Reiter's syndrome has also been broadened considerably, and the clinical spectrum of psoriatic SpA has been better clarified. 'Incomplete' forms of Reiter's syndrome were found to be much more common than the classical triad of arthritis, conjunctivitis, and urethritis. The term 'B27-associated ReA' has been used in recent years to refer to SpA following enteric or urogenital infections, and the disease spectrum includes the clinical picture of typical Reiter's syndrome. Some of the less well defined B27-associated clinical syndromes that have been clarified included seronegative oligoarthritis, polyarthritis, or dactylitis ('sausagelike' toes) of the lower extremities, and heel pain caused by enthesitis (calcaneal and tarsal periostitis, Achilles tendonitis, and plantar fasciitis). These and other undifferentiated forms of SpA had been ignored in previous epidemiological studies because of the inadequacy of the existing classification criteria.

Epidemiological studies, therefore, had been hampered by incomplete definition of the clinical disease spectrum, and there was a need to use broad criteria that will include the patients that had been ignored because their diseases do not fit the current criteria.

The European Spondyloarthropathy Study Group (ESSG) provided the first widely used classification criteria for the whole group of SpA patients, and pointed out their usefulness in encompassing the wider disease spectrum, including those with undifferentiated SpA. These ESSG preliminary criteria for the classification of SpAs are listed in Table 8.1.

Table 8.1 ESSG criteria for spondyloarthropathy

Inflammatory spinal pain	or	Synovitis
		Asymmetrical or
		Predominantly in the lower limbs

And one or more of the following:
Alternate buttock pain
Sacroiliitis
Calcaneal enthesitis
Positive family history
Psoriasis
Inflammatory bowel disease
Urethritis or cervicitis or acute diarrhoea occuring within 1 month before arthritis

Related references **(1)** Amor B, Dougados M, Listrat V, *et al.* Are classification criteria for spondylarthropathies useful as diagnostic criteria? *Rev de Rheumatisme* (English edition) 1995; **6**:10–15.

(2) Khan MA, van der Linden SM, Kushner I, Valkenberg HA, Cats A. Spondylitic disease without radiological evidence of sacroiliitis in relatives of HLA-B27 patients. *Arthritis and Rheumatism* 1985; **28**:40–43.

Key message

The difficulty in clearly categorizing some patients with SpA occurs most often in early stages of these diseases, because their characteristic signs and symptoms may only become manifest after a long follow-up, and may sometimes be aided by family history and examination of the patient's family members. Khan and van der Linden not only pointed out this wider spectrum of SpA, but also emphasized that features typical of SpA may occur in different combinations, and that the existing criteria were too restricted and therefore unable to recognize the wider disease spectrum. The utility of the ESSG criteria have been validated in many countries and ethnic/racial groups.

Why it is important

Spondyloarthropathy (SpA) is a heterogeneous clinical entity that includes AS, the prototype of this group of interrelated disorders, ReA (including Reiter's syndrome), psoriatic arthritis, and arthritis associated with chronic IBDs. It may not always be possible to differentiate clearly between the various forms of SpA, especially in early stages of the disease, because they generally share many clinical features, both skeletal and extra-skeletal. As in other diseases of undetermined aetiology, the diagnosis of these diseases is based on clinical and roentgeno-graphic features.

The studies of Moll, *et al.* and the discovery in 1973 of the association of HLA-B27 with AS and related SpA had clearly demonstrated that these diseases share clinical and radiographic features as well as genetic predisposing factors. HLA-B27 was helpful as a genetic marker for these diseases and the work of many investigators led to the observations that raised questions about our perceptions of the clinical spectrum of SpA. Khan and van der Linden, based on their study, pointed out the wider spectrum of SpA, and that features typical of SpA may occur in different combinations, and that the existing criteria for disease classification and diagnosis were too restricted. Their previously published studies had demonstrated that although radiographically detected sacroiliitis is extremely frequent in AS, it may not be an obligate manifestation, especially in early or atypical forms of the disease. Moreover, arthritis involving the axial skeleton, including the SI joints, can be present in some patients without evidence of erosive disease roentgenographically. The recent advances in radiographic imaging, especially dynamic magnetic resonance imaging, can now help overcome some of the diagnostic difficulties of early roentgenographic sacroiliitis, since these new techniques can visualize both acute and chronic changes in the SI joints at a very early stage. These authors emphasized the usefulness of the ESSG criteria in encompassing the wider spectrum of SpA patients, including those with undifferentiated SpA.

The ESSG criteria are now very widely used and they have been validated in many diverse SpA populations in the world. For example, the clinical utility of these criteria, that were developed based on European patients, has been validated in Mexicans, Brazilians, Turks, Eskimos, Inuits, and other native populations of north America. The ESSG criteria, however, are unable to recognize those patients with SpA who have neither chronic inflammatory back pain nor any oligoarthritis. Some of these patients can be recognized by the Amor's criteria to have SpA (Table 8.2). These two criteria tend to complement each other, and therefore could be used together in tandem to encompass the widest spectrum of SpA patients.

Strengths

1. These papers have provided better disease characterization and definition.
2. They have improved the classification of the diseases grouped under the term SpAs.

Weaknesses

The ESSG criteria are unable to recognize those patients with SpA who do not suffer from chronic inflammatory back pain or any oligoarthritis, yet such patients may meet the Amor's criteria. These two criteria tend to complement each other, and should therefore be used together to encompass the widest possible disease spectrum.

Relevance

The HLA-B27-associated undifferentiated forms of SpA had been ignored in previous epidemiological studies because of the inadequacy of the existing classification criteria, but these clinical syndromes have now been clarified, and the classification criteria for SpA now encompass a much wider spectrum of this group of diseases.

Table 8.2 Amor criteria for spondyloarthropathy

Parameters	Scoring
A. Clinical symptoms or past history of:	
1. Lumbar or dorsal pain at night or morning stiffness of lumbar or dorsal pain	1
2. Asymmetrical oligoarthritis	2
3. Buttock pain	1
or if alternate buttock pain	2
4. Sausage-like digit(s) (fingers or toes)	2
5. Heel pain or other well defined enthesitis pain	2
6. Iritis	2
7. Non-gonococcal urethritis, cervicitis within 1 month before the onset of arthritis	1
8. Acute diarrhoea within 1 month before the onset of arthritis	1
9. Psoriasis, balanitis, or inflammatory bowel disease (ulcerative colitis or Crohn's disease)	2
B. Radiological findings	
10. Sacroiliitis (at least bilateral grade 2 or unilateral grade 3)	2
C. Genetic background	
11. Presence of HLA-B27 and/or family history of ankylosing spondylitis, reactive arthritis, uveitis, psoriasis or inflammatory bowel disease	2
D. Response to treatment	
12. Clearcut improvement within 48 hours after non-steroidal anti-inflammatory drugs (NSAID) intake or rapid relapse of the pain after their discontinuation	2

A patient is considered to be suffering from a spondyloarthropathy if the sum is >6.

Paper 5a

A new approach to defining functional ability in ankylosing spondylitis: the development of the Bath ankylosing spondylitis functional index

Authors

Calin A, Garrett S, Whitelock H, *Kennedy LG, O'Hea J, Mallone P, Jenkinson T*

Reference

Journal of Rheumatology 1994; **21**:2281–2285

Paper 5b

Selection of instruments in the core set for DC-ART, SMARD, physical therapy, and clinical record keeping in ankylosing spondylitis. Progress report of the ASAS Working Group

Authors

Van der Heijde D, Calin A, Dougados M, Khan MA, van der Linden S, Bellamy N, and on behalf of the ASAS Working Group

Reference

Journal of Rheumatology 1999; **26**:951–954

Summary

The clinical assessment of disease activity in patients with AS is often not easy. A few functional indices have now been developed for longitudinal follow-up of AS patients, and for monitoring their response to therapy. The most widely used measures of functional capacity in AS is the Bath ankylosing spondylitis functional index (BASFI) (score 0–10). Disease activity has been assessed by using a self-administered composite index called the Bath ankylosing spondylitis disease activity index (BASDAI) that consists of an evaluation on a visual analogue scale (from 0–10) focusing on axial pain, peripheral joint pain, fatigue/tiredness, enthesitis, and morning stiffness). BASDAI has been found to be a valid and appropriate composite to define disease activity in AS.

There is also a need to develop a reliable, reproducible, and simple radiological scoring method to document radiographic changes in AS. The Bath ankylosing spondylitis radiological index (BASRI) is one such index and it has a moderate-to-good reliability. The radiographs for BASRI are scored using the New York criteria for the SI joints, while the lumbar and cervical spine, and the hip joints are graded 0–4. These scores are added together to give

BASRI-t (total) and if the hips are excluded one gets BASRI-s (spine). There are thus three types of BASRI scores (total, spinal, and hip).

The process of selecting the most appropriate indices needed further standardization. Therefore, a working group called Assessments in Ankylosing Spondylitis (ASAS) was set up for the selection of core sets for the following three different settings: (a) for disease controlling anti-rheumatic therapy (DC-ART); (b) for therapy with symptom modifying anti-rheumatic drugs and for physical therapy (SM-ARD/PT); and (c) for clinical record keeping in daily practice. The instruments that were finally chosen are listed in Table 8.3.

Table 8.3 Specific instruments for each domain in core sets for DC-ART, SM-ARD/PT, and clinical record keeping

Domain	Instrument
Physical function	BASFI *or* Dougados functional index
Pain	Visual analogue scale (VAS)-last week-spine-at night-due to AS *and* VAS-last week-spine-due to AS
Spinal mobility	Chest expansion test *and* modified Schober's test *and* occiput-to-wall distance test
Patient global	VAS-last week
Stiffness	Duration of morning stiffness-spine-last week
Peripheral joints	Number of swollen joints (44 joint count)
Entheses	*No preferred instrument is yet available*
Acute phase reactants	Erythrocyte sedimentation rate
X-ray spine	AP+ Lateral lumbar spine *and* lateral cervical spine *and* x-ray pelvis (sacroiliac and hip joints)
X-ray pelvis	(see under x-ray spine above)
Fatigue	*No preferred instrument is yet available*

The *SM-ARD/PT core set* comprises the following five components:
   Physical function
   Pain
   Spinal mobility
   Patient global
   Stiffness
The additional components for *clinical record keeping* include:
   Peripheral joints
   Entheses
   Acute phase reactants
The *core set for DC-ART*, in addition to the above mentioned 8 components, requires:
   X-ray spine
   X-ray pelvis
   Fatigue

Related references **(1)** Calin A, Nakache J-P, Gueguen A, Zeidler H, Mielants H, Dougados M. Defining disease activity in ankylosing spondylitis: is a combination of variables (Bath ankylosing spondylitis disease activity index) an appropriate instrument? *Rheumatology* 1999; **38**:878–882.

(2) Calin A, Mackay K, Brophy S. A new dimension to outcome: The Bath ankylosing spondylitis radiology index (BASRI). *Journal of Rheumatology* 1999; **26**:998–992.

(3) Garrett S, Jenkinson T, Kennedy LG, Whitelock H, Gaisford P, Calin A. A new approach to defining disease status in ankylosing spondylitis: the Bath ankylosing spondylitis disease activity index. *Journal of Rheumatology* 1994; **21**:2286–2291.

Key message

It is more difficult to assess disease activity of AS than of RA, but the recent studies discussed above provide the proper instruments for assessing disease and functional activity and response to therapy, as well as for clinical record keeping in daily practice.

Why it's important

The clinical status of a disease such as AS can be defined by several components, e.g. pain, function, metrology, and laboratory and radiographic findings. Both erythrocyte sedimentation rate and C-reactive protein are moderately correlated with disease activity and also with damage, but they do not comprehensively represent the disease process in AS. Radiographic evidence of structural damage is an important endpoint in the assessment of AS, and presence of sacroiliitis is a prerequisite for classification according to the (modified) New York criteria.

This process of selecting functional and radiological indices needed further standardization, and there is a general consensus that a clinical outcome measure for use in clinical practice should be simple, brief, easy to score, reliable, valid, and sensitive to change. The OMERACT (Outcome Measures in Rheumatology) group has recently proposed a novel user-friendly paradigm to capture the essential elements of discriminative power (including sensitivity to change), truth, relevance, and feasibility (e.g. applicability and costs). This paradigm is termed the OMERACT filter. The specific instruments selected by the ASAS working group were therefore subjected to the OMERACT filter test for relevance and feasibility.

The ASAS working group has proposed the instruments that need to be used in all research projects in AS. These instruments have now been approved by the OMERACT, the World Health Organization (WHO), and the International League of Associations for Rheumatology (ILAR) for use in clinical research projects in AS, as well as for clinical record keeping in daily practice. They are now called the WHO/ILAR core sets and remission criteria.

Strength

The first set of properly validated instruments to be used in clinical research projects in AS, as well as for clinical record keeping in daily practice.

Weakness

The next step will be to assess the validity of the two measures, entheses and fatigue, which were not accepted by OMERACT because currently no preferred instrument are available for them.

Relevance

A properly validated set of instruments have now been developed for longitudinal follow-up of AS patients, for monitoring their response to therapy, and for clinical record keeping in daily practice. They have been found to be very helpful in fully assessing the dramatic efficacy of anti-TNF-alpha therapy (infliximab and etenercept) in AS and related spondyloarthropathies.

CHAPTER 9

Psoriatic arthritis

Dafna D Gladman

Introduction

The association between arthritis and psoriasis was first made in the 1850s by Alibert (1). However, subsequently it was thought that any inflammatory arthritis that occurred in people with arthritis was a form of rheumatoid arthritis (RA).

The first paper in this selection (Paper 1) is a true 'classic', being the paper in which the late Verna Wright described psoriatic arthritis (PsA) as a separate entity. Baker and colleagues made similar observations a few years later (2), and in 1964 the American Rheumatism Association (ARA) included the disease within its classification of rheumatic diseases for the first time (3). Verna Wright, in conjunction with John Moll and other colleagues made many important contributions to the field, including the discovery of the familial nature of the condition (Paper 2). However, in spite of all their work, a number of authors have continued to question the existence of PsA as a separate entity (4).

Studies on the pathogenesis and genetics have helped to distinguish it as a distinct condition. For example, Veale and colleagues (Paper 3) showed that the reaction in the synovium differs in PsA and RA, and Espinoza and colleagues (Paper 4) found that the fibroblast reaction was abnormal in both the skin and synovium of patients with psoriatic arthropathy. Finally Gladman and her colleagues (Paper 5) have shown that there is a relationship between the expression and severity of PsA and genetic markers in the human leucocyte antigen (HLA) region, although these are different from those seen in rheumatoid disease.

Wright's early descriptions of the disease suggested that it was a relatively mild condition (5), but, as discussed in the section on Paper 1, more recent studies from other countries have suggested that this is not the case (6, 7). There may be genuine differences in expression in different countries, but it seems likely that this is not as benign a disease as was first thought, and patients certainly have problems with disability and employment. Furthermore, Gladman's group have shown that life expectancy is shortened by the condition (Paper 6). Reasons for early mortality, given that this is not a systemic disease, remain to be elucidated.

References

1. Wright V, Moll JHM. *Seronegative polyarthritis*. Amsterdam: North Holland Publishing Company, 1976.
2. Baker H, Golding DN, Thompson M. Psoriasis and arthritis. *Annals of Internal Medicine* 1963; **58**:909–925.
3. Blumberg DS, Bunim JJ, Calkins E, Pirani CL, Zaifler NJ. ARA nomenclature and classification of arthritis and rheumatism. *Arthritis and Rheumatism* 1964; **7**:93–97.
4. Cats A. Is psoriatic arthritis an entity? In: *Rheumatology/85* (Brooks P, York J, (eds.)). Amsterdam: Elsevier, 1985:295–301.
5. Roberts MET, Wright V, Hill AGS, Mehra AC. Psoriatic arthritis. A follow-up study. *Annals of Rheumatic Diseases* 1976; **35**:206–212.
6. Alonso J, Perez A, Castrillo J, Garcia J, Noriega J, Larrea C. Psoriatic arthritis: a clinical, immunological and radiological study of 180 patients. *British Journal of Rheumatology* 1991; **30**:245–250.
7. Gladman D, Stafford-Brady F, Chang C, Lewandowski K, Russell M. Longitudinal study of clinical and radiological progression in psoriatic arthritis. *Journal of Rheumatology* 1990; **17**:809–812.

Paper 1

Psoriasis and arthritis

Author

Wright V

Reference

Annals of Rheumatic Diseases 1956; **15**:348–356

Summary

This study compares 34 patients with psoriasis and erosive arthritis with 55 unselected patients with seropositive RA and with 310 patients with uncomplicated psoriasis. The paper notes the equal male to female ratio of PsA which contrasts with the female preponderance in both RA and uncomplicated psoriasis. The psoriasis usually precedes the arthritis or is synchronous with it in 77% of the cases, but in 23% the arthritis comes first. The clue to the diagnosis of PsA in patients who do not have the psoriasis is a positive family history. Joint changes were more related to nail lesions than to other skin lesions. Nail lesions occur in 87% of patients with PsA and only 25% of patients with uncomplicated psoriasis. Subcutaneous nodules do not occur in PsA. Wright concluded that PsA was milder than RA based on this sample of patients.

Related references

(1) Kammer GM, Soter NA, Gibson DJ, Schur PH. Psoriatic arthritis: a clinical, immunologic and HLA study of 100 patients. *Seminars in Arthritis and Rheumatism* 1979; **9**:75–97.

(2) Gladman DD, Shuckett R, Russell ML, Thorne JC, Schachter RK. Psoriatic arthritis (PSA)–an analysis of 220 patients. *Quarterly Journal of Medicine* 1987; **62**:127–141.

(3) Jones SM, Armas JB, Cohen MG, Lovell CR, Evison G, McHugh NJ. Psoriatic arthritis: outcome of disease subsets and relationship of joint disease to nail and skin disease. *British Journal of Rheumatology* 1994; **33**:834–839.

Key message

There is a specific form of erosive arthritis associated with psoriasis that can be distinguished from RA.

Why it's important

Although previous authors had noted the association between psoriasis and arthritis, the description of PsA as a distinct clinical entity with several clinical patterns is attributed to the late Professor Verna Wright of Leeds. This paper preceded several other contributions from Wright, and Moll and Wright which further developed the concept of PsA and its clinical patterns, including distal joint disease, oligoarthritis, polyarthritis clinically indistinguishable from RA, arthritis mutilans and a SpA. Subsequent studies of large populations of patients with PsA have been published and confirm the existence of these patterns. However, studies that included patients with long-standing disease demonstrate that many patients go on to develop a polyarthritis, and that the disease is not as benign as originally thought (1–3).

Strength

Systematic approach to the evaluation of patients with PsA.

Weaknesses

1. Small number of patients.
2. Short duration of disease.
3. Inclusion of patients with erosive arthritis only.

Relevance

The identification and description of PsA as a distinct entity facilitates correct diagnosis for patients with arthritis and psoriasis and provides a framework for studies of pathogenesis in this condition.

Paper 2

Familial occurrence of psoriatic arthritis

Authors

Moll JM, Wright V

Reference

Annals of Rheumatic Diseases 1973; **32**:181–201

Summary

The authors assessed first and second degree relatives and spouse controls of 88 patients with established PsA and 20 patients with psoriasis and other forms of arthritis (12 RA, seven osteoarthritis (OA), one gout) identified from a hospital population. The prevalence of PsA among the 253 first degree relatives of patients with PsA was 5.5% compared to the calculated prevalence in the UK population of 0.1%. None of the relatives of patients with psoriasis with other forms of arthritis had PsA. The degree of familial aggregation was expressed by the Kellgren factor at 48.8. The prevalence of psoriasis was increased in first degree relatives of probands with either PsA or with psoriasis and other forms of arthritis compared to the population control.

Related reference   (I)   Risch N. Linkage strategies for genetically complex traits. 1. Multilocus model. *American Journal of Human Genetics* 1990; **46**:222–228.

Key message

This study identified the heritability of PsA.

Why it's important

This is a large family investigation which demonstrates unequivocally the role of hereditary factors in PsA. It has paved the way for several other investigations, and provided a rationale to investigate the prevalence of HLA antigens in this disease. It is now clear that there is an association between markers on chromosome 6 and the susceptibility to PsA. Moreover, this family investigation provides impetus for genome-wide studies in this disease. Indeed analyzing Moll and Wright's data with current methodology (1) one finds that the relative risk for first degree relatives (λ_1) of patients with PsA is 55, and for siblings (λs) it is 27.

Strength

This remains the largest family study of PsA to date.

Weakness

Lack of HLA typing for the individuals included in this study.

Relevance

This study confirms that genetic factors are relevant to the susceptibility to PsA. It remains the framework for family studies to date. Several genome-wide studies in psoriasis have been published, and there are current studies looking at families of patients with PsA.

Paper 3

Reduced synovial membrane macrophage numbers, ELAM-1 expression, and lining layer hyperplasia in psoriatic arthritis as compared with rheumatoid arthritis

Authors

Veale D, Yanni G, Rogers S, Barnes L, Bresnihan B, Fitzgerald O

Reference

Arthritis and Rheumatism 1993; **36**:893–900

Summary

Veale and co-workers used monoclonal antibodies to surface molecules to identify cells and vascular endothelium in synovial biopsies from 15 patients with PsA and 15 RA controls matched by age and disease duration. They found that there was less lining layer hyperplasia, fewer macrophages and a greater number of blood vessels in the synovium from PsA patients compared to RA. While ECAM-1 expression was less intense in PsA, there was no difference in the expression of other adhesion molecules. The number of B cells, and T cells and their subsets was similar in the two patient groups.

Key message

There are differences in the synovial changes seen in PsA and RA.

Why it's important

In addition to genetic factors, immunological factors are thought to play an important role in the pathogenesis of PsA. This investigation is the first to compare immunohistological features from matched samples of patients with PsA and RA, and notes that for patients with similar age and disease duration, PsA is associated with an increased vascularity but less inflammatory response than RA synovia.

Strength

Samples matched by age and disease duration.

Weaknesses

1. This is a small study.
2. While patients were not taking disease modifying anti-rheumatic drugs (DMARDs) at the time of study, they had taken some within 3 months. Since some DMARDs may remain in the tissues for prolonged periods the effect of medication on the results is not clear.
3. There were no samples from non-inflammatory arthritis patients.

Relevance

This study supports the role of vascular and immune factors in the pathogenesis of PsA.

Paper 4

Fibroblast function in psoriatic arthritis: I. Alternation of cell kinetics and growth factor responses

Authors

Espinoza LR, Agular JL, Espinoza CG, Cuellar ML, Scopelitis F, Siveira LH

Reference

Journal of Rheumatology 1994; **21**:1502–1506

Summary

The authors investigated the role of fibroblasts in the pathogenesis of PsA. They obtained involved and uninvolved skin and synovial fibroblasts from 10 patients with PsA who were seronegative for rheumatoid factor (RF) and were not on second-line drugs prior to study. Six controls were also studied. Fibroblast cultures were established and cell cycle analysis was performed by flow cytometry. A significant increase in S- and G2-M phase values was observed for psoriatic skin, both involved and uninvolved compared to normal skin, and in psoriatic synovium compared to normal synovium. The abnormalities did not resolve following methotrexate administration despite clinical improvement in the skin lesions. Extracts from fibroblasts were then used to stimulate NIH-3T3 cell line. A marked proliferative response was observed in involved psoriatic fibroblasts compared to controls. A significant increase in kinetic response to growth factors was noted when psoriatic fibroblasts were incubated with growth factors. No correlations with disease duration or severity were noted.

Related reference   **(1)**   Espinoza LR, Espinoza CG, Cuellar ML, Scopelitis E, Silveira LH, Grotendorst GR. Fibroblast function in psoriatic arthritis. II. Increased expression of beta platelet derived growth factor receptors and increased production of growth factors and cytokines. *Journal of Rheumatology* 1994; **21**:1507–1511.

Key message

There is an abnormality in fibroblast activity in both the skin and synovium of patients with PsA.

Why it's important

These studies demonstrate a significant *in vitro* alteration in skin and synovium fibroblasts from patients with PsA. A diffusible factor secreted by the fibroblasts appears to be responsible for these alterations. Alterations in DNA cell cycle and growth factor response of psoriatic fibroblasts in both skin and synovium suggest involvement of this cell type in the pathogenesis of both skin and joint manifestations of the disease. The presence of these abnormalities despite therapy supports an intrinsic role for this abnormality. The authors further demonstrated increased expression of ß- platelet derived growth factor (PDGF) receptor in the psoriatic fibroblasts and increased production of interleukin-1ß and PDGF by psoriatic fibroblasts, providing further support for the role of fibroblasts in the pathogenesis of psoriasis and PsA.

Strengths

1. Clearly demonstrates fibroblast abnormalities from both skin and joint in patients with PsA.
2. Included healthy controls.

Weaknesses

1. Small number of patients were included.
2. All patients had rheumatoid-like arthritis.
3. Disease severity was not defined thus the relationship between the *in vitro* abnormalities and clinical features is difficult to evaluate.

Relevance

The pathogenesis of PsA is unclear. This study provides support for the role of fibroblast abnormality in the development and perpetuation of both skin and joint lesions of the disease.

Paper 5

The role of HLA antigens as indicators of progression in psoriatic arthritis (PsA): multivariate relative risk model

Authors

Gladman DD, Farewell VT

Reference

Arthritis and Rheumatism 1995; **38**:845–850

Summary

An association between HLA antigens and both psoriasis and PsA had been demonstrated. In this study the authors investigated the role of HLA antigens in disease progression in PsA. Disease progression was defined as an increase in clinical damage measured by the number of deformities. The authors developed a model to identify features which would predict disease progression, and had previously demonstrated that among clinical features at the time of first visit five or more swollen joints and a high medication level were predictors for progression, while a low erythrocyte sedimentation rate (ESR) was 'protective'. Applying a similar model but including HLA antigens previously reported to be associated with psoriasis or PsA they identified HLA-B39 as predictive of early progression, HLA-B27 in the presence of HLA-DR7, and HLA-DQw3 in the absence of HLA-DR7 as predictors for clinical progression. Including the clinical features outlined previously in the model they showed that the HLA antigens were stronger than the clinical predictors.

Related references **(1)** Gladman DD, Farewell VT, Nadeau C. Clinical indicators of progression in psoriatic arthritis (PsA): multivariate relative risk model. *Journal of Rheumatology* 1995; **22**:675–679.
(2) Gladman DD, Farewell T, Kopciuk K, Cook RJ. HLA antigens and progression in psoriatic arthritis. *Journal of Rheumatology* 1998; **25**:730–733.

Key message

Genetic markers in the HLA region are important in the expression and progression of PsA.

Why it's important

These studies were the first to use clinical damage as an outcome in PsA and to look for predictors for this outcome While the presence of five or more swollen joints and use of a high level of medication were predictors for progression and a low ESR a 'protector' from such progression, HLA antigens were even stronger predictors. A subsequent study including more patients and all HLA antigens represented in the patient population confirmed the above data and also demonstrated HLA-B22 as protective. Thus the HLA region is important both in the susceptibility and expression of PsA.

Strengths

1. Large number of patients.
2. Good methodology.

Weakness

The study is based on serological typing only.

Relevance

The information gained from this study supports the role for chromosome 6p in the pathogenesis of PsA. It also provides evidence that genetic markers may influence disease progression. Moreover, the identification of markers for disease progression is important in the stratification of patients in therapeutic trials.

Paper 6

Mortality studies in psoriatic arthritis. Results from a single centre. II. Prognostic factors for death

Authors

Gladman DD, Farewell VT, Wong K, Husted J

Reference

Arthritis and Rheumatism 1998; **41**:1103–1110

Summary

The authors set out to investigate prognostic factors associated with mortality in patients with PsA. They had previously demonstrated that patients with PsA were at an increased risk for death compared to the general population. Fifty-three of 428 patients followed prospectively at their PsA clinic between 1978 and 1994 died. The four leading causes of death included diseases of the circulatory system (36.2%), respiratory system (21.3%), malignant neoplasms (17.0%), and injuries/poisoning (14.9%). The overall standardized mortality ratio (SMR) was 1.62. Deaths due to respiratory causes were particularly increased in these patients. Multivariate analysis of potential predictive factors for death present at first visit to clinic revealed that an ESR >15, prior medications, radiological damage and the absence of nail lesions were associated with overall mortality. A gender effect was particularly noted in injuries/poisoning as six of the deaths occurred in males and only one was a female.

Related reference (1)   Wong K, Gladman D, Husted J, Long J, Farewell VT. Mortality studies in psoriatic arthritis. Results from a single centre. I. Risk and causes of death. *Arthritis and Rheumatism* 1997; **40**:1873–1877.

Key message

People with PsA have an increased risk of death which is related to the severity of the disease.

Why it's important

The study demonstrate that patients with PsA are at an increased risk for death compared to the general population. Evidence of previous active and severe disease as manifested by the use of high level of medication and radiological changes as well as an elevated ESR at presentation are prognostic indicators for death. This study further supports the impression that PsA is not a mild disease as originally proposed by Wright (Paper 1).

Strength

This is the first study to demonstrate that patients with PsA are at an increased risk from death.

Weakness

The study is based on a population followed in a speciality clinic and although the clinic includes patients with the full spectrum of the disease, from mild to severe, it may not reflect the severity of PsA in the community.

Relevance

Recognizing that patients with PsA have a severe disease which leads to premature death, and that active and severe disease at presentation are predictive factors in this early mortality will assure that these patients are treated aggressively early in their course to attempt to prevent such an outcome.

CHAPTER 10

Reactive arthritis and Reiter's syndrome

Henning K Zeidler

Introduction

Reactive arthritis (ReA) and Reiter's syndrome are two terms that were used for sometime more or less interchangeably. The latter goes back early in the century and defines a triad or more of clinical manifestations, while the former more recent term relates to the pathophysiological concept of an inflammatory joint process related to an initiating infection elsewhere in the body. Currently ReA is defined as aseptic arthritis triggered by an infectious agent located outside the joint but with non-culturable organisms and/or bacterial components in joint materials (1).

For a long time the classical triad of Reiter's syndrome with conjunctivitis, urethritis and arthritis following diarrhoea or urogenital infection was the hallmark of the disease entity. Later in conjunction with the observation of aseptic arthritis following gut infection with *Yersinia enterocolitica*, mostly in HLA-B27 positive individuals, the new term ReA was proposed, which progressively replaced the previous terms like post-dysenteric, post-venereal and endemic Reiter's syndrome. Moreover, most recently the genetic, clinical and radiographic overlap between ReA, ankylosing spondylitis, and other related diseases, were adapted to be lumped together under the term 'spondarthritides' (2). Due to the complexity surrounding the nomenclature and diagnostic criteria of this group of arthropathies, and due to the lack of standardized diagnostic criteria, Table 10.1 gives an overview of the most frequent terms in use to describe these infection-related diseases. There is an urgent need to further develop our present terminology in the direction of a combined aetiological and clinical terminology (e.g. chlamydia-induced ReA, chlamydia-induced spondarthritis, chlamydia-induced enthesopathy, chlamydia-induced Reiter's syndrome, yersinia-induced ReA, campylobacter-induced ReA, salmonella-induced ReA).

References

1. Kuipers J, Kohler L, Zeidler H. Etiological agents: the molecular biology and phagocyte-host interaction. *Bailliere's Clinical Rheumatology* 1998; **12**:589–609.
2. Calin A, Taurog JD. *The Spondylarthritides*. Oxford: OxfordUniversity Press, 1998.

Table 10.1 Terms used synonymously for reactive arthritis and Reiter's syndrome.

Reactive arthritis (ReA)	Reiter's syndrome
Urogenic:	Incomplete/complete Reiter's syndrome
Urogenic ReA	Fiesinger–Leroy–Reiter's syndrome
Urethritic ReA	Reiter's disease
Post-venereal ReA	Conjunctival–urethral–synovial syndrome
Reactive uroarthritis	
Sexually acquired reactive arthritis (SARA)	
Chlamydia-induced arthritis	
Post-enteric:	
Post-enteric ReA	
Post-dysenteric ReA	
Reactive enteroarthritis	
Enteric ReA	
Yersinia-triggered ReA	
Salmonella-triggered ReA	

Paper Ia

Contribution a l'étude d'une épidemie de dysenterie dans la Somme

Authors

Fiessinger N, Leroy E

Reference

Bulletin de la Société Médicale des Hopitaux de Paris 1916; **40**:2030–2069

Summary

The two French physicians Noel Fiessinger, microbiologist, and Edgar Leroy, military physician, described four cases with a conjunctivo-urethro-synovial syndrome 10 to 20 days after diarrhoea. These patients were part of a very extensive microbiological and clinical analysis of an epidemic of gastroenteritis, which was studied in a military hospital for infectious disease at the Somme, the French part of the First World War front. Although the causative bacteria were not stated, all cases were classified as bacillary dysentery by positive serology, stool culture and exclusion of other causes of gastroenteritis. The joint puncture revealed an inflammatory synovial fluid with many polymorphonuclear cells, but cultures were negative. Nevertheless in the same report in other patients the bacillary dysenteria could be unequivocally attributed by culture to the bacteria shigella, salmonella and yersinia.

Paper Ib

Über eine bisher unerkannte Spirochäteninfektion (Spirochaetosis arthritica)

Author

Reiter H

Reference

Deutsche Medizinische Wochenschrift 1916; **42**:1535–1536

Summary

Hans Reiter reported the case of a young officer serving at the Balkan front who developed, 7 days after acute diarrhoea, an illness characterized by arthritis, urethritis and bilateral conjunctivitis. From the venous blood culture bacteria were grown and classified as a so far unknown bacteria which was considered to be a spirochaete, and the disease was called spirochaetosis arthritica.

Related references (1) Bauer W, Engleman EP. Syndrome of unknown etiology characterized by urethritis, conjunctivitis and arthritis (so-called Reiter's disease). *Transactions of the Association of American Physicians* 1942; **57**: 307–313.

Related references (2) Wallace DJ. Should a war criminal be rewarded with eponymous distinction? The double life of Hans Reiter (1881–1969). *Journal of Clinical Rheumatology* 2000; **6**:49–54.

Key message

Although the clinical association of arthritis and urethritis was described much earlier, both references for the first time described concordantly the clinical picture of the later so-called Reiter's syndrome.

Why it's important

The aetiology of the syndromes were differently attributed as post-infectious following bacillary dysentery and spirochaetosis arthritica, respectively. Both publications appeared at nearly the same time – December 8 (1) and 14 (2) 1916, but for language and other reasons the denomination as Reiter's disease or Reiter's syndrome were adopted in the German and English speaking medical literature and textbooks. Therefore the publication of Reiter is mostly quoted as the first report and the most frequent cited paper, but the French speaking medical society more correctly gave credit to all first observers of the 'Fiessinger-Leroy-Reiter-Syndrome'.

Strengths

1. Clear and simple observation of a clinical arthritic syndrome in association with a preceeding enteritic infection.
2. An example of a good clinical observation.
3. Over the whole century stimulated the thinking and research on association between bacterial infection and arthritis.

Weakness

The description of a spirochaete by Reiter was never confirmed.

Relevance

Although Reiter's paper made only a negligible and some what misleading contribution to the subject, the eponym Reiter's syndrome has been retained in the literature and textbook up to recent years because of a wide usage and the preference for the German and English languages in the medical literature of this century. Moreover, the urethra-conjunctiva-synovial syndrome was described before the report of Hans Reiter and the French authors. Both papers for the first time made a distinction between gonorrhoea and the newly described suspected causative bacteria. The French authors clearly described the association with dysentery and added the microbiological identification of enteric bacteria like salmonella and shigella. Therefore the French description is the first one really to establish the association of bacterial enteric infection and the syndrome. Hans Reiter wrongly attributed the syndrome to a spirochaetal organism. Most importantly, Reiter was a fanatic anti-Semite and a vocal proponent of the eugenics movements of the Nazi regime (2).

Altogether, for historical and ethical reasons it is certainly time to rename the syndrome and no longer include Reiter's name. To be in line with the classical clinical triad cited in many textbooks the name 'urethra-conjunctiva-synovial syndrome' should be preferred to the term 'reactive cutaneo-arthropathy', which now is classified as one clinical manifestation or subtype of the whole spectrum of the group of reactive arthritides.

Paper 2

Isolation of bedsoniae from the joints of patients with Reiter's syndrome

Authors

Schachter J, Barnes MG, Jones JP, Engleman EP, Meyer KF

Reference

Proceedings of the Society for Experimental Biology (New York) 1966; **122**:283–285

Summary

The study investigated 16 patients with Reiter's syndrome all of whom had arthritis and urethritis and/or conjunctivitis. Specimens (synovial membrane, synovial fluid, urethra, conjunctiva) for bedsoniae isolation attempts were obtained from eight patients. Bedsoniae were cultured in four patients from synovial material (two synovial membrane, one synovial fluid, one from both sources), in two patients from urethra, and in one patient from conjunctiva. In total five patients were positive for one or more of the investigated samples. Bedsoniae were not isolated from synovial samples of 15 control patients with osteoarthritis (OA) or rheumatoid arthritis (RA).

Related references (1)   Dunlop EMO, Harper IA, Jones BR. Seronegative polyarthritis: the bedsonia (chlamydia) group of agents and Reiter's disease. *Annals of Rheumatic Diseases* 1968; **27**:234–240.

(2)   Engleman EP, Schachter J, Gilbert RJ, Smith DE, Meyer KF. Bedsonia and Reiter's syndrome: a progress report. *Arthritis and Rheumatism* 1969; **12**:292 (abstract).

(3)   Gordon FB, Quan AL, Steinman TI, Philips RN. Chlamydial isolates from Reiter's syndrome. *British Journal of Venereal Diseases* 1973; **49**:376–380.

(4)   Keat AC, Thomas BJ, Dixey J, Osborne MF, Sonnex C, Taylor-Robinson D. *Chlamydia trachomatis* and reactive arthritis – the missing link. *The Lancet* 1987; **1**:72–74.

Key message

First isolation of bedsoniae from synovial material of patients with Reiter's syndrome, the psittacosis-lymphogranuloma venerum-trachoma agent later classified as *Chlamydia trachomatis*. This report lends support to the hypothesis that this agent plays an aetiological role and can be cultured from the joint, urethra and conjunctiva.

Why it's important

Although the infectious aetiology of post-venereal Reiter's syndrome had been suggested for a long time, and two earlier reports described the isolation of large trachoma-like organisms and of inclusion conjunctivitis agents, respectively, from the urethra of patients with Reiter's syndrome and male patients with nonseptic urethritis, the observation of Schachter, *et al.* for the first time definitely identified bedsoniae by culture from the joint.

More importantly in three patients the microorganisms were grown from two different sources (one synovial membrane and synovial fluid, one synovial membrane and urethra, one urethra and conjunctiva) indicating the multilocular presence of the bacterial agents. In all cases in which positive results were obtained, the patients were studied during the initial attack of the diseases, although detailed information on the presentation are missing and the exact duration of the symptoms in the investigated population were not given. All samples from 15 control patients with OA and RA were negative for bedsoniae, which indicated a putative causative role of the agent. Most importantly, the authors also refer to preliminary studies, in which intraperitoneal infection with yolk-sac suspensions of the isolates in guinea pigs produced arthritis in some instances, and of greater significance, arthritis has been regularly produced by intra-articular injection of the isolate into subhuman primates.

Surprizingly, only a few studies using the original yolk-sac culture method confirmed the positive isolation from patients with Reiter's syndrome (1, 2). In contrast, more recent investigations using new cell culture techniques sensitive for *C. trachomatis* were not successful in culturing live replicating bacteria (3, 4). Therefore, the question of the presence and persistence of live culturable chlamydia in the joint is not finally resolved, although new molecular biology data demonstrate short-lived chlamydial RNA in the synovial membrane, indicating the persistence of live organisms.

Strengths

1. Comprehensive search for one putative causative organism in different relevant clinical samples (joint, urethra, conjunctiva).
2. All controls negative.
3. Stimulated the rheumatological research community to look more intensively for the role of chlamydia in patients with arthritis.

Weaknesses

1. No exact description of the clinical presentation, symptoms and disease duration.
2. More recent cell culture techniques were not successful in culturing live replicating bacteria.

Relevance

First isolation of chlamydia, formerly termed bedsoniae, from joint material, urethra and conjunctiva of patients with Reiter's syndrome. Although later studies with cell culture techniques failed to isolate the organisms, currently the intra-articular presence of chlamydia has been convincingly shown. Future investigations have definitively to elucidate whether only inapparent non-culturable but live bacteria can be isolated, or replicating chlamydia only culturable by sophisticated methods.

Paper 3

Arthritis associated with Yersinia enterocolitica *infection*

Authors

Ahvonen P, Sievers K, Aho K

References

Acta Rheumatologica Scandinavica 1969; **15**:232–253

Summary

During a 3 month period in 1968, 3875 unselected sera sent in for rheumatoid factor (RF) test were screened for agglutination antibodies against *Yersinia enterocolitica* types 3 and 8. Nineteen of the 46 patients with a significant titre of 160 or higher had polyarthritis with acute onset. Of the remaining 27 patients 11 had erythema nodosum and febrile diarrhoea, usually associated with some symptoms in joints. Most of the patients with acute polyarthritis had preceding fever and gastrointestinal symptoms, five patients had urinary symptoms or signs, and three also had conjunctivitis. The joints most often involved were fingers, knees, and ankles. Three patients had acute sacroiliitis and some others back pain or severe myalgia.

Related references **(1)** Terrti R, Granfors K, Lehtonen O-P, Mertsola J, Makela AL, Valimaki I, Hanninen P, Toivanen A. An outbreak of yersinia pseudotuberculosis infection. *Journal of Infectious Diseases* 1984; **149**:245–250.

(2) Winblad S. Arthritis associated with *Yersinia enterocolitica* infections. *Scandinavian Journal of Infectious Diseases* 1975; **7**:191–195.

Key message

First serological study convincingly describing the association of *Yersinia enterocolitica* infections with arthritis and other musculoskeletal symptoms.

Why it's important

Although these and others authors earlier observed a few cases of arthritis, arthralgia, and Reiter's syndrome in patients with positive *Yersinia enterocolitica* serology or stool cultures, the present study is the first one definitely describing the association with this infection as well as a spectrum of rheumatological manifestations including arthritis, sacroiliitis, back pain, gastroenteritis, erythema nodosum, fever, urinary symptoms, and conjunctivitis.

Strengths

1. Comprehensive clinical, serological and laboratory investigation.
2. Large population with rheumatic symptoms screened for yersinia antibodies.

Weaknesses

1. Most of the patients had been admitted to hospital because of the severity of the disease, thus a selective series, comprising only moderate to severe cases.
2. Possibly did not include cases with short duration or mild symptoms.

Relevance

The diagnosis of yersina-associated arthritis was based on serological evidence and was supported to some extent by epidemiological data and by exclusion of other possible causes. All cases had negative serology for brucella and salmonella infection (Widal test), RF (Waaler-Rose and Latex test) and anti-streptolysin 0 titre. Specimens for yersinia stool culture were obtained relatively late and in all cases after or during antibiotic therapy, the possible reason why in none of the patients yersinia could be isolated from the stool.

Altogether the study not only described yersinia as an enteric infectious agent triggering arthritis, but for the first time used the term ReA and also made the point that *Y. enterocolitica* arthritis should be differentiated from rheumatic fever, arthritis associated with salmonella, shigella, brucella and gonococcal infections and finally, if protracted, from RA.

Paper 4

Reiter's disease and HL-A27

Authors

Brewerton DA, Caffrey M, Nicholls A, Walters D, Oates JK, James DCO

Reference

The Lancet 1973 ;**ii**:996–998

Summary

HL-A27 has been found in 25 out of 33 patients (76%) with Reiter's disease, but only three out of 33 patients (9%) with non-specific urethritis and two out of 33 controls (6%). When all patients with sacroiliitis or spondylitis were excluded, HL-A27 was present in 15 out of 33 patients (65%) with peripheral involvement alone. The eight patients who were HL-A27 negative did not differ clinically from those who did, except that they did not have sacroiliitis or spondylitis.

Related references (1) Brewerton D, Caffrey M, Nicholls A, Walter D, James DCO. Acute anterior uveitis and HL-A27. *The Lancet* 1973; **ii**:994–996.

(2) Moll JMH, Haslock J, Macrae JF, Wright V. Associations between ankylosing spondylitis, psoriatic arthritis, Reiter's disease, the intestinal arthropathies and Behçet's syndrome. *Medicine 1974;* **53**: 343–364.

(3) Aho K, Ahvonen P, Lassus A, Sievers K, Tiilikainen A. HL-A antigen 27 and reactive arthritis. *The Lancet* 1973; **ii**:157.

Key message

The high frequency of HLA-B27 (initially termed HL-A27) was reported first in patients with ankylosing spondylitis and their relatives. The present paper and a related study in acute anterior uveitis and the diseases associated with it (1) extend this observation and clearly indicate that a group of rheumatic diseases with common clinical features are also interrelated by a common background.

Why it's important

Clinically, ReA (Reiter's syndrome) follows venereally-aquired non-specific urethritis or it follows dysentery or diarrhoea. Before the discovery of the association with HLA-B27 it was not known why only a small proportion of those who contact infection develop the disease. The repeated finding of HLA-B27 in ankylosing spondylitis, Reiter's syndrome and other related diseases has put forward the hypothesis that one factor in pathogenesis is inherited, related to different triggered infections, and closely associated with the histocompatibility system.

Strengths

1. Only those patients were included in the study who had an acute episode of peripheral arthritis of typical distribution for which no other cause could be found, occurring soon after an attack of urethritis.
2. Patients selection was agreed before the HLA-B27 results were known.
3. Careful subanalysis of the frequency of HLA-B27 according to clinical presentations and manifestations.

Relevance

The concordant high frequency of HLA-B27 in Reiter's syndrome, ankylosing spondylitis and other related diseases support the concept of seronegative spondarthritis developed by Moll and Wright from clinical, serological, and radiological evidence (2). Moreover, the relationship of Reiter's disease with triggering infections by various infective agents opened the view to suggest a common underlying process contributing to the pathogenesis of a wide group of clinical disorders. In fact, the earlier reports of yersinia arthritis also indicated the association between a bacterial infection, HLA-B27, and arthritis (3).

Paper 5

Followup study of patients with Reiter's disease and reactive arthritis with special reference to HLA-B27

Authors

Leirisalo M, Skylv C, Kousa M, Voipio-Pulkki L-M, Souranta H, Nissila M, Hvidman L, Nielsen ED, Svejgaard A, Tiilikainen A, Laitinen O

Reference

Arthritis and Rheumatism 1982; **25**:249–259

Summary

The study reports the follow-up of patients with Reiter's syndrome (n = 160), yersinia arthritis (n = 144), and salmonella arthritis (n = 8). After a follow-up period of a mean time of 65, 52, and 32 months, respectively in the different diagnostic categories, chronic back pain and joint symptoms were frequent in all patients groups. Patients with yersinia arthritis who were HLA-B27 positive had more severe acute disease (more frequent back pain, urological symptoms, mucocutaneous manifestations, and a longer duration of the disease) and more frequent chronic back pain and sacroiliitis. In contrast, in Reiter's syndrome the follow-up revealed no difference in the occurrence of any single chronic symptom between B27 positive and B27 negative patients.

Related references

(1) Csonka GW. The course of Reiter's syndrome. *British Medical Journal* 1958; **1**:1088–1090.

(2) Leirisalo-Repo M, Suorenta H. Ten-year follow-up study of patients with yersinia arthritis. *Arthritis and Rheumatism* 1988; **31**:533–537.

(3) Sairanen E, Paronen I, Mahonen H. Reiter's syndrome: a follow-up study. *Acta Medica Scandinavica* 1969; **185**:57–63.

Key message

Chronic and recurrent joint symptoms and back pain, although usually mild, occur in a considerable number of patients, and even radiological sacroiliitis develops in some patients. Contrary to yersinia arthritis, the presence of B27 in Reiter's syndrome has no influence on the clinical picture of the disease.

Why it's important

A large study following the disease course of different subgroups of patients with ReA, which most importantly also include HLA-B27 tissue typing.

Strengths

1. Comparison of different subgroups of ReA.
2. Extended analysis of the association of HLA-B27 with disease manifestations in clinical course.

Weaknesses

1. Not a prospective study, therefore, large variability of follow-up.
2. Patients were collected in hospitals, which may restrict the generalizability of the results because of selection bias.
3. Only a very small number with salmonella arthritis.

Relevance

Although previous studies have addressed the question of prognosis of Reiter's syndrome (1, 3) and yersinia arthritis, the present study is a very large one, which for the first time directly compared different subgroups of ReA with different triggering infective agents, and most importantly, included HLA-typing in the analysis of the acute disease and follow-up. The main conclusions were that the HLA-B27 in ReA is highly variable, absent in many patients with Reiter's syndrome and not obligatory for the disease development, but so far in yersinia arthritis is of prognostic relevance indicating more severe disease and more frequent late sequelae (see also 2).

Paper 6

Chlamydia trachomatis *and reactive arthritis: the missing link*

Authors

Keat A, Thomas B, Dixey J, Osborn M, Sonnex C, Taylor-Robinson D

Reference

The Lancet 1987; **i**:72–74

Summary

Synovium, synovial fluid cells, or both from eight patients with sexually acquired ReA (SARA) were examined by means of a fluorescence labelled antibody to *Chlamydia trachomatis* (*C. tr.*). Chlamydial particles were seen in five of the 8 patients with SARA but in none of the controls (n = 8) with other rheumatic diseases. All five patients had high titres of serum chlamydial antibodies.

Related references

(1) Granfors K, Jalkanen S, von Essen R, Lahesmaa-Rantala R, Isomaki O, Pekkola-Heino K, Merilahti-Palo R, Saario R, Isomaki H, Toivanen A. Yersinia antigen in synovial-fluid cells from patients with reactive arthritis. *New England Journal of Medicine* 1989; **320**:216–221.

(2) Schumacher HR Jr, Magge S, Cherian PV, Sleckman J, Rothfuss S, Clayburne G, Sieck M. Light and electron microscopic studies on the synovial membrane in Reiter's syndrome. *Arthritis and Rheumatism* 1988; **31**:937–946.

(3) Taylor-Robinson D, Thomas BJ, Dixey J, Osborne MF, Furr PM, Keat AC. Evidence that *Chlamydia trachomatis* causes seronegative arthritis in woman. *Annals of Rheumatic Diseases* 1988; **47**:295–299.

Key message

Identification of fluorescent chlamydial particles in joint samples of patients with SARA indicating that the synovitis may result directly from the intra-articular presence of chlamydia.

Why it's important

Although *C.tr.* has been implicated for long time as a triggering infection in Reiter's syndrome and SARA, earlier isolations of the bacteria from the joint have been questioned and not replicated (Paper 2). Therefore, the present study was a major step towards the acceptance that chlamydial antigen and/or chlamydial particles are present in the joint of patients with post-urethritic ReA. The authors concluded that renewed efforts to culture the organisms are essential and that early treatment with an appropriate antibiotic therapy might alter or thwart the progress of disease. Unfortunately, both suggestions although so promising have not been realized up to today, especially as all efforts to cure ReA by short- or long-term antibiotic treatment have failed.

Strengths

1. The fluorescence monoclonal antibody method is well established for diagnosis of *C.tr.* in urogenital swabs.
2. The method is as least as sensitive as culture.
3. With the same antibody chlamydial particles have been seen in preparations from mouse joints after experimental intra-articular inoculation of *C.tr.*

Weaknesses

1. The identified fluorescent particles were classified as elementary body without any morphological confirmation; other possible forms like reticulate body, intermediate body or aberrant forms were not excluded.
2. Only limited information on the demographics of the patients.
3. No comprehensive descriptions of the clinical signs and symptoms of the patients.

Relevance

The study has been widely accepted as the missing link to confirm that *C.tr.* is the causative agent of post-urethritic ReA and that the intra-articular presence of the organism may directly result in the synovitis, instead of the long-time favoured hypothesis of an extra-articular infection causing the arthritic immune reaction. The observation of the intra-articular presence of *C.tr.* not only changed the concept of pathogenesis of ReA but also stimulated intensive research activities to elucidate the question of whether *C.tr.* is viable or dead in the joint.

Paper 7a

Chlamydial rRNA in the joints of patients with chlamydia-induced arthritis and undifferentiated arthritis

Authors

Hammer M, Nettelnbreker E, Hopf S, Schmitz E, Porschke K, Zeidler H

Reference

Clinical and Experimental Rheumatology 1992; **10**:63–66

Summary

In one of 11 patients with chlamydia-induced arthritis (CIA) and three of 24 patients with undifferentiated arthritis (UndA), but none of 16 controls (post-enteric ReA, n = 4; Lyme arthritis, n = 3; RA, n = 8) chlamydial rRNA was found in the synovial fluid using a commercially available nucleic acid hybridization test based on a isotopic (^{125}J) conjugated single stranded DNA-probe (GEN-PROBE). In one additional patient with CIA the synovial membranes were positive for chlamydial rRNA.

Paper 7b

Molecular evidence for the presence of chlamydia in the synovium of patients with Reiter's syndrome

Authors

Rahman MU, Cheema MA, Schumacher HR, Hudson AP

Reference

Arthritis and Rheumatism 1992; **35**:521–529

Summary

Seven of 9 patients with Reiter's syndrome were found positive in synovial biopsy samples for chlamydial rRNA with a molecular hybridization technique using a cloned 466-basepair DNA fragment encoding the 5'-most portion of *Chlamydia trachomatis* (serovar L$_2$) 16sRNA gene. Three of 13 patients with other mostly incompletely explained arthritis were also positive for chlamydial RNA.

Related references (1)   Wordsworth BP, Hughes RA, Allan I, Keat AC, Bell JI. Chlamydial DNA is absent from the joint of patients with sexually acquired reactive arthritis. *British Journal of Rheumatology* 1990; **29**:208–210.

Related references (2) Kuipers JG, Jurgens-Saathoff B, Bialowons A, Wollenhaupt J, Zeidler H. Detection of *Chlamydia trachomatis* in peripheral blood leucocytes of reactive arthritis patients by polymerase chain reaction. *Arthritis and Rheumatism* 1998; **48**:1894–1895.

(3) Gaston JSH, Cox C, Granfors K. Clinical and experimental evidence for persistent yersinia infection in reactive arthritis. *Arthritis and Rheumatism* 1999; **42**:2239–2242.

Key message

Both studies for the first time identified by molecular hybridization techniques chlamydial RNA in joint samples of patients with Reiter's syndrome, post-urethritic ReA and unclassified arthritis.

Why it's important

The detection of chlamydial RNA in combination with previous findings of chlamydia-like particles and/or chlamydial antigens in synovium and synovial fluid of patients with Reiter's syndrome and ReA suggest that whole, live bacterial organisms are present in inflamed joints. In contrast, an earlier search for chlamydial DNA in synovial fluid of patients with SARA had failed (1).

It is now well accepted that aberrant, live bacteria are persisting in synovial cells especially in macrophages. Most recently chlamydia has also been identified in the blood in patients with CIA indicating the bacterial dissemination from the entry site via the bloodstream into the joint (2). Therefore, the definition of ReA at least for CIA now has to be modified in the sense that it is no longer a sterile immune-mediated inflammatory process occurring distant to a primary focus of infection, but rather bacteria driven disease with persistence of the agent in the joint for a longer time. If this holds true for other forms of ReA (e.g. induced by yersinia, salmonella or shigella) has to be elucidated in the future. Only recently, yersinia DNA was found in chronic remittent ReA in the joint, whereas for a long time yersinia antigens (lipopolysaccharide) have been shown in the joint and circulation (3).

Strength

Both studies although varying in the applied techniques, prevailing samples (synovial fluid versus synovium) and diagnostic categories concordantly identified chlamydial RNA in joint material.

Weaknesses

1. The data provide no insight into the detailed biological state of chlamydia in the joint, i.e. whether it is actively, if slowly, dividing, or whether vegetative growth has been suspended.
2. In the study of Hammer, *et al.* the commercially available nucleic acid hybridization test GEN-PROBE was of low sensitivity although of good specificity.

Relevance

The identification of chlamydial RNA by simple hybridization techniques indicated the intra-articular persistence of intact, possibly viable chlamydia because in general RNA is degraded soon after lysis of bacterial cells. This observation stimulated further studies to demonstrate chlamydial DNA, short lived RNA and other genetic material proving the presence of whole, metabolically active chlamydia in joint material.

CHAPTER 11

Lupus

Graham RV Hughes and Munther Khamashta

Introduction

The second half of the 20th century saw a revolution in the perception and treatment of many major diseases, none more so than lupus. In the 1950s, 1960s and even (in some countries) the 1970s, lupus was considered a rare 'small print' disease. Not a part of 'main-stream' rheumatology. A fatal disease which required life-long steroids. No pregnancies allowed. A kidney disease.

Now, we have dedicated lupus centres run by physicians with the proper skills and training in dermatology, in medical aspects of pregnancy, in the neurology of lupus, and more. All countries recognize the huge increase in the frequency of new lupus cases, a prevalence figure in many studies far exceeding that of better known diseases such as multiple sclerosis and leukaemia.

This chapter selects five articles which have contributed to this change; the early clinical studies of Edmund Dubois, the introduction of anti-DNA testing, the description of the antiphospholipid syndrome (APS), and an example of the changing pattern of treatment, the use of pulse-cyclophosphamide regimes. Finally, a paper, which in pointing out the increased late coronary risk in lupus, paved the way for a whole new role for lupus, that of a dIsease model for accelerated atheroma.

In the 1950s there were few large published series of lupus patients. One man changed all that, Dr E.L. Dubois of Los Angeles. His clinical description of 520 cases provided the baseline for the majority of later clinical series. They contributed to our understanding of the breadth of features of systemic lupus erythematosus (SLE), notably, for example, highlighting the importance of central nervous system (CNS) involvement in the disease. Finally, this series provided the basis for his monumental textbook on lupus, the first 'Bible' of the disease.

In Dubois' time, steroids were the dominant treatment for lupus, with doses of over 80 mg daily given by some physicians. The introduction of pulsed intravenous (I.V.) cyclophosphamide regimes by the National Institutes of Health (NIH) group in the early 1970s proved a major advance, largely in allowing the use of lower steroid doses. The NIH regime, although considered over-aggressive by some workers (including ourselves) has, with modification stood the test of time and has undoubtedly improved the prognosis of lupus nephritis out of all recognition.

Of the multiplicity of antibodies found in lupus, two have achieved over-riding importance, anti-DNA antibody testing (the benchmark test for lupus, a test remarkable in its specificity for the disease), and antiphospholipid antibodies. It is our belief that the description of the APS will have implications far beyond lupus. In cerebral disease, for example cases of idiopathic stroke, of 'atypical multiple sclerosis' and of severe migraine are being attributed to the pro-coagulant state associated with antiphospholipid antibodies, and being treated successfully with anticoagulants.

The syndrome is probably the single most important treatable cause of 'idiopathic' recurrent foetal loss. One of the results of studies of antiphospholipid antibodies has been an important link with accelerated arterial disease. This discovery has opened up a new dimension in the study of disease models of arterial disease.

While 40 years ago, the causes of mortality in lupus were renal disease, steroid overdosage and infection, the disease pattern has changed. The last of our five classic papers goes back to the early clinical observation that there might be another 'late' threat, arterial disease. Lupus and the APS are now important models for the study of accelerated atheroma, another lateral move for those who treat and think about these diseases.

Paper I

Clinical manifestations of systemic lupus erythematosus. Computer analysis of 520 cases

Authors

Dubois EL, Tuffanelli DL

Reference

Journal of the American Medical Association 1964; **190**:104–111

Summary

Diagnosis of SLE was confirmed by the presence of lupus erythematosus (LE) cells in 75.7% of the patients, findings of skin biopsies in 6.0% and of renal biopsies in 1.2%, and by the clinical picture alone in 17.1%. Blacks comprised 34% of the subjects. Spontaneous remissions occurred in 35% of the patients. Proven familial SLE occurred in 2%. Myalgia was present in 48.2%. No history of cutaneous involvement at any time was found in 28%. Classic skin lesions of chronic discoid lupus at the onset of their illness were present in 10.8%. Urinary abnormalities were noted in only 46.1%. Uremia caused 34% of the 135 deaths and progressive CNS involvement caused 18.4%. The prognosis has markedly improved. The mean duration is now 94.8 months for the entire series versus 38.5 months in an untreated control group.

Related references (1) Wallace DJ, Hahn BH (eds.). *Dubois' Lupus Erythematosus*. 5th edition. Baltimore: Williams & Wilkins, 1997.

(2) Lahita R (ed.). *Systemic Lupus Erythematosus*. 3rd edition. San Diego: Academic Press, 1998.

Key message

This paper summarized the clinical diversity of SLE, as studied by an individual clinician.

Why it's important

After the initial clinical descriptions of lupus by Osler and others, a century ago, no single physician contributed more to the broadening of the clinical concept of lupus. Dubois' huge clinical experience, based on his private practice, would probably not now be accepted for publication, an example if ever one were needed, of 'eminence-based medicine' rather than 'evidence-based medicine'. His Los Angeles observations began with eight patients who all had a positive lupus erythematosus cell test, and ended with the world's largest lupus centre, with over 500 patients.

His clinical observations were numerous, notably the highlighting of the importance of CNS involvement in lupus, the linking of avascular necrosis of bone with SLE, his pioneering of treatment protocols, and, especially, his championing of the use of antimalarials in lupus.

He encouraged many, many physicians (including strong personal encouragement for me, Graham Hughes) to study this disease, at that time widely regarded as 'rare' and 'small print'. His work spawned the first 'classic' textbook on lupus, an almost single-handed tome, now together with Lahita's textbook, one of the two 'Bibles' of the disease.

Strength

The clinical observations of one man, heavily and directly involved in the practice of medicine.

Weakness

Many of his patients would now come under different diagnostic labels, chronic active hepatitis, Sjögren's syndrome and so on, but the evolution of these subsets came later with the development of newer immunoassays.

Relevance

The series which, more than any other, portrayed the broad sweep of clinical features of SLE.

Paper 2

Therapy of lupus nephritis: controlled trial of prednisone and cytotoxic drugs

Authors

Austin HA, Klippel JH, Balow JE, Le Riche NGH, Steinberg AD, Plotz PH, Decker JL

Reference

New England Journal of Medicine 1986; **314**: 614–119

Summary

We evaluated renal function in 107 patients with active lupus nephritis who participated in long-term randomized therapeutic trials (median follow-up, 7 years). For patients taking oral prednisone alone, the probability of renal failure began to increase substantially after 5 years of observation. Renal function was better preserved in patients who received various cytotoxic drug therapies, but the difference was statistically significant only for I.V. cyclophosphamide plus low-dose prednisone as compared with high-dose prednisone alone (p = 0.027). The advantage of treatment with I.V. cyclophosphamide over oral prednisone alone was particularly apparent in the high-risk subgroup of patients who had chronic histological changes on renal biopsy at study entry. Patients treated with I.V. cyclophosphamide have not experienced haemorrhagic cystitis, cancer or a disproportionate number of major infections. We conclude that, as compared with high-dose oral prednisone alone, treatment of lupus glomerulonephritis with I.V. cyclophosphamide reduces the risk of end-stage renal failure with few serious complications.

Related references (1) Klippel JH. Indications for and use of, cytotoxic agents in SLE. *Balliere's Clinical Rheumatology* 1998; **12**:511–527.

(2) D'Cruz D, Cuadrado MJ, Mujic F, Tungekar MF, Taub M, Lloyd M, Khamashta MA, Hughes GRV. Immunosuppressive therapy in lupus nephritis.*Clinical and Experimental Rheumatology* 1997; **15**:275–282.

Key message

Bolus I.V. cyclophosphamide together with corticosteroids, plays a key role in the management of severe SLE, notably nephritis.

Why it's important

The diagnosis of lupus was once a password for routine long-term high-dose steroid therapy. In the 1970s and early 1980s, immunosuppressives became more widely used as 'steroid-sparing' agents, azathioprine for milder cases, cyclophosphamide for more severely ill patients. The side-effects of long-term oral cyclophosphamide, notably cystitis, amenorrhoea and infections, severely limited the use of this drug in most young lupus patients. The group at the NIH deserves the credit not only for the introduction and championing of intermittent 'pulse' regimes, but for their dogged perseverance in following the treatment sub-groups of patients for many years. They have shown that intermittent pulses combined with steroids is far superior in improving overall prognosis in lupus nephritis than steroids alone (1).

Over the past decade, a number of groups, including ours have modified the somewhat strong original NIH dose regimes, resulting in similar success in the majority of patients, but with far fewer adverse effects, notably the almost total eradication of amenorrhoea (2).

Strength

Intermittent 'pulse' regimes are well tolerated and improve compliance.

Weakness

I.V. administration requires regular close out-patient monitoring.

Relevance

Intermittent I.V. cyclophosphamide regimes are well tolerated, are beneficial in severe lupus, and have contributed directly to improved prognosis in SLE.

Paper 3

Complement fixation with cell nuclei and DNA in lupus erythematosus

Authors

Robbins WC, Holman HR, Deicher H, Kunkel HG

Reference

Proceedings of the Society for Experimental Biology and Medicine 1957; **96**:575–579

Summary

Sera from patients with active LE fixed complement with a wide variety of nuclei from different organs and species, with calf thymus nucleo-protein, and in two instances with histone. Isolated calf thymus, salmon sperm, human leucocyte and pneumococcal DNA also fixed complement with many of these sera. Similar reactions were not encountered in a limited control series including normal individuals and other pathological states.

Most active LE sera fixed complement with both nuclei and DNA in roughly parallel titre. However, exceptions were encountered and one serum reacted strongly with nuclei but failed to react with DNA. Cross-absorption experiments with nuclei and DNA suggested the presence of two distinct serum factors.

The LE factor appeared to be related to the factor responsible for complement fixation with nuclei but distinct from that responsible for DNA fixation. The significance of these findings with respect to antibodies against unclear constituents is discussed.

Related references **(1)** Pincus T, Schur PH, Rose JA, Decker JL, Talal N. Measurement of serum DNA-binding activity in SLE. *New England Journal of Medicine* 1969; **281**:701–703.

(2) Hughes GRV. Significance of anti-DNA antibodies in SLE. *The Lancet* 1971; 861.

Key message

Four papers, published almost simultaneously in 1957, followed up on earlier observations that lupus sera contained specific antibodies against nuclear constituents. Lupus serum antibodies could react against DNA.

Why it's important

The finding of anti-DNA antibodies in serum has proved to be one of the most abidingly specific in medicine, and proved vital in distinguishing anti-nuclear antibody (ANA) specificity in lupus from that in other autoimmune diseases. It is exceptionally rare to find antibodies against double-stranded (ds) DNA in any condition other than lupus.

The clinical studies by Pincus and colleagues in 1969 and by Cohen, Hughes and Christian in 1970, showed that not only could an immunoassay for anti-dsDNA be diagnostically important, but that the level of antibody could provide a rough indicator of disease activity. Although some clinicians make therapeutic decisions based on antibody titre, we consider the practice too imprecise. Anti-DNA antibodies measured either by immunoassay, immunofluorescence (Crithidia) or ELISA are now the standard test for lupus, and have directly contributed to the growth in prevalence of lupus world-wide, changing it from a rare, 'small print' disease to a major illness, overtaking RA in some countries.

Strength

Measurement of anti-dsDNA is the specific test for lupus.

Weakness

Some lupus patients (notably some with skin disease) remain persistently anti-dsDNA negative.

Relevance

The application of anti-DNA testing to connective tissue diseasess has provided both a diagnostic test for lupus, and a rough guide to disease severity.

Paper 4

Thrombosis, abortion, cerebral disease and the lupus anticoagulant

Author

Hughes GRV

Reference

British Medical Journal 1983; **287**:1088–1089

Summary

Systemic lupus erythematosus, with its broad range of clinical and immunological abnormalities continues to provide lessons relevant to research in a wider variety of disciplines and diseases. In some patients three apparently unrelated clinical features of SLE, recurrent venous thrombosis, CNS disease (including myelitis), and recurrent abortions, may, it seems, have common pathogenic mechanisms. Clinicians have suspected as much for some time; those dealing with many patients with SLE recognize a group of women who have as features of their disease multiple (even a dozen or more) spontaneous abortions, multiple deep vein and other thromboses, and neurological abnormalities including either putative cerebral thrombosis or myelitis or both. Interestingly, some of these patients have negative test results for ANA. Recent studies from the Hammersmith Hospital, London have confirmed and extended the association of the lupus anticoagulant with thrombosis.

Harris, *et al.* have developed a sensitive solid phase radioimmunoassay for anticardiolipin antibodies some 200–400 times more sensitive than, for example, the precipitation method used in the Venereal Disease Research Laboratory test. There was a strong correlation between raised titres of anticardiolipin antibodies and venous and arterial thrombosis. Of the 15 patients with the highest anticardiolipin antibody titres, six had a history of venous thrombosis and five had cerebral thrombosis without other predisposing factors. Two each had pulmonary hypertension and multiple abortions. For those of us hardened into nihilism by years of study of various autoantibodies in SLE, there is a rare sense of excitement at the implications of the associations now being reported.

Related references   **(1)**   Harris EN, Gharavi AE, Boey ML, Patel BM, Mackworth-Young CG, Loizou S, Hughes GRV. Anticardiolipin antibodies: detection by radioimmunoassay and association with thrombosis in systemic lupus erythematosus. *The Lancet* 1983; **ii**:1211–1214.

  (2)   Hughes GRV. Hughes' syndrome: the antiphospholipid syndrome. A historical review. *Lupus* 1998; **7**(suppl.2) S1–S3.

Key message

Antiphospholipid antibodies, detected by sensitive immunoassays, are a strong risk-marker for a syndrome characterized by venous and arterial thrombosis (especially strokes), and recurrent abortion.

Why it's important

Originally described in our lupus clinic patients, it quickly became clear that many patients with the APS have no evidence of lupus, indeed it is likely that the so-called primary APS, or Hughes' syndrome, far exceeds the prevalence of lupus itself. Five examples of the importance of the syndrome in internal medicine are given:

- It is an important, and potentially preventable cause of stroke, up to 20% of strokes in the under-40s being due to Hughes' syndrome.
- It is now recognized as one of the most important causes of repeated pregnancy loss.
- Treatment of pregnant APS women has improved pregnancy success rates from under 20% to over 70%.
- It is a potentially treatable cause of a number of common medical conditions including migraine, epilepsy, memory loss, multiple sclerosis and deep vein thrombosis.
- In lupus, management has been profoundly altered by the recognition that some features, notably many aspects of CNS lupus, are due to thrombosis rather than inflammation.

Strength

An easy-to-perform test now picks up a group of individuals susceptible to thrombosis.

Weakness

Many, possibly the majority of antibody-positive individuals do not thrombose. Other factors, as yet unknown, may be involved.

Relevance

A pro-thrombotic syndrome, identified by the presence of antiphospholipid antibodies, which has clinical implications not only in rheumatology, but also in fields as diverse as obstetrics, neurology and cardiology.

Paper 5

The bimodal mortality pattern of systemic lupus erythematosus

Authors

Urowitz MB, Bookman AAM, Koehler BE, Gordon DA, Smythe HA, Ogryzlo MA

Reference

American Journal of Medicine 1976; **60**:221–225

Summary

The changing pattern of mortality in SLE led to an examination of the deaths in a long-term systematic analysis of 81 patients followed for 5 years at the University of Toronto Rheumatic Disease Unit. During the follow-up 11 patients died, six patients died within the first year after diagnosis (group I) and five patients died an average of 8.6 years (from 2.5 to 19.5 years) after diagnosis (group II). In those who died early the SLE was active clinically and serologically, and nephritis was present in four. Their mean prednisone dose was 53.3 mg/day. In four patients a major septic episode contributed to their death. In those who died late in the course of the disease, only one patient had active lupus and none had active lupus nephritis. Their mean prednisone dose was 10.1 mg/day taken for a mean of 7.2 years. In none was sepsis a contributing factor to their death. All five of these patients had had a recent myocardial infarction at the time of death; in four, it was the primary cause of death. Mortality in SLE follows a bimodal pattern. Patients who die early in the course of their disease, die with active lupus, receive large doses of steroids and have a remarkable incidence of infection. In those who die late in the course of the disease, death is associated with inactive lupus, long duration of steroid therapy and a striking incidence of myocardial infarction due to atherosclerotic heart disease.

Related references **(1)** Vaarala O, Alfthan G, Jauhiainen M, *et al.* Cross-reaction between antibodies to oxidised low-density lipoprotein and to cardiolipin in systemic lupus erythematosus. *The Lancet* 1993; **341**:923–925.

(2) Shoenfeld Y. The anti-phospholipid (Hughes) syndrome: a crossroads of autoimmunity and atherosclerosis. *Lupus* 1997; **6**:559–560.

Key message

Lupus is now a major disease model for the study of accelerated vascular disease.

Why it's important

Traditionally, most epidemiological studies of lupus had listed renal disease and infection as the major cause of death. The Toronto publication in 1976 was the first major study to show a bimodal mortality pattern. While it was widely recognized that the statistical prognosis of lupus improved with each decade, this study highlighted a second mortality peak from coronary and arterial disease.

The number of studies confirming this observation is now becoming a flood, with estimates of as high as a 50-fold increase in coronary artery disease in lupus patients. The causes of this phenomenon are still being studied. Hypercholesterolaemia, nephrotic syndrome, steroid treatment and hypertension are all candidates, but clearly do not provide the whole solution.

The discovery of the APS opened up a new line of investigation. It was clear that strokes, coronary artery disease and accelerated atheroma were a feature in many patients with APS, patients who had never received steroids or suffered renal disease, for example. In 1993, Vaarala and her colleagues in Finland published an important study suggesting that some antiphospholipid antibodies were capable of cross-reacting with oxidised low-density lipoproteins (oxLDL) (1). A subsequent study suggested that anti-oxLDL were in turn more closely associated with arterial than with venous thrombosis.

These observations have opened up a major research effort in the immunology of atheroma, with a focus on the role of antibodies in the development of oxidation-mediated endothelial injury. Many workers both in cardiovascular medicine and lupus are now collaborating in this area (reviewed in 2), shifting the emphasis from lipids, through inflammatory processes, to immunology. Lupus and Hughes syndrome are now important models for the study of atheroma.

Strength

These observations have already shifted the emphasis of management of lupus patients towards prophylaxis of risk factors for coronary artery disease. They have also provided a new disease model for the study of atheroma.

Weaknesses

1. Arterial disease in lupus and Hughes syndrome is almost certainly multifactorial.
2. The importance of antibody-mediated disease remains unknown.

Relevance

Coronary and cerebral vascular diseases are an important causes of death in lupus. New clues involving immunological mechanisms may lead to a modification of treatment and prophylaxis.

CHAPTER 12

Scleroderma (systemic sclerosis)

E Carwile LeRoy

Introduction

Reviewing a century of progress in the understanding of a disease as cryptic as scleroderma (systemic sclerosis, SSc) is daunting. In one sense direct involvement in SSc research for the last three decades of the century places one perhaps too close to be objective; in another sense not being around for the first seven decades creates a distance which, while enhancing objectivity, reduces the awareness gained by direct involvement. Nonetheless, a perspective in SSc understanding gained in the 20th century can perhaps best be begun by examining briefly the contributions of earlier times.

In Naples, Italy, in 1753 Carlo Curzio, a physician, described a young woman whose skin became hardened over the entire body. This has been taken by some as the first reported case of SSc. Doubt is cast by Curzio's reported follow-up that complete remission followed symptomatic management, suggesting as an alternative diagnosis the self-remitting scleredema of Bushke which follows bacterial infections of the neck and throat. Little else of note is recorded which can be traced to the 18th century.

In contrast, the 19th century, with major medical centres in London, Edinburgh, Berlin, Paris, Vienna and both the Middle and Far East, recorded numerous reports of a wasting condition associated with hard skin. Physicians were wont to derive their own Latin and Greek based terms for this uncommon disease, some of which are listed in Table 12.1. Many well-recognized physicians, including Wernike, Addison, Kaposi, Osler, and Raynaud contributed descriptions which introduced the multisystemic nature of SSc. Publications by Horteloup and Gintrac are recommended (1, 2). This period is reviewed thoroughly by Rodnan and Benedek (3).

Table 12.1 Alternative terms for scleroderma.

Endurcissement du tissue cellulaire	Oedématie concrète
Sclérème en placards	Sclérème lardacée
Sclerostenosis cutanea	Morphée
Rheumatische Sclerose des Unterhautz-ellgewebes	Sclérème simple ou nonoedémateux
Sclerma or pachydermateous disease	Cacimus eburneus
Cutis tensa chronica	Elephantiasis sclerosa
Sclerosis corii	Sclerosis telae cellularis et adiposae
Trophoneurosis disseminata	Cicatrisirendes Hautsclerom
Scleriasis	Hautsclerom
Keloid	Sclérème des adultes
Textus cellularis duritiens	Scleroma
Sclerema	Scirrhosarca

Rodnan GP, Benedek TG. *Annals of Internal Medicine* 1962; **57**:305–318.

References

1. Horteloup P. *De la Sclerodermie.* Paris: P. Asselin, 1865.
2. Gintrac E. Note sur la sclerodermie. *Review Medicin Chirurgie* (Paris) 1847 **2**:263.
3. Rodnan GP, Benedek TG. An historical account of the study of progressive systemic sclerosis (diffuse scleroderma). *Annals of Internal Medicine* 1962; **57**:305–318.

Paper I

Survival with systemic sclerosis (scleroderma). A life-table analysis of clinical and demographic factors in 309 patients

Authors

Medsger TA Jr, Masi AT, Rodnan GP, Benedek TG, Robinson H

Reference

Annals of Internal Medicine 1971; **75**:369–376

Abstract

A life-table analysis of survivorship with SSc was performed, using 223 patients diagnosed in Pittsburgh, Pennsylvania, and 86 patients in Memphis, Tennessee. The demographic and clinical characteristics of the two series were similar, thus allowing for both comparison of the two groups and analysis of the total 309 patients. A follow-up during 1970 was successful in 94% of all patients. No difference in survival was found between the two patient groups, the combined 7 year cumulative survivorship being 35%. Significantly decreased survival was found in older patients of both series after allowance was made for the natural increase of mortality with age. Males had significantly worse survival than females. Negroes had significantly worse survival than whites during the first year of follow-up of all patients. When no internal organ involvement was detected at entry to study, the negro prognosis was significantly worse throughout a 7 year follow-up period. Renal, cardiac, and pulmonary involvement were each independently correlated with decreased survival.

Summary

Two major centres combined their hospital case records to analyze >300 SSc patients. With an overall 7 year survivorship of 35%, a progressively poorer prognosis was noted with no internal involvement, lung, heart or kidney involvement, respectively, and survival dropped below 50% at 4 years for lung, at 2 years for heart, and at less than 1 year for kidney involvement. This report placed the prognosis of SSc on a firm foundation for the first time.

Citation count

225

Related references

(1) Goetz RH. Pathology of progressive systemic sclerosis (generalized scleroderma) with special reference to changes in the viscera. *Clinical Proceedings (South Africa)* 1945; **4**:337–392.

(2) Tuffanelli DL, Winkelmann RK. Systemic scleroderma. A clinical study of 727 cases. *Archives of Dermatology* 1961; **84**:359–371.

Key message

Internal organ involvement predicts the survival of SSc patients.

Why it's important

This was the first study in which patients were evaluated uniformly for internal organ involvement.

Strengths

1. Records from multiple hospitals were used.
2. Patient selection techniques were standardized.
3. Statistical analysis was careful and complete.
4. Authors were experienced sclerodermologists.

Weaknesses

1. Survival onset began at diagnosis, not at symptom onset.
2. Retrospective, dependent on physician who completed hospital records.

Relevance

A new era of outcome prediction in SSc began with this article. Figure 12.1 (Figure 5 in original paper), showing a progressive worsening of prognosis with lung, heart, and kidney failure, has become a landmark in SSc thinking and spurred organ-specific and vascular studies of pathogenesis and management.

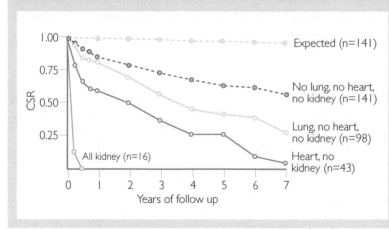

Figure 12.1 Observed cumulative survival rates (CSR) for scleroderma patients with lung, heart, or kidney involvement and observed and expected CSR for patients with none of these involvements at entry to study.

Paper 2

The relationship of hypertension and renal failure in scleroderma (progressive systemic sclerosis) to structural and functional abnormalities of the renal cortical circulation

Authors

Cannon PJ, Hassar M, Case DB, Casarella WJ, Sommers SC, LeRoy EC

Reference

Medicine 1974; **53**:1–46

Abstract

A clinicopathological review of 210 patients with SSc seen in one institution with emphasis on renal (94 patients) involvement, the vascular lesions and the outcome (autopsies in 40 patients), all in the era prior to the introduction of angiotensin-converting enzyme (ACE) inhibitors, which dramatically changed the natural history of scleroderma renal crisis (SRC), characterized by oliguria, proteinuria, hyperreninemia, and renal cortical infarction with renal insufficiency.

Summary

Proteinuria, azotemia and hypertension were used as clinical markers of renal involvement in a survey of 210 SSc patients who were seen at Columbia-Presbyterian Medical Center (CPMC) over a 20 year period. One or more markers were observed in 94 patients, an incidence of renal involvement of 45%. Proteinuria occurred in 36%, azotemia in 19% and the syndrome of 'malignant' hypertension in 7%. The mean onset of renal markers was within 3 years of onset of the disease. No particular subsets of patients (age, sex, race) showed increased susceptibility to renal involvement (diffuse and limited subsets of SSc were not evaluated).

The onset of hypertension in SSc was not related to corticosteroid administration. Two clinical patterns were observed: 'malignant' hypertension, and mild chronic hypertension which terminated abruptly with renal failure. In the latter group, as in the 10 normotensive SSc patients who developed oliguric renal failure, the onset of azotemia was usually preceded by episodes of heart failure, pericardial effusion, dehydration or abdominal surgery.

Only 10% of the SSc patients without clinical markers died during the 20 years, whereas 60% of those with renal involvement died during the same period. The relative incidence of death in patients with different markers was: proteinuria 63%, hypertension 66%, azotemia 77% and 'malignant' hypertension 80%. The incidence of markers in the patients that died (82%) was higher than in the total population (45%). Among the 40 patients autopsied at CPMC, renal involvement was the leading cause of death (43%). Two-thirds of all deaths and 76% of deaths from renal involvement by SSc occurred in fall and winter. The mean time from onset of a clinical marker to death in this group was: hypertension, 13 months; proteinuria, 7 months; 'malignant' hypertension and azotemia, 1 month.

Ninety percent of autopsied patients exhibited histological renal abnormalities; in 63% a lesion was found in the interlobular arteries which appeared different from the vascular changes seen in hypertensive disease. In the smaller arteries, arterioles and glomeruli the abnormalities found ('fibrinoid' necrosis, arteriosclerosis, capillary thrombi, glomerular hyperlobulation and endothelial swelling), were similar in normotensive and hypertensive SSc patients and mimicked those of essential and 'malignant' hypertension. Patients with renal failure exhibited focal areas of cortical necrosis.

The studies indicate the prognostic importance of the kidney vascular lesions in SSc. A hypothesis is proposed that the structural and functional changes in the renal cortical circulation contribute to the pathogenesis of both hypertension and oliguric renal failure in this disorder. Possible therapeutic roles for renal vasodilators and for dialysis and renal transplantation in SSc are suggested.

Citation count

228

Related references

(1)   Klemperer P, Pollack AD, Baehr G. Diffuse collagen disease. Acute disseminated lupus erythematosus and diffuse scleroderma. *Journal of the American Medical Association* 1942; **119**:331–332.

(2)   Weiss S, Stead EA Jr, Warren JV, Bailey OT. Scleroderma heart disease with a consideration of certain other visceral manifestations of scleroderma. *Archives of Internal Medicine* 1943; **71**:749–776.

Key message

Simple clinical surrogate markers (proteinuria, azotemia, microangiopathic haemolytic anaemia) can identify a population of SSc patients at risk for SRC. Without sensitive detection and appropriate therapy (ACE inhibitors), SRC is a lethal feature of SSc. All SSc patients should be screened for SRC.

Strengths

1. Coordinates clinical evaluation with renal cortical blood flow measurements (^{133}Xe), outcomes, and renal histopathology.
2. Because therapy was ineffective in the era before 1974, these patients represent the natural history of SRC.
3. In general, these patients were thoroughly evaluated.

Weaknesses

1. Retrospective.
2. Experience of one institution.

Relevance

In the 1970s, SRC was the most lethal of the features of SSc. This article brings clinical, physiological, radiographic, and histopathological studies together to define the renal involvement of SSc.

Paper 3

Scleroderma (systemic sclerosis): classification, subsets and pathogenesis

Authors

LeRoy EC, Black C, Fleischmajer R, Jablonska S, Krieg T, Medsger TA Jr, Rowell N, Wollheim F

Reference

Journal of Rheumatology 1988; **15**:202–205

Abstract

A subclassification of SSc patients is proposed by a group of experienced investigators. The subsets are defined by skin involvement with limited cutaneous SSc (lcSSc) patients having no taut skin proximal to the knees, elbows or clavicles and diffuse cutaneous SSc (dcSSc) patients having truncal skin tautness.

Summary

A two-subset classification was proposed which is justified by survival data from the published studies of other investigators (Table 12.2).

Table 12.2 Survival in SSc (%) *

	1 year	6 years	12 years
lcSSc	98	80	50
dcSSc	80	30	15

*Adapted from Giordano M, Valentini G, Migliaresi S, *et al.* Different antibody patterns and different prognoses in patients with scleroderma with various extent of skin sclerosis. *Journal of Rheumatology* 1986; **13**:911–920.

Citation count

384

Related references **(1)** Masi AT, Rodnan GP, Medsger TA, *et al.* Subcommittee for Scleroderma Criteria of the American Rheumatism Association Diagnostic and Therapeutic Criteria Committee: Preliminary criteria for the classification of systemic sclerosis (scleroderma). *Arthritis and Rheumatism* 1980; **23**:581–590.

(2) Littlejohn GO, Barnett A, Miller M. Survival study of patients with scleroderma diagnosed over 30 years (1953–1983). The value of a cutaneous classification in the early stage of the disease. *Journal of Rheumatology* 1988; **15**:276–283.

Key message

Subsets defined by skin involvement can be instructive in overall prognosis, implying that skin and internal organ involvement in SSc are related to the same pathophysiological mechanism.

Why it's important

These guidelines have proved helpful to the physician in the evaluation of individual patients and to investigators in the classification of patient populations.

Strength

The consensus experience of the authors.

Weakness

Not subjected to a rigorous prospective study of new patients from multiple geographic areas.

Relevance

A consensus definition of two useful subsets of SSc.

Paper 4

Identification of a nuclear protein (Scl-70) as a unique target of human antinuclear antibodies in scleroderma

Authors

Douvas AS, Achten M, Tan EM

Reference

Journal of Biological Chemistry 1979; **254**:10514–10522

Abstract

The initial observations concerning an SSc-specific autoantigen, herein called Scl-70 from its size (partially degraded), which turned out to be topoisomerase I, a ubiquitous nuclear enzyme.

Summary

This is a careful immunohistochemical analysis of SSc-specific (both false positive and false negative examples are rare) and diffuse SSc-selective autoantibodies later shown to recognize the nuclear enzyme topoisomerase I. Other SSc-selective autoantibodies include anti-centromere, anti-RNA polymerase III, and anti-fibrillin I. Overlap syndromes have different autoimmune profiles. When careful autoimmune serology was combined with immunogenetic studies (HLA and allotypy), the very strong association between sequence-specific HLA haplotypes and autoantibodies of a specific type was realized to be the rule in human autoimmune disease. Often the HLA haplotype was more closely associated with the autoimmune pattern than was the clinical disease profile or outcome.

Citation count

207

Related references

(1) Rothfield NF, Rodnan GP. Serum antinuclear antibodies in progressive systemic sclerosis (scleroderma). *Arthritis and Rheumatism* 1968; **11**:607–617.

(2) Arnett FC. HLA and autoimmunity in scleroderma (systemic sclerosis). *Intern Rev Immunol* 1995; **12**:107–128.

Key message

With precise technique, autoantibodies can be useful in the diagnosis, subset staging, and prognosis in SSc.

Why it's important

This study provides a broad base of information regarding an important autoantibody in the SSc clinical armamentarium, touching on clinical issues and providing detailed immunochemical evaluation of the nature of the antigen by classical techniques.

Strengths

1. Immunochemical expertise.
2. Experience comparing other autoantibody reactions.

Weakness

Molecular genetic techniques, unavailable at the time of this study, could have provided full antigen identification.

Relevance

This study represents major progress in the precise definition of the autoimmune response of patients with SSc.

Paper 5

Connective tissue synthesis by scleroderma skin fibroblasts in cell culture

Author

LeRoy EC

Reference

Journal of Experimental Medicine 1972; **135**:1351–1362

Abstract

Skin fibroblasts are propagated by monolayer-explant tissue culture techniques from wrist and fore-arm biopsies of clinically and histologically involved skin from nine patients with SSc and grown as pairs with controls from skin biopsies from healthy donors matched for biopsy site, age, gender, and ethnicity. Hydroxyproline measurements showed 3-fold greater soluble collagen in media and 2.5-fold greater insoluble collagen in cell pellets from the SSc fibroblasts in the paired mass cell cultures. Glycoprotein production was also increased, based on sialic acid measurements.

Summary

Skin fibroblasts from subjects with SSc and control subjects were grown in tissue culture to compare the characteristics of connective tissue metabolism. A striking increase in soluble collagen (media hydroxyproline) was observed in eight of nine SSc cultures when they were compared with identically handled control cultures matched for age, sex, and the anatomic site of donor skin. Glycoprotein content as estimated by hexosamine and sialic acid was also significantly increased in the SSc cultures. Estimations of protein-polysaccharide content by uronic acid determinations were low in all cultures and not significantly increased in SSc cultures.

This report demonstrated the feasibility of using fibroblast cell cultures to study chronic rheumatic and connective tissue disorders (CTD). The initial results suggest a net increase in collagen and glycoprotein synthesis in SSc fibroblast cultures. The implications of an abnormality of connective tissue metabolism by skin fibroblasts propagated *in vitro* in the acquired disorder SSc are discussed.

Citation count

150

Related references

(1) Uitto J, Bauer EA, Eisen AZ. Scleroderma: increased biosynthesis of triple-helical type I and type III procollagens associated with unaltered expression of collagenase by skin fibroblasts in culture. *Journal of Clinical Investigation* 1979; **64**:921–930.

(2) Jimenez SA, Feldman G, Bashey RI, Bienkowski R, Rosenbloom J. Co-ordinate increase in the expression of type I and type III collagen genes in progressive systemic sclerosis fibroblasts. *Biochemical Journal* 1986; **237**:837–843.

Why it's important

The first demonstration of increased collagen production by cells from an involved organ of patients with SSc (or any other diffuse CTD), providing solid biochemical evidence to support the designation 30 years before that SSc (and others) was a 'collagen' disease. Subsequently, many other characteristics of the activated state of the SSc fibroblast have been determined.

Strengths

1. The first demonstration of an abnormality of collagen production in the fibrotic disease SSc.
2. An example of the value of direct cellular studies from lesional biopsies of patients with autoimmune disease.

Weaknesses

1. Collagen was not characterized as to type.
2. Mechanism of increased production was not delineated as to transcription, translation, or post-translational regulation.

Relevance

Increased levels of collagen production by fibroblasts from skin biopsies of involved skin of SSc patients early in their course of skin involvement was first observed here. This observation spawned an intense and continuing investigation by many laboratories of the characteristics of the activated SSc fibroblast and the regulation of the extracellular matrix in SSc and other fibrotic diseases.

Paper 6

Variable response to oral angiotensin-converting enzyme blockade in hypertensive scleroderma patients

Authors

Whitman HH III, Case DB, Laragh JH, Christian CL, Botstein G, Maricq H, LeRoy EC

Reference

Arthritis and Rheumatism 1982; **25**:241–8

Abstract

Twelve SSc patients with hypertension, seven of whom had malignant hypertension and renal failure or SRC, were treated with captopril. The first dose lowered mean pressure in all patients by 2.84 kPa (21.3 mmHg); in six patients it relieved encephalopathy. Blood pressure was controlled in all patients. Two of seven patients with SRC had improvement in renal function; the five patients who did not have malignant hypertension improved or stabilized. Despite good pressure control, however, renal failure developed in five patients with SRC. The data indicated that captopril is effective antihypertensive therapy in SSc and, when given early, may prevent renal failure and death.

Citation count

51

Related references

(1) D'Angelo WA, Fries JF, Masi AT, Shulman LE. Pathologic observations in systemic sclerosis (scleroderma). *American Journal of Medicine* 1969; **46**:428–440.

(2) Lopez-Overjero JA, Saal SD, D'Angelo WA, Cheigh JS, Stenzel KH, Laragh JH. Reversal of vascular and renal crisis of scleroderma by oral angiotensin-converting-enzyme blockade. *New England Journal of Medicine* 1979; **300**:1417–1419.

Why it's important

This study of twelve SSc patients with SRC treated with the first ACE inhibitor (captopril) demonstrated the efficacy of early detection and treatment, probably before renal cortical infarction had become complete.

Strength

An effective therapy for the often fatal SRC.

Weaknesses

1. Uncontrolled, not blinded, open study.
2. Relatively short follow up.

Relevance

Captopril and other ACE inhibitors have significantly prolonged life in SSc patients by preventing the sudden, severe renal insufficiency which half or so of SSc patients were at risk to develop. On ACE inhibitors, renal failure occurs rarely, and it is much more chronic and insidious in its course when compared with the pre-ACE inhibitor era.

Paper 7

Diagnostic potential of in vivo capillary microscopy in scleroderma and related disorders

Authors

Maricq HR, LeRoy EC, D'Angelo WA, Medsger TA Jr, Rodnan GP, Sharp GC, Wolfe JF

Reference

Arthritis and Rheumatism 1980; **23**:183–9

Abstract

The prevalence of scleroderma-type capillary abnormalities, as observed by in vivo microscopy, was determined in 173 patients from three rheumatic disease centres. The patients had a variety of CTDs: SSc 50; systemic lupus erythematosus (SLE) 60; mixed connective tissue disease (MCTD) 26; Raynaud's disease 11; other rheumatic disorders 26. Enlarged and deformed capillary loops surrounded by relatively avascular areas, most prominently in the nailfolds, were found in 82% of patients with SSc and in 54% with MCTD. The rarity of these abnormalities in SLE (2%) despite the presence of Raynaud's phenomenon suggests that they are not an expression of the Raynaud's phenomenon frequently associated with SSc and MCTD. The single patient with Raynaud's disease and scleroderma-type capillary changes subsequently developed SSc.

Summary

Maricq, et al. adapted widefield microscopy to study the capillaries of the nailfold. These studies, over 25 years, have helped to distinguish SSc subsets, have served as a guide to disease activity, and to separate the varieties of fasciitis from the major groups of limited and diffuse SSc (diffuse fasciitis with eosinophilia, eosinophilia myalgia syndrome, toxic oil syndrome), as well as MCTD patients at risk for pulmonary hypertension and localized SSc, by either the presence or absence of nailfold capillary changes of SSc type (dilatation and avascular areas).

Citation count

163

Related references **(1)** Brown GE, O'Leary PA. Skin capillaries in scleroderma. *Archives of Internal Medicine* 1925; **36**:73–88.

(2) Lewis T. Experiments relating to the peripheral mechanism involved in spasmodic arrest of the circulation in the fingers, a variety of Raynaud's Disease. *Heart* 1929; **15**:7–101.

(3) Banks BM. Is there a common denominator in scleroderma, dermatomyositis, disseminated lupus erythematosus, The Libman-Sacks Syndrome and polyarteritis nodosa. *New England Journal of Medicine* 1941; **225**:433–444.

Key message

A safe and user friendly technique provides significant clinical information early in the course of CTD syndromes, with implications as to diagnosis, subset delineation, activity assessment and prognosis.

Why it's important

Both generalist and specialist physicians have access in their office or clinic to the few tools necessary (low power microscope, epillumination, immersion oil, camera for reimbursement documentation) to evaluate all patients with Raynaud's phenomenon (5–20% of adult population) for early features of CTD.

Strengths

1. Adaptable to office practice.
2. Non-invasive, thus user friendly.
3. Inexpensive.
4. In SSc, dilated capillaries remain constant; thus test is reproducible.

Weaknesses

1. Requires modest training and experience on part of examiner.
2. Photography adds significant complexity.

Relevance

Widefield nailfold capillaroscopy for CTD has stood the test of time and widespread physician use. Hand in hand with SSc-selective serology (anti-centromere, topoisomerase I, RNA polymerase III and Th/To) it is the best screening procedure available. In fact, nailfold capillary patterns with serology constitute and define the most limited form of lcSSc (formerly CREST).

CHAPTER 13

Systemic vasculitis

David GI Scott

Introduction

The systemic vasculitides are a heterogeneous group of diseases that appear to be becoming commoner (or are recognized more frequently) in the last 5–10 years. Vasculitis can occur *de novo* (primary vasculitis) including diseases such as Wegener's granulomatosis, polyarteritis nodosa and Churg–Strauss syndrome, or can also be due to infections (especially viral), malignancy and chronic connective tissue diseases, such as rheumatoid arthritis (RA) and systemic lupus erythematosus (SLE).

The first description of systemic vasculitis is usually attributed to Kussmaul and Maier (1866) (1) though there were earlier descriptions by Rokitansky (2) and others. From this time until the early 1950s almost all vasculitides were called peri- (poly-) arteritis nodosa. The first author to rationally subdivide the many different clinical syndromes encompassing systemic vasculitis was Pearl Zeek who in a seminal review in the *American Journal of Clinical Pathology* in 1952 (Paper 1) classified vasculitis into five distinct subgroups. Classification systems have evolved over the ensuing 50 years but most are based on Zeek's original system. Classification criteria were first published in 1990 by the American College of Rheumatology (ACR) (3) who compared clinical features of eight different vasculitic syndromes and developed criteria which were useful only in distinguishing one type of vasculitis from another. A consensus was reached on the nomenclature to be used for vasculitis and definitions of specific vasculitides at a consensus conference in Chapel Hill in 1992 (published in 1994, Paper 2). These definitions and classifications have allowed more accurate recording on the epidemiology of vasculitis. The primary systemic vasculitides, though rare, probably occur in approximately 20/million/year, but when all primary and secondary vasculitides are included the incidence is probably in excess of 200/million/year.

The aetiology of vasculitis is poorly understood. Early studies in animal models examined the role of allergy and serum sickness. More recently there have been links with infections (hepatitis B and hepatitis C) and the link with autoantibodies has been established following the description of antibodies to anti-neutrophil cytoplasmic antigens (ANCA) in 1984 by van der Woude and colleagues (Paper 3). ANCA are now established in clinical practice to aid diagnosis and prognosis of systemic vasculitides, particularly Wegener's granulomatosis.

Corticosteroids improved the survival of patients with primary systemic vasculitis from approximately 10 to 50% at 2 years, though had less of an effect on Wegener's granulomatosis. The introduction of cyclophosphamide in the 1970s to treat systemic vasculitis has dramatically improved outcome significantly further (Paper 4). Cyclophosphamide is now the gold standard treatment for systemic vasculitis and current research is examining different ways of delivering cyclophosphamide or similar immunosuppressive drugs to reduce toxicity. This improved outcome has resulted in vasculitides now being thought of as chronic autoimmune diseases with many of the physical and psychological consequences seen in other rheumatic conditions such as RA and SLE.

References

1. Kaussmaul A, Maier R. Über eine bisher nicht beschreibene eigenthümliche Arterienerkrankung (Periarteritis nodosa), die mit Morbus Bright und rapid fortschreitender allgemeiner Muskellhmung einhergeht. *Deutsche Archive Klinical Medizin* 1886; **1**:484–514.

2. Rokitansky K. Ueber einige der wichtigsten Krankheiten der Arterien. Deukschriften der Kais. *Akademie der Wissenschaften Besonders Abgedrucket* 1852; **4**:49.

3. Fries JF, Hunder GG, Block DA, *et al.* The American College of Rheumatology 1990 criteria for the classification of vasculitis: summary. *Arthritis and Rheumatism* 1990; **33**:1135–1136.

Paper I

Periarteritis nodosa: a critical review

Author

Zeek PM

Reference

American Journal of Clinical Pathology 1952; **22**:777–790

Summary

This paper reviews literature from 1866–1952 in three eras, 1866–1900, 1900–1925 and 1925–1952. It covers clinical descriptions of vasculitis concentrating on putative aetiologies and the descriptions of vasculitis in animal models. In the early periods allergy and immunization, including serum sickness, were thought to be important factors. Clinical and histological descriptions appeared to include a number of different types of vasculitis which Zeek summarized and classified into five different types: (a) hypersensitivity angiitis, (b) allergic granulomatous angiitis, (c) rheumatic arteritis, (d) periarteritis nodosa, and (e) temporal arteritis.

Related references **(1)** Lie JT. Classification and immunodiagnosis of vasculitis: a new solution or promises unfulfilled? (Editorial). *Journal of Rheumatology* 1988; **15**:5.

(2) Scott DGI, Watts RA. Classification and epidemiology of systemic vasculitis. *British Journal of Rheumatology* 1994; **33**:897–899.

Key message

The first description/classification of vasculitis into five different types recognizing differences in clinical and histological features and outcome.

Why it's important

Prior to this review the term peri- (poly-) arteritis nodosa was used to describe a wide range of different diseases ranging from relatively benign small vessel vasculitis to potentially fatal systemic vasculitis (polyarteritis) and temporal arteritis, diseases which are now recognized to have very different aetiologies and outcomes. Zeek summarized the different putative aetiologies in some detail recognizing previous work on the potential role of allergy and serum sickness.

This important careful review of the literature on vasculitis up to 1952 explained not only the different clinical patterns but grouped together different types of vasculitis into five distinct patterns which has formed the basis for all current classification systems. The basis of Zeek's diseases can, for example, be seen in the classification systems described by Fauci and colleagues in the 1970s (Paper 4), Lie in the 1980s (1), the Chapel Hill consensus definitions (Paper 2) and Scott and Watts in the 1990s (2). It is interesting to note that only in the last 6 years has polyarteritis nodosa been clearly separated into microscopic polyangiitis and 'classic' polyarteritis nodosa in a way that has now been accepted internationally. Zeek in fact undertook this separation to some degree in her review.

Strengths

1. A comprehensive view of the literature.
2. A logical classification which formed the basis of future classifications.

Weaknesses

1. A review article and, therefore, contains no original research data.
2. Takayasu arteritis and Wegener's granulomatosis, though previously described, were not included.

Relevance

Zeek's classification of vasculitis has formed the basis of our understanding of the different vasculitic diseases. This paper was the first to acknowledge properly the different clinical and histological expressions of vasculitis and their prognosis, which was to become particularly relevant with concurrent introduction of corticosteroid treatment.

Paper 2

Nomenclature of systemic vasculitides: proposal of an international consensus conference

Authors

Jennette JC, Falk RJ, Andrassy K, Bacon PA, Churg J, Gross WL, Hagen EC, Hoffman GS, Hunder GG, Kallenberg CGM, McCluskey RT, Sinico RA, Rees AJ, van Es LA, Waldherr R, Wiik A

Reference

Arthritis and Rheumatism 1994; **37**:187–192

Summary

An *ad hoc* committee comprising clinicians and pathologists from six countries and multiple medical disciplines convened in Chapel Hill, North Carolina, with the aim of reaching a consensus on the names of the most common forms of non-infectious systemic vasculitis and to construct root definitions of the vasculitides so named. This publication includes a classification of vasculitis as well as definitions based on classical, clinical and pathological features of the commoner vasculitides linking them to vessel size.

Related references (1) Fries JF, Hunder GG, Block DA, *et al.* The American College of Rheumatology 1990 criteria for the classification of vasculitis: summary. *Arthritis and Rheumatism* 1990; **33**:1135–1136.

(2) Scott DGI, Watts RA. Classification and epidemiology of systemic vasculitis. *British Journal of Rheumatology* 1994; **33**:897–899.

Key message

The current nomenclature of vasculitis requires standardization. Definitions, if adopted internationally, will improve our understanding of these diseases.

Why it's important

In 1990 the ACR (1) published data describing classification criteria of eight different vasculitides based on an analysis collected prospectively from approximately 1000 patients with clinically well-defined vasculitis. Criteria were developed to separate one type of vasculitis from another. There were, however, no standard definitions for making the initial diagnosis. The ACR data did not, therefore, resolve many of the basic nomenclature problems surrounding systemic vasculitis and the classification criteria are only helpful in differentiating one type of vasculitis from another.

This paper provided the basic framework in terms of nomenclature for systemic vasculitis in that:

- It was the first to recognize microscopic polyangiitis within the overall classification system of vasculitis.
- It was the first to link putative aetiological factors (e.g. ANCA) with definitions.
- It redefined classical polyarteritis nodosa.

The distinction between polyarteritis nodosa and microscopic polyangiitis initially caused controversy but these descriptions have stood the test of time (so far).

Strengths

1. The definitions are clear and succinct and easy to apply in the clinical setting.
2. The consensus came from a wide spectrum of specialities.
3. These definitions are now widely used internationally.

Weaknesses

1. The definitions are subjective but have been (mis)used as classification criteria.
2. The international experts were to some degree self-selected.
3. The classification grouped together a disparate group of small vessel vasculitides ranging from potentially fatal Wegener's granulomatosis to benign cutaneous vasculitis. A more logical classification would separate Wegener's granulomatosis, Churg–Strauss syndrome and microscopic polyangiitis as being not only associated with ANCA, but also strongly associated with glomerulonephritis and more responsive to cyclophosphamide treatment, whereas Henoch Schonlein purpura, essential cryoglobulinaemia and cutaneous leucocytoclastic angiitis are associated with immune complex deposition rather than ANCA, cause less, if any, renal disease and rarely require aggressive immunosuppressive treatment (see Scott and Watts (2)).

Relevance

The definition of the different vasculitic diseases allows the international community to use a common language. This paper changed our understanding of polyarteritis nodosa and clearly identified differences between classic polyarteritis nodosa and microscopic polyangiitis (which had previously been included under the group hypersensitivity vasculitis). The ACR review found this group to have the poorest specificity and sensitivity in terms of classification criteria.

Paper 3

Autoantibodies against neutrophils and monocytes: tool for diagnosis and marker of disease activity and marker of disease activity in Wegener's granulomatosis

Authors

Van der Woude FJ, Lobatto S, Permin H, van der Giessen M, Rasmussen N, Wiik A, van Es LA, van der Hem GK, The TH

Reference

The Lancet 1985; **i**(February 23):425–429

Summary

Immunoglobulin G (IgG) autoantibodies against extra-nuclear components of polymorphonuclear granulocytes were detected in 25 of 27 serum samples from patients with active Wegener's granulomatosis and in only four of 32 samples from patients without signs of disease activity (Figure 13.1). In a prospective study these antibodies proved to be better markers of disease activity than several other laboratory measurements used previously. The autoantibodies were disease specific. This autoantibody may have a pathogenetic role in Wegener's granulomatosis. The detection of this antibody is valuable for diagnosis and estimation of disease activity.

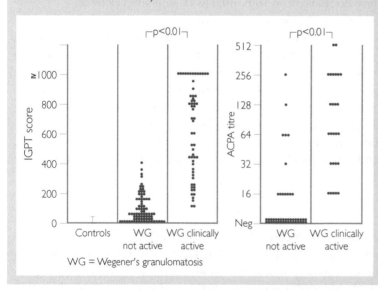

Figure 13.1 Relation of IgG ACPA titres and IGPT scores with disease activity.

Key message

This is the first description of a specific antibody associated with primary systemic vasculitis particularly Wegener' s granulomatosis.

Why it's important

Prior to this paper the aetiology of vasculitis was poorly understood. Vasculitis had often been considered amongst the connective tissue diseases but was notable for the absence of any obvious immune response. Indeed, the differentiation by histology between inflammation of the kidney due to connective tissue diseases such as lupus and the primary vasculitides was the absence of specific immune deposition in the primary vasculitides.

This paper was the first to recognize the link between these antibodies (which had only recently been described) and systemic vasculitis. The characterization of the antibody which evolved from this paper has resulted in an industry of research linking autoantibodies, neutrophils and endothelial cells in the pathogenesis of vasculitis. The first ANCA workshop meet in Copenhagen with 40 interested clinicians and pathologists. This has resulted in regular meetings, the last being the 9th ANCA workshop in Groningen including over 275 delegates. These antibodies are currently used to aid diagnosis and assess prognosis of primary systemic vasculitis, especially Wegener's granulomatosis. Subsequent studies have shown that in Wegener's the antibody has specificity against proteinase 3 (PR3). ANCA are also now used in the classification of vasculitis and link three diseases, Wegener's granulomatosis, microscopic polyangiitis and Churg–Strauss syndrome. The latter two are usually associated with a perinuclear staining with antibodies directed against myeloperoxidase, whereas Wegener's granulomatosis is associated with antibodies against PR3.

Strengths

1. Relatively large numbers of patients with classical Wegener's granulomatosis.
2. Wide range of normal and disease controls.
3. Clear message linking presence of the antibody to the disease.

Weaknesses

1. Disease activity criteria were only applied to the patient group.
2. Disease activity scores were applied retrospectively in many of the patients.

Relevance

Anti-nuclear cytoplasmic antibodies are now recognized as the most useful laboratory test in the diagnosis of systemic vasculitis. The link between specific antibodies against PR3 and Wegener's granulomatosis has been confirmed in many subsequent studies. The description of this antibody has led to huge expansion in the understanding of the relationship between autoimmunity, neutrophil and endothelial cell interactions leading to potentially new and exciting therapeutic targets.

Paper 4

Cyclophosphamide therapy of severe systemic necrotizing vasculitis

Authors

Fauci AS, Katz P, Barton MD, Haynes BF, Wolff SM

Reference

New England Journal of Medicine 1979; **301**(5):235–238

Summary

Seventeen patients with severe systemic vasculitis were studied over an 11 year period. Sixteen were treated daily with cyclophosphamide (2 mg/kg/day) and one with azathioprine. Before entering the study all patients had active and progressive disease even though 16 patients had been receiving corticosteroids that had caused severe and often incapacitating toxic effects. Three patients died during the study. Complete and often dramatic remissions occurred in the surviving 14 patients who were then placed on alternate-day corticosteroid treatment with continuation of cyclophosphamide. The mean duration of remission was 22 months (range 2–61).

Key message

First description of cyclophosphamide treatment for a wide range of systemic vasculitides in significant numbers showing a dramatic improvement in outcome.

Why it's important

Prior to the use of cyclophosphamide, the prognosis of systemic vasculitis, particularly Wegener's granulomatosis, was poor with a median survival in Wegener's with renal involvement of only 5 months. The overall mortality at 2 years for all diseases was less than 15% and even with corticosteroids this had only improved to 48%. The use of corticosteroids was also associated with significant toxicity. Previous descriptions of the use of immunosuppressive treatments was restricted to case reports of one or two patients only.

This paper established cyclophosphamide as the standard treatment for severe systemic vasculitis. The regime described by this group became known as the Fauci regime and was until only a few years ago the gold standard against which all other treatments were judged. Current international studies looking at new treatments of systemic vasculitis still use oral cyclophosphamide in most cases, though the length of treatment has been shortened owing to the discovery of significant long-term bladder toxicity with prolonged oral treatment.

Strengths

1. Large numbers of patients (when compared to previous studies).
2. Clear message showing clinical benefit in patients with severe disease.

Weaknesses

1. Patients studied over quite a long period of time in an uncontrolled fashion.
2. Varied clinical diagnoses included rheumatoid vasculitis, polyarteritis nodosa, microscopic polyangiitis and Wegener's granulomatosis.

Relevance

Vasculitis was transformed from a fatal disease to a treatable, though not always curable disease, with the use of cyclophosphamide which was introduced by Fauci and his colleagues from the National Institutes of Health. The outcome of these serious diseases was dramatically altered by a treatment which over the ensuing 20 years was consider the 'gold standard'.

CHAPTER 14

Sjögren's syndrome

Roland Jonsson

Introduction

Sjögren's syndrome (SS) is a chronic inflammatory and lymphoproliferative disease affecting ~0.5% of the population with autoimmune features and characterized by a progressive mononuclear cell infiltration of exocrine glands, notably the lacrimal and salivary glands (autoimmune exocrinopathy). These lymphoid infiltrations leads to dryness of the eyes (keratoconjunctivitis sicca), dryness of the mouth (xerostomia), and very frequently dryness of the nose, throat, vagina and skin. SS is associated with the production of autoantibodies since B cell activation is a consistent immue-regulatory abnormality. The spectrum of the disease extends from an organ-specific autoimmune disorder to a systemic process (musculoskeletal, pulmonary, gastric, haematological, dermatological, renal, and nervous system involvement). SS may develop alone (primary) or in association with almost any of the autoimmune rheumatic diseases (secondary), the most frequent being rheumatoid arthritis (RA) and systemic lupus erythematosus (SLE). SS is also associated with an increased risk of B cell lymphoma development. Current therapy provides only marginal symptomatic relief.

Sjögren's syndrome was described during the 19th century in a number of case reports with various combinations of dry mouth, dry eyes and chronic arthritis between the years of 1882 and 1924 (in 1). In 1892, Mikulicz reported a man with bilateral parotid and lachrymal gland enlargement associated with massive round cell infiltration (2). Gourgerot, in 1926, described three patients with salivary and mucous gland atrophy and insufficiency (3). In 1927 Mulock Houwer reported the association of filamentary keratitis, the major ocular manifestation of the syndrome, with chronic arthritis (in 1). In 1933 Henrik Sjögren, a Swedish opthalmologist, reported in his classical doctoral dissertation detailed clinical and histological findings in 19 women with xerostomia and keratoconjunctivitis sicca, of whom 13 had chronic arthritis (4). Later, in 1953, Morgan and Castleman established that SS and Mikulicz disease were the same entity (5). The link between SS and malignant lymphoma was described in a classical paper in 1964 (6). The distinction between primary and secondary SS was suggested in 1965 (7) and later verified (8, 9). From the diagnostic point of view the first histological grading assessing the infiltration of labial glands was described in 1968 (10). The SS associated (Ro/SSA) autoantibodies in the sera were described in 1969 (11). SS in families was described in a subsequent study (12). Gene interaction and complementation of the immune response was shown for human leucocyte antigen (HLA) and the RNA proteins Ro/SSA and La/SSB (13). A set of preliminary classification criteria was identified by a European Concerted Action group in 1993, which has been widely accepted (14).

The future challenge will be to further clarify the disease process including genetic and environmental influences. For this purpose, SS is a useful disease model to study the mechanisms of autoimmunity perhaps applicable to other autoimmune diseases.

References

1. Jonsson R, Haga H-J, Gordon T. Sjögren's syndrome. In: *Arthritis and Allied Conditions - A Textbook of Rheumatology* (Koopman WJ, ed.), 4th edition. Philadelphia: Williams & Wilkins, 2001: pp 1736–1759.

2. Mikulicz J. Über eine eigenartige symmetrische erkrankung der tränen- und mundspeicheldrüsen. *Beitr z Chir Festscr f Theodor Billrodt*, Stuttgart, 1892: 610–630.

3. Gourgerot H. Insufficance progresive et atrophie des glands salivaires et muqueuses de la bouche, des conjonctives (et parfois des muqueuses nasale, laryngée, vulvaire) sécheresse de la bouche, des conjonctives. *Bull Méd (Paris)* 1926; **40**:360–368.

4. Sjögren H. Zur kenntnis der keratoconjunctivis sicca. *Acta Opthalmologica* 1933; **11**(suppl. II):1–151.

5. Morgan WS, Castleman B. A clinicopathologic study of 'Mikulicz's disease'. *American Journal of Pathology* 1953; **29**:471–503.

6. Talal N, Bunim JJ. Development of malignant lymphoma in the course of Sjögren's syndrome. *American Journal of Medicine* 1964; **36**:529–540.

7. Bloch KJ, Buchanan WW, Wohl MJ, *et al.* Sjögren's syndrome: a clinical, pathological and serological study of sixty-two cases. *Medicine* 1965; **44**:187–231.

8. Moutsopoulos HM, Webber BL, Vlagopoulos TP, *et al.* Differences in the clinical manifestations of sicca syndrome in the presence and absence of rheumatoid arthritis. *American Journal of Medicine* 1979; **66**:733–736.

9. Moutsopoulos HM, Mann DL, Johnson AH, *et al.* Genetic differences between primary and secondary sicca syndrome. *New England Journal of Medicine* 1979; **301**:761–763.

10. Chisholm DM, Mason DK. Labial salivary gland biopsy in Sjögren's disease. *Journal of Clinical Pathology* 1968; **21**:656–660.

11. Clark G, Reichlin M, Tomasi TB. Characterization of a soluble cytoplasmic antigen reactive with sera from patients with systemic lupus erythematosus. *Journal of Immunology* 1969; **102**:117–122.

12. Reveille JD, Wilson RW, Provost TT, *et al.* Primary Sjögren's syndrome and other autoimmune diseases in families. Prevalence and immunogenetic studies in six kindreds. *Annals of Internal Medicine* 1984; **101**:748–756.

13. Harley JB, Reichlin M, Arnett FC, *et al.* Gene interaction at HLA-DQ enhances autoantibody production in primary Sjögren's syndrome. *Science* 1986; **232**:1145–1147.

14. Vitali C, Bombardieri S, Moutsopoulos H, *et al.* Preliminary criteria for the classification of Sjögren's syndrome: results of a prospective concerted action supported by the European Community. *Arthritis and Rheumatism* 1993; **36**:340–347.

Paper I

Zur kenntnis der keratoconjunctivis sicca: Keratitis filiformis bei hypofunktion der tränendrüsen

Author

Sjögren H

Reference

Acta Opthalmologica 1933; **11**(suppl.II):1–151

Summary

The first detailed description of 19 female patients with xerostomia and keratoconjunctivitis sicca, of whom 13 had chronic arthritis. Careful clinical and ophthalmological examinations are presented, which included microscopic examination of the lachrymal glands in 10 and parts of conjunctivae/corneae in 12 patients. In one patient who died, an autopsy was performed, which also included an examination of the salivary glands. Infiltration of round cells (mononuclear cells) in glandular parenchyma was described and found to be accumulated/focal in nature. The study laid the ground for the designation of a syndrome.

Related references (1) Mikulicz J. Über eine eigenartige symmetrische erkrankung der tränen–und mundspeicheldrüsen. *Beitr z Chir Festscr f Theodor Billrodt*, Stuttgart, 1892: 610–630.

(2) Gourgerot H. Insufficance progresive et atrophie des glands salivaires et muqueuses de la bouche, des conjonctives (et parfois des muqueuses nasale, laryngée, vulvaire) sécheresse de la bouche, des conjonctives. *Bull Méd (Paris)* 1926; **40**:360–368.

(3) Morgan WS, Castleman B. A clinicopathologic study of 'Mikulicz's disease'. *American Journal of Pathology* 1953; **29**:471–503.

Key message

The first detailed description of a fairly large number of patients, all women with xerostomia and keratoconjunctivitis sicca, of whom 13 had chronic arthritis, thereby establishing the name of the syndrome, and its association with RA.

Why it's important

At the time when Henrik Sjögren presented his dissertation he was well aware that each separate condition had been described before (1), i.e. keratitis filiformis by Leber already in 1882 (in reference1, Introduction), dry mouth (xerostomia) by Hadden in 1888 (in reference 1, Introduction) and the combination by the French dermatologist Henri Gourgerot in 1926 (2). In 1927, Muloch Houwer described joint symptoms in connection with keratitis filiformis, and Houwer in fact found that one case report had been published by the German Erich Fischer already in 1889 (in reference 1, Introduction).

In 1933, Henrik Sjögren had collected a total of 19 cases, all female aged 29–72 years. He had conducted careful clinical and ophthalmological studies, which included microscopic examination of the lachrymal glands and parts of conjunctivae/corneae and in one patient examination of the salivary glands. This made up the basis of Henrik Sjögren's classical doctoral dissertation. Further, Sjögren coined the expression 'keratoconjunctivitis sicca' and he had previously carefully described a method to stain the damaged cells in the conjunctiva and cornea by using 1% Bengal rose, a staining similar to that seen in 'keratitis filiformis'.

Strengths

1. The first detailed description of a fairly large number of patients with xerostomia and keratoconjunctivitis sicca.
2. Definition of keratoconjunctivitis sicca.
3. The suggestion that SS was part of a systemic disease.

Weaknesses

1. The thesis was published in German and thus gained limited initial recognition.
2. Salivary gland tissue was examined in only one patient.

Relevance

The thesis increased the awareness of SS as a systemic disease in particular after it was translated to English by Dr Bruce Hamilton in 1943. It also laid the foundation for future studies in the field (3), which started predominantly in the 1960s.

Paper 2

Development of malignant lymphoma in the course of Sjögren's syndrome

Authors

Talal N, Bunim JJ

Reference

American Journal of Medicine 1964; **36**:529–540

Summary

Of 58 patients with SS followed at the National Institute of Arthritis and Metabolic Diseases, reticulum cell sarcomas developed in three, and lesions resembling Waldenström's macroglobulinaemia in a fourth. These changes were present in lymph nodes and organs exclusive of the salivary and lacrimal glands. These patients have certain clinical and laboratory features in common which distinguish them from patients with the usual benign cases of SS. These features include a relatively high incidence of splenomegaly, purpura, vasculitis, leukopenia, lymphopenia and hypogammaglobulinaemia. The gamma globulin abnormalities have been investigated by immunoelectrophoretic analysis, utracentrifugation and fluorescent antibody techniques. In one patient, gamma globulin decreased from elevated to markedly low levels; the rheumatoid factor (RF) and tissue antibodies disappeared as reticulum cell sarcoma developed. In another patient, lymph nodes were populated with an abnormally large proportion of cells containing 19S macroglobulin, and several cells exhibited unusual intranuclear inclusions, which stained positive with periodic acid-Schiff stain. The relationship between connective tissue diseases, gamma globulin abnormalities, thymomas and malignant lymphomas is discussed. The hypothesis is presented that in SS the chronic state of immunological hyperactivity and the proliferation of immunologically competent cells producing abnormal tissue antibodies predispose to the relatively frequent development of malignant lymphoma.

Related references (1) Bunim JJ, Talal N. The association of malignant lymphoma with Sjögren's syndrome. *Transactions of the Association of American Physicians* 1963; **76**:45–56.

(2) Kassan S, Thomas T, Moutsopoulos HM. Increased risk of lymphoma in sicca syndrome. *Annals of Internal Medicine* 1978; **89**:888–892.

(3) Voulgarelis M, Dafni UG, Isenberg DA, Moutsopoulos HM and Members of the European Concerted Action on SS: Jonsson R, Haga H-J, *et al.* Malignant lymphoma in primary Sjögren's syndrome – A multicenter, retrospective, clinical study by the European Concerted Action on Sjögren's syndrome. *Arthritis and Rheumatism* 1999; **42**:1765–1772.

Key message

The paper illustrates development of malignant lymphoma, the most severe outcome/complication of SS.

Why it's important

Sjögren's syndrome is considered a benign but systemic condition characterized by infiltration of the salivary and lacrimal glands with lymphoid cells, by hypergammaglobulinaemia and by the presence of multiple circulating antibodies directed against various tissue components. It is clear from the sequence of the clinical pathological events described in the paper that the occurrence of SS and the enhanced immunological reactivity preceded by several years the development of malignant lymphomas. It seems reasonable to speculate that the chronic state of immunological hyperactivity and presumably, the associated proliferation of lymphoid cells predispose to the development of malignant lymphoma. It is possible, although unlikely, that SS is actually an early manifestation of an occult lymphoma. However, this appears unlikely due to the following: (a) the benign lesions present in the biopsy specimens of salivary glands; (b) the long course of illness, and (c) the frequency of purpura, vasculitis and abnormal tissue antibodies.

Strengths

1. Documentation of a severe complication in SS.
2. The study comprises well characterized patients.

Weaknesses

1. The report is only a collection of cases and without a control/comparative group.
2. The prevalence and relative risk of lymphoma development is not presented.

Relevance

The awareness that malignant lymphoma can develop in the course of SS is of fundamental clinical importantance (1, 2). One of the risk factors is parotid swelling. Other frequent accompanying clinical presentations are skin vasculitis, peripheral nerve involvement, anaemia, and lymphopenia (3). The clinical and laboratory data suggest that SS is a disease of unusually aggressive B cell activation which begins in the salivary glands and later becomes extra-glandular with a strong propensity to malignant transformation at any time in its course. The finding of monoclonal immunoglobulins or light chains in many SS patients suggests that a monoclonal process is present very early and coexists with the polyclonal B cell disorder.

Paper 3

Sjögren's syndrome: a clinical, pathological and serological study of sixty-two cases

Authors

Bloch KJ, Buchanan WW, Wohl MJ, Bunim JJ

Reference

Medicine 1965; **44**:187–231

Summary

The clinical, serological, and pathological characteristics of five different subgroups of patients with SS are reported. These groups consisted of 30 patients in whom the sicca complex was associated with definite or classical RA (Group A), two with 'probable' RA (Group B), three with progressive systemic sclerosis (Group C), and four patients with polymyositis (Group D). In addition, 23 patients had the sicca complex in the absence of an associated connective tissue disease (Group E).

Histological examinations of salivary glands from 20 patients in this series (16 biopsy and five post-mortem specimens) presented a fairly wide spectrum of changes from acinar atrophy with adipose replacement and relatively sparse lymphocytic infiltration, to massive lymphocytic infiltration and replacement of acinar by lymphoid tissue. Proliferative changes in the duct-lining cells were noted in 70% of specimens, but in only 45% had these progressed to epi-myo-epithelial islands. Germinal centres were found in six biopsies. The integrity of lobular architecture was preserved in all cases. Patients with SS, particularly those in Group E, frequently had hypergammaglobulinemia, and RFs were demonstrated in the serum of nearly all patients in this series regardless of the absence of rheumatoid joint disease. Rheumatoid factors occurred in Group E with a frequency found in only one other condition, RA accompanied by subcutaneous nodules. Antibodies directed against several nuclear and cytoplasmic antigens were detected, especially in the serum of patients in Group E. It was not possible to demonstrate antibodies directed specifically against lacrimal or salivary gland constituents. Reticulum-cell sarcoma developed in three patients several years after the onset of SS and one patient developed extensive abnormal but not malignant lymphoid infiltrates in several organs. The relationship between radiation therapy directed at the salivary and lacrimal glands and the development of these lesions was discussed.

Methylcellulose is the drug of choice for keratoconjunctivitis sicca. Although systemic corticosteroid administration does cause a reduction in size of enlarged lacrimal and salivary glands, it does not increase secretion and is therefore not indicated as treatment of SS. Antimalarial drugs have not been effective. Radiation therapy to enlarged glands cannot be recommended. Neuropathy in one patient associated with arteritis but not with RA, responded well to corticosteroid therapy.

Related references **(1)** Moutsopoulos HM, Webber BL, Vlagopoulos TP, Chused TM, Decker JL. Differences in the clinical manifestations of sicca syndrome in the presence and absence of rheumatoid arthritis. *American Journal of Medicine* 1979; **66**:733–736.

(2) Moutsopoulos HM, Mann DL, Johnson AH, Chused TM. Genetic differences between primary and secondary sicca syndrome. *New England Journal of Medicine* 1979; **301**:761–763.

Key message

The study offered the first and current definition of SS as a triad of keratoconjunctivitis sicca, xerostomia and another connective tissue disease with two of three components considered sufficient for diagnosis.

Why it's important

Much interest has been focussed on the clinical and immunological derangements in the connective tissue diseases, which have in common the presence of circulating autoantibodies against one or several tissues or proteins. The present study delineated and characterized several clinical subgroups of SS. About one-half of the patients had RA associated with the sicca syndrome. In the majority of these, widespread and destructive joint disease was evident. The coexistence of the sicca syndrome in such patients suggests an association with more fully expressed RA. From a wide spectrum of clinical manifestations and course an ordered definition is presented. Such clinical information is highly appreciated. Altogether, this was an early paper which was the first comprehensive study of SS.

Strengths

1. A clear and concise definition of SS is presented.
2. Description of diseases to exclude.

Weaknesses

1. Imperfect definition of xerostomia.
2. The study lacks analysis of anti-Ro/SSA and anti-La/SSB.

Relevance

The definition of SS together with the distinction of one primary and one secondary form to a great extent increased the attention of this enigmatic and distressing syndrome. Subsequent studies delineated further both the clinical manifestations (1) as well as the genetic differences (2) between primary and secondary SS. These early clinical studies laid the ground for subsequent attempts to further define the genetics behind the disease as well as defining diagnostic and classification criteria for SS.

Paper 4

Labial salivary gland biopsy in Sjögren's disease

Authors

Chisholm DM, Mason DK

Reference

Journal of Clinical Pathology 1968; **21**:656–660

Summary

A labial biopsy technique is described and was used to study 40 patients with connective tissue disease and 60 post-mortem subjects. More than one focus of lymphocytes per 4 mm^2 (0.08 in^2) of minor salivary tissue (grade 4) was found to be a consistent finding in patients with SS. The labial biopsy is shown to be a further valuable investigative procedure in such patients.

Related references **(1)** Greenspan JS, Daniels TM, Talal N, Sylvester RA. The histopathology of Sjögren's syndrome in labial salivary gland biopsies. *Oral Surgery, Oral Medicine and Oral Pathology* 1974; **37**:217–229.

(2) Daniels TE. Labial salivary gland biopsy in Sjögren's syndrome. Assessment as a diagnostic criterion in 362 suspected cases. *Arthritis and Rheumatism* 1984; **27**:147–156.

(3) Daniels TE, Whitcher JP. Association of patterns of labial salivary gland inflammation with keratoconjunctivitis sicca. Analysis of 618 patients with suspected Sjögren's syndrome. *Arthritis and Rheumatism* 1994; **37**:869–877.

Key message

The labial salivary gland biopsy is shown to be a valuable diagnostic tool in SS.

Why it's important

A useful and internationally agreed definition of the disease exists (reference 7, Introduction) but there are no fully agreed criteria for diagnosing SS. The oral component of SS begins with lymphocytic infiltration of the major and minor salivary glands, causing various oral symptoms, insidious decrease in resting and stimulated salivary flow, and changes in the composition and physical characteristics of saliva. Occasional enlargements of major glands in SS usually represent the histopathological entity called '(benign) lymphoepithelial lesion', which is a firm, non-tender swelling that usually affects the entire gland. The presence of a benign lymphoepithelial lesion in a major salivary gland or sufficient focal lymphocytic sialadenitis (Figure 14.1) in a minor salivary gland biopsy specimen provides objective, disease-associated evidence of the salivary component of SS. This paper was the first to describe that the severity of infiltration in minor glands can be graded. Further, the subsequent suggestion of a focus scoring (1–3) of sialadenitis can provide a threshhold for individual diagnosis representing a semi-quantitative assessment.

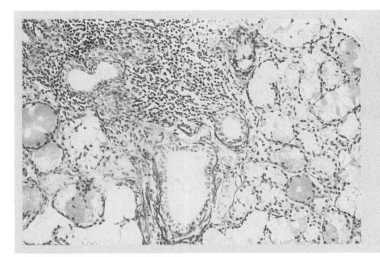

Figure 14.1 Focal sialadenitis in a labial salivary gland biopsy.

Strengths

1. Introduced focal lymphocytic sialadenitis in the minor salivary glands as an important diagnostic tool.
2. Established a semi-quantitative significance threshold for patients at >1 lymphocytic focus/4 mm^2 (0.08 in^2) glandular tissue.
3. Correlation with post-mortem specimens.

Weaknesses

1. Related focal sialadenitis to only a few other clinical manifestations of the syndrome.
2. Rather small sample material.

Relevance

There is great need for internationally accepted diagnostic criteria for both primary and secondary SS, but such criteria need to be as disease-specific as possible. There is no current diagnostic gold standard against which to calculate accurately the sensitivity and specificity values for diagnostic tests in SS, or for any other syndrome. Based on the strong association between focal sialadenitis in an adequate labial salivary gland biopsy specimen and consistent and rigorous tests for keratoconjunctivitis sicca (2, 3), proposed tests can be assessed against the histological criterion. Alternative tests in the diagnosis of SS should be proposed to be included in the criteria only when it is clear that all such tests are diagnostically equivalent.

Paper 5

Characterization of a soluble cytoplasmic antigen reactive with sera from patients with systemic lupus erythematosus

Authors

Clark G, Reichlin M, Tomasi TB

Reference

Journal of Immunology 1969; **102**:117–122

Summary

A tissue antigen reactive with sera from SLE patients has been partially characterized. The antigen is a soluble cytoplasmic component which is present in a variety of human tissues and is distinct from known nuclear antigens. It is an acidic macromolecule which has the electrophoretic mobility of an alpha$_1$ globulin and is resistant to most proteolytic enzymes including trypsin, pepsin and chymotrypsin. Antigenicity is destroyed by 0.02 M periodate and by 0.001 M parahydroxy mercuribenzoate. Antibodies to this antigen have been found in 40% of unselected SLE sera and were absent from a large number of sera from normal persons and from the sera of patients with other connective tissue disorders.

Related references   **(1)**   Anderson JR, Gray KG, Beck JS, Kinnear WF. Precipitating autoantibodies in Sjögren's syndrome. *The Lancet* 1961; **ii**:456–460.

(2)   Mattioloi M, Reichlin M. Heterogeneity of RNA protein antigens reactive with the sera in systemic lupus erythematosus. Description of a cytoplasmic non-ribosomal antigen. *Arthritis and Rheumatism* 1974; **17**:421–429.

(3)   Alspaugh MA, Tan EM. Antibodies to cellular antigens in Sjögren's syndrome. *Journal of Clinical Investigation* 1975; **55**:1067–1073.

(4)   Tengnér P, Halse A-K, Haga H-J, Jonsson R, Wahren-Herlenius M. Detection of anti-Ro/SSA and anti-La/SSB autoantibody producing cells in salivary glands from patients with Sjögren's syndrome. *Arthritis and Rheumatism* 1998; **41**:2238–2248.

Key message

Present the first characterization of a tissue antigen, Ro, which reacts with many Sjögren's syndrome sera.

Why it's important

The results from this study show the Ro antigen to be distinct from the nuclear antigens thus far described (1) (Figure 14.2). The antigen is derived primarily from the soluble cytoplasmic fraction of a human tissue homogenate (2). It is present in many human organs as well as tissues of some other species. The Ro peptide is a 60 kD single chain protein. Peptides derived from Ro retain a portion of immune reactivity.

Antibodies to the Ro antigen were found in SS and SLE (3) and have not been detected in normal sera or in significant numbers in sera of patients with scleroderma, polymyositis, RA, myeloma and other diseases. Together with La, these autoantibodies established SS as an autoimmune disease (3). The clinical relationships of autoantibodies to forms of disease expression are the most powerful evidence that they are involved in the immunopathogenesis of SS.

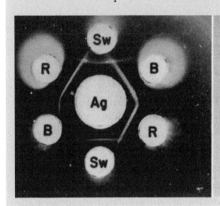 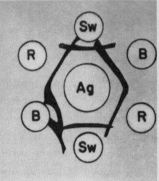

Figure 14.2 Ouchterlony agar diffusion demonstrating the Ro antigen (from reference 11, Introduction).

Strengths

1. First characterization of the Ro antigen.
2. Established SS as an autoimmune disease.

Weakness

No molecular forms (e.g. Ro52) were analysed separately.

Relevance

Like RF and anti-nuclear antibody (ANA), anti-Ro but also anti-La cannot be considered specific for SS. There is also some variation in presented figures for positivity depending on laboratory techniques for detection as well as patient cohort sampling and referrals (in reference 1, Introduction). Over 60% of patients with subacute cutaneous lupus have Ro and half of whom also have La precipitins. Approximately 30 and 10% of SLE have Ro and La precipitins, respectively. Anti-Ro is also common in neonatal lupus. The figures for SS are 60–75% positive for Ro and about 40% positive for La.

Though autoantibodies are clearly at least associated with extraglandular manifestations such as vasculitis, purpura and leukopenia there is less convincing evidence that they are directly involved in the destruction of the salivary (4) and lacrimal glands. However, this paper started the autoantibody/autoimmune parade for SS and served to illustrate the close relationship between lupus and SS.

Paper 6

Primary Sjögren's syndrome and other autoimmune diseases in families. Prevalence and immunogenetic studies in six kindreds

Authors

Reveille JD, Wilson RW, Provost TT, Bias WB, Arnett FC

Reference

*Annals of Internal Medicine*1984; **101**:748–756

Summary

The relationship of HLA and heavy chain immunoglobulin (Gm) haplotypes to disease and autoantibody expression were examined in six large kindreds, each having one or more members with primary SS. Various other autoimmune diseases and autoantibodies occurred among the 117 relatives in these families. The HLA and Gm haplotypes did not necessarily segregate persons into those with SS, other autoimmune disorders, or serological abnormalities, but HLA alleles DR3 and DR2 occurred in significant excess in relatives with SS, irrespective of HLA haplotype. Segregation analysis suggested a Mendelian dominant genetic defect common to the many autoimmune diseases and serological reactions that was not linked to HLA or Gm. A significant effect of female sex was also documented. These studies suggest that SS results from the interaction of several HLA-linked and non-HLA genes.

Related references (1) Provost TT, Talal N, Harley JB, Reichlin M, Alexander E. The relationship between anti-Ro (SS-A) antibody positive Sjögren's syndrome and anti-Ro (SS-A) antibody-positive lupus erythematosus. *Archives of Dermatology* 1988; **124**:63–71.

(2) Provost TT, Talal N, Bias W, Harley JB, Reichlin M, Alexander E. Ro (SS-A) positive Sjögren's/lupus erythematosus (SS/LE) overlap patients are associated with the HLA-DR3 and/or DRw6 phenotypes. *Journal of Investigative Dermatology* 1988; **91**:369–371.

(3) Rischmueller M, Lester S, Chen Z, Champion G, Van Den Berg R, Beer R, Coates T, McCluskey J, Gordon T. HLA class II phenotype controls diversification of the autoantibody response in primary Sjögren's syndrome. *Clinical and Experimental Immunology* 1998; **111**:365–371.

Key message

The study suggests that SS results from the interaction of several HLA-linked but also genes outside the HLA system.

Why it's important

The occurrence of SS as well as other autoimmune diseases in family members of patients with this syndrome has previously been well described but most often as case reports. This paper was one of the first indications that autoimmunity in general tends to aggregate in families. A survey of family histories in 98 unrelated patients with SS has shown similar high frequencies of sicca syndrome as well as other diseases of autoimmunity. Twelve percent of 51 patients with primary SS had at least one other relative with the same disorder. Interestingly, this 12% familiar clustering of primary is comparable to that reported for SLE. In fact, this study suggests intimate relationships between primary and SLE in that these two disorders tended to cluster in the same families. The study presented a future-looking idea, since the studies to check this out are only now just underway.

Strengths

1. The relationships of HLA to disease and autoantibody expression is presented.
2. A significant effect of female sex was documented.
3. Clustering of SS and SLE in families.

Weaknesses

1. Twin studies are lacking.
2. The study is fairly descriptive.
3. Full genome scanning is lacking (but not available at that time).

Relevance

The apparent excess of SS and other autoimmune diseases in relatives of patients with SS suggests an heriditary predisposition. Relatives with SS, other disorders, or serological abnormalities (1) do not necessarily need to share HLA haplotypes. Thus, a simple model of Mendelian inheritance linked to HLA seems unlikely. However, the inheritance of a certain HLA allele, HLA-DR3, appears to occur independently of HLA haplotypes shared with other affected relatives (2). Mechanisms underlying certain HLA effects are also unknown, although some studies have suggested that HLA alleles are more strongly associated with the production of a particular antibody response in these disorders (3). Altogether, these studies suggest that SS and the other autoimmune diseases seen in families result from many genetics effects and are multifactorial.

Paper 7

Gene interaction at HLA-DQ enhances autoantibody production in primary Sjögren's syndrome

Authors

Harley JB, Reichlin M, Arnett FC, Alexander E, Bias WB, Provost TT

Reference

Science 1986; **232**:1145–1147

Summary

Primary SS is an autoimmune disorder characterized by dryness of the mouth and eyes. The HLA locus DQ is related to the primary SS autoantibodies that bind the RNA proteins Ro/SSA and La/SSB. Both DQ1 and DQ2 alleles are associated with high concentrations of these autoantibodies. An analysis of all possible combinations at DQ has shown that the entire effect was due to heterozygotes expressing the DQ1 and DQ2 alleles. These data suggest that gene interaction between DQ1 and DQ2 (or alleles at associated loci), possibly from gene complementation of trans-associated surface molecules, influences the autoimmune response in primary SS.

Related references (1) Hamilton RG, Harley JB, Bias WB, Roebber M, Reichlin M, Hochberg MC, Arnett FC. Two Ro (SS-A) autoantibody responses in systemic lupus erythematosus. Correlation of HLA-DR/DQ specificities with quantitative expression of Ro (SS-A) autoantibody. *Arthritis and Rheumatism* 1988; **31**:496–505.

(2) Scofield RH, Frank MB, Neas BR, Horowitz RM, Hardgrave KL, Fujisaku A, McArthur R, Harley JB. Cooperative association of T cell beta receptor and HLA-DQ alleles in the production of anti-Ro in systemic lupus erythematosus. *Clinical Immunology and Immunopathology* 1994; **72**:335–341.

(3) Fujisaku A, Frank MB, Neas B, Reichlin M, Harley JB. HLA-DQ gene complementation and other histocompatibility relationships in man with the anti-Ro/SSA autoantibody response of systemic lupus erythematosus. *Journal of Clinical Investigation* 1990; **86**:606–611.

Key message

Gene interaction between two HLA loci suggest gene complementation.

Why it's important

The genetic composition at the HLA locus DQ has been shown to have an important effect upon the relative quantitative concentrations of autoantibodies present in sera from patients with primary SS. Patients who are heterozygous at the HLA-DQ for the alleles DQ1 and DQ2 have much higher levels of anti-Ro/SSA, anti-La/SSB, RF and ANA. Gene interaction at HLA-DQ then contributes to higher levels of autoantibodies. The most intriguing possibility is that this data does indeed reflect gene complementation by the physical association of multiple polymorphic gene products. This paper shows that the HLA relationships are complicated and that they operate at the level of risk for disease as well as at the level of probability of anti-Ro and anti-La antibodies in SS. Later work confirmed these relationships for anti-Ro in SLE (1) and also implicated the T cell receptor (2).

Strengths

1. Illustrates clearly the HLA linkage in SS.
2. Gene complementation gives raised autoantibody levels.

Weakness

Used serology for HLA-typing (the only available method in 1986).

Relevance

In a subsequent study it was shown that the anti-Ro response had gene complementation in SLE (3) consistent with what had been observed in SS. However, this time it was done at the DNA level using an approach which revealed more of the polymorphic richness of the HLA. The pathogenic mechanisms and disease perpetuation/chronicity in SS remains unknown. The most urgent issues for understanding SS are consequently studies of aetiology and detailed pathogenic processes. The roles that genetic factors and autoantibodies play will be of utmost importance for progress in this field.

Paper 8

Preliminary criteria for the classification of Sjögren's syndrome: results of a prospective concerted action supported by the European Community

Authors

Vitali C, Bombardieri S, Moutsopoulos H, *et al.*

Reference

Arthritis and Rheumatism 1993; **36**:34–347

Summary

Objective. Different sets of diagnostic criteria have been proposed for SS, but none have been validated with a large series of patients or in a multicentre study. We conducted the present study involving 26 centres from 12 countries (11 in Europe, plus Israel), with the goals of reaching a consensus on the diagnostic procedures for SS and defining classification criteria to be used in epidemiological surveys and adopted by the scientific community.

Methods: The study protocol was subdivided into two parts. For part 1, questionnaires regarding both ocular and oral involvement were developed; they included 13 questions and seven questions, respectively. For part II a limited set of diagnostic tests was selected, and the exact procedure to be followed in performing these tests was defined. Part 1 of the study included 240 patients with primary SS and 240 age- and sex-matched controls. Two hundred and forty-six patients with primary SS, 201 with secondary SS, 113 with connective tissue diseases but without associated SS, and 133 control patients were studied in part II.

Results: The study resulted in (a) the validation of a simple six-item questionnaire for determination of dry eyes and dry mouth, which showed good discriminant power between patients and controls, to be used in the initial screening for sicca syndrome, and (b) the definition of a new set of criteria for the classification of SS. The sensitivity and specificity of the criteria in correctly identifying patients with either the primary or the secondary variant of SS were also determined.

Conclusion: Using the findings of this prospective multicentre European study, general agreement can be reached on the diagnostic procedures to be used for patient with SS. Final validation of the preliminary classification criteria for SS is underway.

Related references (1) Daniels TE, Silverman S, Michalski JP, Greenspan JS, Sylvester RA, Talal N. The oral component of Sjögren's syndrome. *Oral Surgery, Oral Medicine and Oral Pathology* 1975; **39**:875–885.

(2) Manthorpe R, Frost-Larsen K, Isager H, Prause JU. Sjögren's syndrome. A review with emphasis on immunlogical features. *Allergy* 1981; **36**:139–153.

(3) Fox RI, Robinson CA, Curd JG, Kozin F, Howell FV. Sjögren's syndrome: proposed criteria for classification. *Arthritis and Rheumatism* 1986; **29**:577–585.

Related references   (4)   Vitali C, Moutsopoulos HM, Bombardieri S, *et al*. The European
community study group on diagnostic criteria for Sjögren's syn-
drome. Sensitivity and specificity of tests for ocular and oral
involvement in Sjögren's syndrome. *Annals of Rheumatic Diseases*
1994; **53**:637–647.

Key message

Definition and validation of simple tools that may be used to measure the prevalence of SS in
the general population, and to reach agreement on classification criteria for this disease.

Why it's important

Although there has been a useful and internationally agreed-upon definition of SS available
for more than 30 years (Paper 3), there has been shortage of fully agreed criteria for diagnosing it. Understanding the clinical spectrum for SS and the various tests used to diagnose
its components (1) provides a basis for further refinement of potential criteria (2, 3). The
spectrum of the presentation of the disorder is very broad, ranging from the local consequences of exocrine gland dysfunction to major, life-threatening systemic complications.
Although SS was once thought to be rare, recent data suggest that the prevalence of this condition may approach or even exceed that of RA. Up to now, patients with SS have been
missed at diagnosis or uncorrectly classified, due to both great variability at disease presentation and to the lack of well-defined and commonly accepted diagnostic criteria. Thus, this
study report the results of a multicentre study performed in Europe and supported by the
European Commission.

Strengths

1. Use of diagnostic sensitivity and specificity calculations for each symptom and test.
2. The study was a multicentre procedure.

Weaknesses

1. The criteria are too inclusive by including subjective symptoms and having few/no exclusions.
2. Each test was performed on only 26–90% of the patients studied.
3. Thus, the sensitivity and specificity calculations might not be methodologically sound.

Relevance

The main accomplishments of the study were: (a) the validation of a simple questionnaire
for dry eyes and dry mouth, to be used as the first step in the selection of potential patients
with SS, and (b) the definition of a set of classification criteria that is both highly specific and
highly sensitive (4) in discriminating patients with primary or secondary SS from controls
and from patients with connective tissue disease but without SS (Figure 14.3, overleaf).
There is clearly a need for internationally accepted diagnostic criteria for this disorder, but
those criteria must be as disease-specific as possible. The diagnosis of SS is significant for at
least two reasons: (a) clinically, a diagnosis of SS commits the patient to living with the spec-
tre of an incurable and potentially progressive disease; (b) scientifically, if patients are
included in studies of SS on the basis of subjective or less-specific criteria, some will be
included who do not have a systemic and immunological mediated disease. Our ability to
increase knowledge on the genetic background, the epidemiology and the pathogenesis of
this clinically and scientifically important entity will thus be hampered.

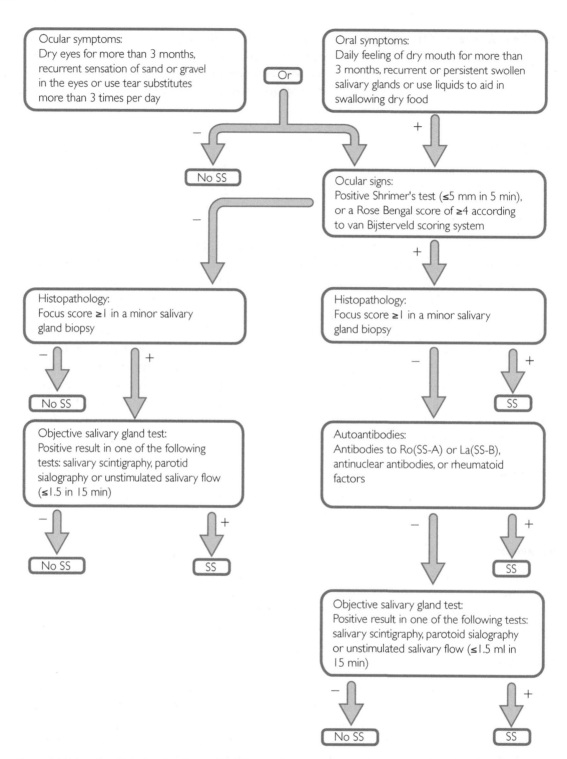

Figure 14.3 An algorithm for the diagnosis of Sjögren's syndrome based on the European criteria (reference 14, Introduction).

Acknowledgements

The following experts on Sjögren's syndrome and rheumatic disease selection of papers and the content and are hereby acknowledged: Anne Isine Bolstad, Troy Daniels, Tom P Gordon, Hans-Jacob Haga, John B Harley, Haralampos Moutsopoulos, Norman Talal, Claudio Vitali, Kate Frøland and Karl Brokstad are acknowledged for editorial assistance. R.J. is supported by EU grants BMH4-CT96-0595, BMH4-CT98-3489, The NorFA grant # 98.15.022-0 and the Research Council of Norway grant # 115563/320.

CHAPTER 15

Myositis

Frederick W Miller and Paul H Plotz

Introduction

We have selected six key publications for this review which have helped to mould our current understanding of a rare but increasingly recognized group of syndromes characterized by chronic idiopathic muscle inflammation. These classic papers include: the first scholarly review of the then known myositis cases; the first use of methotrexate in steroid-resistant patients; the first careful delineation of diagnostic criteria and clinical groups; the best descriptions of immunopathological differences among dermatomyositis (DM), polymyositis (PM), and inclusion body myositis (IBM); the clearest description of the phenotypic and prognostic distinctiveness of IBM, and finally a large study documenting the recent discovery that myositis can be divided into clinically useful groups by the use of the myositis-specific autoantibodies.

Although cases of myositis were described in Europe in the latter part of the 19th century, Steiner's detailed and scholarly report of a case of DM in 1903 (Paper 1) introduced the disease to the English-speaking world. Just as the concept of rheumatoid arthritis (RA) as a condition separate from its phenocopies did not become clear until several decades into this century, so too did PM, the subtler cousin of DM, not crystallize as a distinct entity until the publication of Walton and Adams' wonderful monograph in the 1950s (1). In our view, the separation of the inflammatory myopathies from the genetic dystrophies remains incomplete today. Some cases of 'limb girdle dystrophy' do respond well to anti-inflammatory therapy, and some cases of 'polymyositis' are highly resistant to it. Thus, nosology is still a living issue in the inflammatory myopathies.

The rarity and heterogeneity of the myositis syndromes has resulted in little information to guide physicians in the treatment of myositis. The beneficial effects of corticosteroids in myositis were recognized early, but the discovery of the benefits of methotrexate by Malaviya and his associates in 1968 (Paper 2) antedates recognition of its usefulness in other inflammatory conditions. Subsequently the roles of azathioprine, high dose intravenous gamma globulin, and combination chemotherapy in the treatment of myositis have been demonstrated, but a real therapeutic breakthrough has not yet occurred.

Diagnostic criteria and the categorization of myositis into five more homogenous groups were two major legacies of Bohan and coworkers (Paper 3). Among the important areas in which recent progress has been made in extensions of this work are juvenile and cancer-associated myositis. A large, careful study of juvenile myositis is just now being undertaken by a consortium of clinics. The relationship of cancer to myositis is real, but biologically impenetrable. Several excellent studies, most especially the large controlled investigation by Sigurgeirsson and colleagues (2), however, have at least quantitated the risk and pointed the way for practitioners who must decide how deeply to search for cancer when they first encounter a new patient with myositis.

The meticulous immunopathological observations of A. Engel and his collaborators (Paper 4) set the stage for understanding the mechanisms of muscle damage. When the new biological agents are applied to myositis, the therapeutic rationale will have been derived from those beautiful studies. The recognition of IBM represents a milestone on a still unfinished road. The description of IBM did not come abruptly, and we have included here not the first hints of the illness (3, 4), but the landmark clinical and laboratory description (Paper 5). The exact bounds of this entity remain uncertain for several reasons. Sporadic IBM does not always show inflammation, and anti-inflammatory therapy has been only marginally effective when inflammation is present. Thus, here too nosology remains alive, and the role of interacting genetic predispositions is likely to be increasingly recognized.

The pathological as well as clinical distinction between DM and PM has been supplemented recently by the discovery that certain autoantibodies, which are wholly disease-specific for myositis, delineate distinct clinical entities. Mathews and Bernstein (5) identified the enzymes that join an amino acid to the correct tRNA as myositis-specific targets of autoimmunity, and Love and her colleagues (Paper 6) expanded the observations of others to show that myositis is really a complex family of diseases. This latter work was an important and necessary step in understanding pathogenesis and in grouping patients into appropriate subsets for therapeutic and genetic studies.

We are only beginning our exploration of the myositis syndromes, and the millennium ahead holds unimaginable milestones on the path toward discovery of how these sign-symptom-laboratory complexes we so poorly understand today can be defined, cured, or even prevented.

References

1. Walton JN, Adams RD. *Polymyositis*. Edinburgh and London: E. & S. Livingstone Ltd, 1958.
2. Sigurgeirsson B, Lindelof B, Edhag O, Allander E. Risk of cancer in patients with dermatomyositis or polymyositis. A population-based study. *New England Journal of Medicine* 1992; **326**(6):363–367.
3. Chou SM. Myxovirus-like structures and accompanying nuclear changes in chronic polymyositis. *Archives of Pathology* 1968; **86**:649–658.
4. Yunis EJ, Samaha FJ. Inclusion body myositis. *Laboratory Investigations* 1971; **25**:240–248.
5. Mathews MB, Bernstein RM. Myositis autoantibody inhibits histidyl-tRNA synthetase: a model for autoimmunity. *Nature* 1983 Jul 14–20; **304**(5922):177–179.

Paper I

Dermatomyositis with report of a case which presented a rare muscle anomaly but once described in man

Author

Steiner WJ

Reference

Journal of Experimental Medicine 1903; **6**:407–442

Summary

After a thorough analytical summary of all previously described cases of similar illnesses, Steiner here describes a patient with myositis whom he examined and whose biopsy he describes. He notes many features of the clinical illness and of the histologic changes still considered central to the diagnosis, and he separates it from trichinosis, infective myositis, syphilitic myositis, and, most importantly, from 'neuromyositis'–that is myopathy accompanying neurologic disease. 'Dermatomyositis', he wrote, 'may be defined as an acute, subacute, or chronic disease of unknown origin, characterized by a gradual onset with vague and indefinite prodromata, followed by oedema, dermatitis, and a multiple muscle inflammation.'

Key message

This is a convenient starting point for the modern conception of myositis as an idiopathic, non-infectious inflammation primarily limited to the skeletal muscles and skin with an acute, sub-acute, or chronic course. Although rash was not a significant feature of this case, Steiner recognized the resemblance to cases with dermatitis. The delineation of PM and its separation from the dystrophies only became clear (and is still occasionally obscure) with the publication of Walton and Adams' beautiful monograph in 1958 (reference 1, Introduction).

Why it's important

When Steiner was a Medical House Officer under Osler at Johns Hopkins in 1899, he cared for a 31-year-old labourer from the stone quarries who presented with sore, swollen, and weak muscles. Despite a diet that included raw sausage, the patient did not have trichinosis (no worms in the teased biopsy and a normal eosinophil count). He also had dyspnoea, but no dermatitis. Distal as well as proximal muscles were clinically involved, and the biopsy described in detail (five pages of text) was from a gastrocnemius muscle. Neurological examination was normal, except of the muscles. An extensive electrical examination consisted entirely of a description of the gross response to electrical stimulation of the muscles rather than the spontaneous discharge pattern, which is central now.

In his careful summary of earlier descriptions, combined with his own observations, Steiner recognized the relationship to the disease now called PM, to scleroderma, and to vasculitis and a number of epidemiological features which still hold. His summary of the previously described pathological features, even more than the description of his own case, closely matches what are still recognized as central features: 'parenchymous and interstitial inflammation...being either focal and diffuse;' muscle fibres separated by oedema and inflammatory cells; perivascular inflammation; degeneration including the loss of striations, and regeneration. Of the clinical findings, he particularly noted the course of spontaneous remission and relapse; the variable occurrence of dermatitis which may be succeeded by hyperpigmentation; the involvement of the respiratory muscles, and the ominous implication of dysphagia. He also discussed the possibility that infection and toxins have an aetiological role, and comes to the same uncertain conclusion we would today.

Strengths, weaknesses, and relevance

In assessing the earliest descriptions of familiar diseases, one must always confront the fact that the first cases are almost invariably the severest. Nevertheless, they offer a glimpse of the natural history, and consequently a view of the aetiology and pathogenesis, which early recognition and aggressive intervention obscure. Like most cases of all its autoinflammatory relatives, myositis has a natural cycle of relapse and remission – a fact which should not be forgotten. With the publication of this classic, Steiner's paper defined the field.

Paper 2

Treatment of dermatomyositis with methotrexate

Authors

Malaviya AN, Many A, Schwartz RS

Reference

The Lancet 1968; **2**(7566):485–488

Summary

Four patients with DM were treated with intravenous methotrexate. Three of them were refractory to corticosteroids, and one had received no other treatment. Each patient was bed-ridden by severe muscular weakness before treatment, and one was in the terminal phases of the disease. All patients responded to methotrexate with improvement of muscular strength to normal or near normal and disappearance of the rash. Concomitantly, laboratory abnormalities indicative of muscle disease disappeared.

Key message

Prior to the publication of this paper, the effective management of the debilitating weakness and troublesome rash of DM had been limited to corticosteroids. Malaviya, *et al.* realized that dermatomyositis was closely enough associated with other diseases recognized as immunological in origin and was occasionally accompanied by serological abnormalities so that it might respond to the anti-metabolite methotrexate. The remarkable success in their first four patients reported in this paper not only introduced what is now known to be one of the most efficacious treatments, but also strengthened the place of this illness in the family of autoimmune rheumatological diseases.

Related references **(1)** Sokoloff MC, Goldberg LS, Pearson CM. Treatment of corticosteroid-resistant polymyositis with methotrexate, *The Lancet* 1971; 1:14–16.

(2) Villalba L, Hicks JE, Adams EH, Sherman JB, Gourley MF, Leff RL, Thornton BC, Burgess SH, Plotz PH, Miller FW. Treatment of refractory myositis: A randomized crossover study of two new cytotoxic regimens. *Arthritis and Rheumatism* 1998; **41**:392–399.

Why it's important

The introduction of corticosteroids for the treatment of RA eclipsed the slightly earlier observations on the efficacy of the anti-metabolite aminopterin in refractory arthritis and it took decades for rheumatologists to re-discover the benefits of methotrexate in RA. Well before that re-discovery, however, Malaviya, *et al.*, faced with the hopeless case of a boy dying of DM despite corticosteroids, drew the analogy between DM and other diseases which had responded to methotrexate, supposedly because immunological events were involved in pathogenesis, and tried methotrexate. The boy recovered dramatically. It was a year before they tried it again, and again they achieved an apparently durable remission in a patient with cancer-associated DM who was failing on corticosteroids. Two years later, faced with a fresh case of DM, they moved first to methotrexate and induced a remission without ever exposing the patient to corticosteroids.

A confirmatory paper by Sokoloff, Goldberg, and Pearson in 1971 (1) extended the observations to patients with PM and reported two failures in seven patients treated, bringing the state of knowledge of the place of methotrexate in the treatment of the idiopathic inflammatory myopathies almost to the point where it remains today. The recognition that methotrexate by mouth could be as effective was the most important remaining step, along with the proof that methotrexate could achieve substantial improvement when given with azathioprine and corticosteroids in patients who had failed to respond to steroids and either of the cytotoxics alone (2). It is now becoming common to use methotrexate or azathioprine along with corticosteroids as the first-line of therapy in patients with severe disease or poor prognostic features to spare the toxicities of prolonged, high dose steroids.

Strengths, weaknesses, and relevance

We are no longer so sure that we understand the mode of action of this useful drug. The failure of high intravenous doses in the range commonly used to treat malignancy to improve upon low oral doses certainly suggests that the pharmacological mechanisms in the two families of diseases are different. It is not even clear that an effect on immune mechanisms is the dominant one at play in the therapy of myositis or arthritis, but the bold leap of the Tufts group was a great advance that has stood the test of time.

Paper 3

A computer-assisted analysis of 153 patients with polymyositis and dermatomyositis

Authors

Bohan A, Peter JB, Bowman RL, Pearson CM

Reference

Medicine 1977; **56**(4):255–286

Summary

Diagnostic criteria and a classification scheme were developed by an empirical analysis of a large number of well-studied patients with PM-DM. Diagnosis was based upon a combined clinical-laboratory-pathological evaluation. The most useful criteria for diagnosis were found to be: 'a) proximal muscle weakness; b) elevation of serum enzymes; c) the characteristic electromyographic triad; d) typical muscle biopsy histopathology, and e) the classical skin rash of dermatomyositis'. The most sensitive diagnostic criteria were CPK, aldolase, and proximal muscle weakness. Definitions were developed for possible, probable and definite disease. The myositis syndromes were further classified into five distinct groups of patients: PM, DM, cancer-associated myositis, childhood myositis, and myositis syndromes in association with other connective tissue diseases (overlap myositis).

Key message

Five criteria were found to diagnose probable or definite disease in nearly 99% of clinically-defined PM-DM patients. Furthermore, the myositis syndromes defined by these criteria could be divided into five homogeneous groups based upon a number of clinical features.

Related references **(1)** Wagner E. Fall einer seltenen Muskelkrankheit. *Arch Heilkd* 1863; **IV**:282.

(2) Unverricht H. Dermatomyositis acuta. *Deutsche Medizinische Wochenschrift* 1891; **17**:41–49.

(3) Hoffman GS, Franck WA, Raddatz DA, *et al*, Presentation, treatment, and prognosis of idiopathic inflammatory muscle disease in a rural hospital, *American Journal of Medicine* 1983; **75**:433–438.

Why it's important

Although PM and DM had been recognized for a century before the publication of this paper (1, 2), no well-accepted criteria for the diagnosis or classification of these syndromes existed before this work. This study has stood the test of time, in that decades later, these approaches defined by Bohan, *et al.* are still the most frequently utilized for the diagnosis and classification of myositis. The generalized acceptance of these criteria resulted in much needed consistency among the clinical, pathogenic and therapeutic studies that followed and allowed for more reliable meta-analyses of studies so necessary for rare diseases.

In addition to defining practical criteria and classifications, this study included detailed descriptions of the clinical, electromyographic, pathological, serological, and prognostic features of the largest cohort of patients published up to that time. It condensed 15 years of experience by this major centre for the study of myopathies into a clinically useful summary that remains one of the best descriptions of disease in one of the largest populations of myositis patients ever studied. A number of aspects of the inflammatory myopathies, later confirmed by other investigations, first emerged from this study. These include the findings that: persistently normal serum enzymes, normal EMGs and normal muscle biopsies are seen in some patients with clinically obvious PM-DM; the paraspinal muscles are likely to be the most sensitive for EMG assessments; malignancy is associated with both DM and PM and is the leading cause of death (71%) in this group, and responses to treatment cannot be defined by muscle enzymes alone.

While we now know that additional clinical groups, including IBM, are important components of the idiopathic inflammatory myopathies (Paper 5), and that the serological classification of these diseases also adds useful information (Paper 6), the comprehensive and careful description and analysis of this large group of patients served as the classic foundation for defining and classifying these diseases.

Strengths, weaknesses, and relevance

This is the best-documented description of myositis in almost all of its clinically relevant aspects that we have, but, like all but a handful (3) of other descriptions of myositis, it portrays the most seriously affected patients and probably therefore must be considered still incomplete. Knowledge of the actual spectrum of the idiopathic inflammatory myopathies awaits the elucidation of the pathogeneses of the myositis syndromes and the many other myopathies that mimic these disorders.

Paper 4

Mononuclear cells in myopathies

Authors

Engel AG, Arahata K

Reference

Human Pathology 1986; **17**:704–721

Summary

Detailed immuno-phenotyping of all the inflammatory cells in inflammatory myopathies demonstrated that gradients of B cells and CD4+ T cells declined and the gradient of CD8+ T cells rose from perivascular to perimysial to endomysial areas of inflamed muscle in biopsies from DM, PM, and IBM patients, but there were marked differences in the proportion of cells in the various locations. In DM, B cells and CD4+ T cells were generally found together, there was a high CD4+/CD8+ ratio, and there was a relatively greater perivascular infiltrate. Few T cells were found abutting or invading non-necrotic muscle fibres. In both PM and IBM, activated CD8+ T cells were commonly found invading non-necrotic muscle cells at endomysial sites. Macrophages were common and NK cells rare in all three diseases. Two major processes are proposed. In DM, the predominant process is humoral immunity, whereas in PM and IBM, the predominant process is a cytotoxic T cell attack on muscle cells which appears to be antigen driven and major histocompatibility complex (MHC) restricted.

Key message

At least two major immunopathogenic processes are evident in the inflammatory myopathies: a humoral and vascular-based process which dominates DM and a cytotoxic cellular process which dominates PM and IBM, although both processes may be at play in a given patient. The close resemblance of immunopathogenic findings in PM and IBM is striking given their clinical and serological differences, and in both, non-necrotic muscle cells are invaded by activated cytotoxic T cells.

Related reference (1) Banker BO, Victor M. Dermatomyositis (systemic angiopathy) of childhood. *Medicine* 1966; **45**:261.

Why it's important

Over many years, scattered observations on the immunopathogenesis of the inflammatory myopathies had been gathered by a number of groups, but no clear picture had emerged (1). In part, of course, this was due to the only gradual emergence of the now canonical separation of lymphocyte cell types using immunological cell surface markers. At the time of this study, the main cell types and some of the cytokines that regulate immune function were known and good reagents were available. Engel and Arahata applied exquisitely careful and comprehensive studies using combinations of markers to identify the location, the cell type, and the state of activation of all the inflammatory cells in many muscle biopsies from all the major inflammatory myopathies.

They could document the vasculocentric and humoral process most commonly found in both adults and children with DM by demonstrating the dominance of B and CD4+ T cells in the inflammation at perivascular and perimysial areas. In PM, although some of these features were present, a major process was the presence of activated CD8+ T cells at endomysial locations and within non-necrotic muscle cells (Figure 15.1). NK cells were virtually absent and macrophages were widely dispersed in both types of inflammation. IBM strikingly resembled PM, echoing the imprecise clinical boundary between treatment-resistant PM and IBM in older adults. The significant up-regulation of MHC Class I on non-necrotic muscle cells and the paucity of pro-inflammatory cytokines have also emerged as characteristic parts of the pathogenic picture.

Additional observations on the inflammatory infiltrate of Duchenne dystrophy document the qualitative resemblance to, but wide quantitative difference from, PM and reinforce the role that the reversal of inflammation may play in the partial response dystrophy patients may experience from anti-inflammatory treatment. Just as the autoantibodies and the rashes mark different groups of myositis patients, so do the basic immunopathological processes. The kind of understanding of this family of diseases that will one day allow a rational and sharply targeted approach to therapy was substantially advanced by the painstaking observations in this paper, and it set an extremely high standard for future quantitative immunohistological studies.

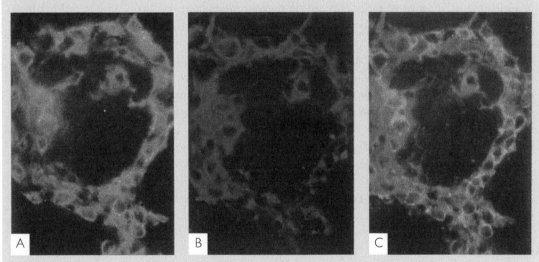

Figure 15.1 Non-necrotic muscle fibres surrounded and invaded by mononuclear cells in polymyositis: (A) CD8+ cytotoxic T cells are visualized by green fluorescence. (B) HLA DR+ activated cells are demonstrated by red fluorescence. (C) Double exposure of A and B reveals that many of the CD8+ T cells are also activated as shown by their yellow colour.

Strengths, weaknesses, and relevance

This study and others by Engel, Arahata, and their colleagues defined the anatomy and cell surface markers in the inflammatory myopathies, but those markers alone do not define the immunopathogenesis. Later studies, building upon this work, are continuing to refine and deepen understanding of the pathogenesis of myositis.

Paper 5

Inclusion body myositis. Observations in 40 patients

Authors

Lotz BP, Engel AG, Nishino H, Steven JC, Litchy WJ

Reference

Brain 1989; **112**(3):727–747

Summary

The histopathological, ultrastructural, and clinical features of IBM were defined in 48 of 170 consecutive myositis patients in whom the diagnosis was suspected on light microscopic grounds. 'One or more vacuoles containing membranous material, groups of atrophic fibres, and an autoaggressive endomysial inflammatory exudate occurred in 100%, 96% and 92% of the muscle biopsy specimens.' Filamentous inclusions, typically near vacuoles, were seen by electron microscopy in 40 of 48 patients and distinguished IBM from other inflammatory myopathies. 'The typical clinical features in patients diagnosed by histological criteria as IBM were: insidious onset after age 50 years with painless, proximal lower extremity weakness; slow but relentless progression with selectively severe involvement of the quadriceps, iliopsoas, tibialis anterior, biceps and triceps muscles; relatively early depression of the knee reflexes, and a normal or mildly elevated serum creatine kinase level. The male: female ratio was 3:1. Distal weakness occurred in about 50%, but only in 35% was it as great or greater than proximal weakness.' Prednisone failed to prevent disease progression in patients observed for 2 or more years. IBM is a clinically and pathologically distinct form of idiopathic inflammatory myopathy.

Key message

IBM is a unique form of myositis, defined by a combination of clinical, histological and ultrastructural features, with poor responses to prednisone.

Related reference   **(I)**   Yunis EJ, Samaha FJ. Inclusion body myositis. *Laboratory Investigations* 1971; **25**:240–248.

Why it's important

In 1968, Chou described a 66-year old man with progressive weakness of all muscles, dysphagia, pronounced atrophy of the shoulder girdle and quadriceps muscles, myopathic electromyograms, myonecrosis and mononuclear cell infiltrates in muscle biopsies, and unusual muscle ultrastructural features, including myxovirus-like intranuclear and intracytoplasmic filaments (reference 3, Introduction). In 1971, Yunis and Samaha (1) coined the term 'inclusion body myositis' to describe a 26 year old white woman with an 8 year history of weakness, normal creatine kinase levels, wasting of the abductors and adductors of the thigh but normal quadriceps muscles, inflammatory infiltrates on muscle biopsy, and similar fibrillar nuclear and cytoplasmic inclusions on electron microscopic examination. Other case reports and case series followed these initial publications.

Lotz and his colleagues, however, were the first to assemble what is still the largest published cohort of IBM patients, and define the extended clinical and pathological spectrum of this illness. A number of distinguishing and clinically important aspects of IBM, which have been subsequently confirmed by others, were emphasized in this paper. These include: the elderly male predominance; the insidious onset; the slowly progressive, painless weakness; quadriceps atrophy and the frequent involvement of distal muscles; the presence of certain neurogenic features and dysphagia in some patients but few other extramuscular symptoms; normal or relatively low serum levels of creatine kinase; the lack of a distinguishing electromyographic pattern; occasional associations with other autoimmune disorders and malignancy, and poor responses to corticosteroids.

Strengths, weaknesses, and relevance

We now know that the IBMs are a heterogeneous group of inflammatory and non-inflammatory, and hereditary and sporadic conditions which share the common feature of characteristic purplish rimmed vacuoles on trichrome staining and paired helical filamentous inclusions on ultrastructural evaluation of muscle biopsies. Much of this progress in understanding IBM, as well as the increased awareness by physicians that has resulted in the recognition that IBM is the most common myopathy in persons greater than 50 years of age, can be traced to the careful delineation of this fascinating entity by the authors of this paper.

Paper 6

A new approach to the classification of idiopathic inflammatory mypathy: myositis-specific autoantibodies define useful homogeneous patient groups

Authors

Love LA, Leff RL, Fraser DD, Targoff IN, Dalakas M, Plotz PH, Miller FW

Reference

Medicine (Baltimore) 1991; **70**;360–374

Summary

Idiopathic inflammatory myopathies (IIM) are a heterogeneous group of systemic rheumatic diseases which share common features. A number of classification schemes have been proposed for them. We compared the usefulness of myositis-specific autoantibodies to the standard clinical categories in predicting clinical signs and symptoms, human leucocyte antigen (HLA) types and prognosis in 212 adult IIM patients. Although patients with IBM (n = 26) differed, there were few other significant differences among other clinical groups. In contrast, autoantibody status defined distinct sets of patients and each patient had only one myositis-specific autoantibody. Patients with anti-aminoacyl-tRNA synthetase autoantibodies (n = 47) had significantly more arthritis, fever, interstitial lung disease and 'mechanic's hands', were taking more prednisone and cytotoxic drugs, had higher death rates, and frequently had HLA-DRw52. Those with anti-signal recognition particle antibodies (n = 7) had increased palpitations, myalgias, severe refractory disease with high death rates, and were frequently DR5, DRw52 +ve. Patients with anti-Mi-2 autoantibodies (n = 10) had increased 'v-sign' and 'shawl-sign' rashes, cuticular overgrowth, and a good response to therapy, and were often DR7 and DRw53+ve. The two patients with anti-MAS antibodies were the only ones to have rhabdomyolysis preceding myositis; both had insulin dependent diabetes, and both had HLA-B60, -C3, -DR4 and -DRw53.

Key message

The presence of myositis-specific antibodies help with the interpretation of symptoms and signs in myositis patients, and in the prediction of their clinical course and prognosis.

Related reference **(1)** Plotz PH, Dalakas M, Leff RL, Love LA, Miller FW, Cronin ME. Current concepts in idiopathic inflammatory myopathies: polymyositis, dermatomyositis and related disorders. *Annals of Internal Medicine* 1989; **111**:143–157.

Why it's important

This work, amongst others, has helped to make it abundantly clear that myositis includes a complex family of different diseases. The standard clinical grouping is into primary PM, primary DM, myositis with another connective tissue diseae, myositis associated with a diagnosis of cancer, and IBM. However, the authors of this paper showed that of these five categories, only IBM stands out as being different in its clinical manifestations. In contrast, they showed that the single, specific type of autoantibody that each patient has is a good predictor of the clinical features, course and outcome of the disease (Table 15.1). This, along with the HLA associations, suggests that there are specific immunogenetics and immune responses linked to specific clinical features in this family of diseases. If this is the case, then these findings should lead onto our being able to distinguish and treat specific pathological pathways responsible for disease in different groups of patients. The authors of this article therefore proposed an adjunct classification of IIM, based on antibody status, which they recommend should be incorporated into all future studies of epidemiology, aetiology and therapy of IIM.

Table 15.1 Disease profiles of patients with idiopathic inflammatory myositis.

IIM group	Synthetase+	SRP+	Mi-2	MAS+	IBM
Gender (M:F)	2.7	6	1.2	1	0.5
Age at onset	41.3	36.5	46.3	36.5	51.8
Onset	Acute	Very acute	Acute	Acute	Insidious
Major symptoms and signs	Interstitial lung disease, dyspnoea on exertion, fevers, arthritis, 'mechanic's hand'	Palpitations, cardiac disease, severe weakness	'V sign' rash, 'shawl sign' rash, cuticular overgrowth	Alcoholic rhabdomyolitis	Falling, atrophy distal and asymmetric weakness
HLA associations	DR3 DRw52	DR5 DRw52	DR7 DRw53	DR4 DRw53	DR3 DRw52
Clinical group	Jo-1, PM > DM, others DM >> PM	PM	DM	PM	Not DM
Prognosis:					
Steroid response	Moderate	Poor	Good	Good	Poor
Response to taper	Flare	Flare	Good	Good	Little
Mortality (%)	21	43	11	0	0

Strengths, weaknesses and relevance

This excellent study is based on a relatively large sample of patients (212). However, they all came from the National Institutes for Health, which is a tertiary referral centre, and may represent a more severe group of IIM patients than those seen in other practices or in the community. Furthermore, some of the rarer clinical groups, such as juvenile DM, were not included. However, it seems likely that the proposed new classification will stand the test of time, and the fact that each patient with IIM has a single autoantibody, which acts as a marker of a specific clinical expression, course and outcome, is a finding of huge potential importance–not only to our understanding of IIM, but to all autoimmune disease.

CHAPTER 16

Arthritis and infection

Andrew Keat and Ralph C Williams, Jr

Introduction

Bone and joint sepsis has been described in the medical literature from the times of ancient Greece and Rome, and generalized infectious diseases which can affect joints, such as gonorrhoea and tuberculosis, have been common for centuries. Infections of bones and joints were probably relatively common and frequently fatal prior to the introduction of antibiotics. However, it is of interest to note that there is paleopathological evidence for long survival of some people with severe osteomyelitis long before the germ theory of disease or antibiotics were thought of (1). Chemotherapy was first used for osteomyelitis in 1936 (2, 3), and the subsequent use of antibiotics for joint and other infections has reduced the severity and frequency of septic arthritis as well as osteomyelitis.

However, in the second half of the 20th century arthritis and infection became very important again, for two different reasons. First it became apparent that infections could trigger certain forms of rheumatic disease, such as reactive arthritis (see chapter 10) and the search for the 'immaculate infection' which might be the cause of rheumatoid arthritis (RA) continues today. Secondly, infection became a major issue in relation to the development of joint replacement surgery.

There are many different types of joint infection, and the choice of just eight classic papers in this field proved very difficult. One of the early classical descriptions of joint pathology in septic arthritis has been included (Paper 1). The author and editors agreed on one other paper that dates from the first half of the 20th century, which is a classical description of gonoccocal arthritis which includes a very early description of the dramatic response of this condition to sulphanilimide (Paper 2). Septic arthritis is more likely to occur in patients who are immunosuppressed or in those with other rheumatic diseases, including RA and systemic lupus erythematosus (SLE). The third paper describes the condition in RA patients, pointing out how features of sepsis may be masked in RA. The importance of John Chanley's work on joint prostheses is mentioned in the chapter on osteoarthritis (chapter 17); here we celebrate his contribution to the understanding of how post-operative and prosthetic infection rates could be reduced (Paper 4).

The last three papers are concerned with different sorts of relationships between infections and joint disease. Paper 5 is the first description of an arthritis being caused by immune complex disease triggered by an infection (meningococcal). Paper 6 describes the arthritis seen in adults in response to parvovirus infection, and Paper 7 relates to the recent but classical work of Alan Steere and his colleagues on Lyme disease. Finally we have included two classical contributions on rheumatic fever (Paper 8, reviewed by Ralph Williams). There are several other conditions that we would like to have included, such as mycoplasmal septic arthritis (4), hepatitis B (5, 6), tuberculosis (7) and syphilis.

References

1. Rogers J, Dieppe P. Lessons from paleopathology. *The Practitioner* 1983; **227**: 1191–1199.

2. Le Cocq JF, Le Cocq E. Use of neoarsphenamine in treatment of acute *S. aureus* septicaemia and osteomyelitis. *Journal of Bone and Joint Surgery* 1941; **23**:596–597.

3. Hedstrom SA, Lidgren L. Septic arthritis and osteomyelitis. In: *Rheumatology* (Klippel J, Dieppe P. eds.). 2nd edition, London: Mosby, 6.2.1–6.2.10.

4. Furr PM, Taylor-Robinson D, Webster ADB. Mycoplasmas and ureaplasmas in patients with hypogammaglobulinemia and their role in arthritis: microbiological observations over twenty years. *Annals of Rheumatic Diseases* 1994; **53**;183–187.

5. Duffy J, Lidsky MD, Sharp JT, Dans JS, Pearson DA, Hollinger FB, Min KW. Polyarthritis, polyarteritis and hepatitis B. *Medicine (Baltimore)* 1976; **55**:19–37.

6. Schumacher HR, Gall EP. Arthritis in acute hepatitis and chronic active hepatitis. Pathology of the synovial membrane with evidence for the presence of Australia antigen in synovial membranes. *American Journal of Medicine* 1974; **57**:655–64.

7. Chapman M, Murray RO, Stoker DJ. Tuberculosis of bones and joints. *Seminars in Roentgenology* 1979; **14**:266–282.

Paper 1

Histological changes in the knee joint in various infections

Authors

Keefer CS, Parker F, Myers WK

Reference

Archives of Pathology 1934; **18**:199–215

Summary

The pathological lesions of eight cases of infective arthritis due to streptococcic, gonococcic, meningococcic and pneumococcic infections and to an unidentified gram-negative coccus are reported. The character of the change varied with the mode of infection which occurred in one of three ways: (a) by the bloodstream; (b) by direct extension from osteomyelitis; (c) by direct extension from the skin overlying the joint.

In the cases in which the infection of the joints occurred as a result of haematogenous infection, the process began in the synovial connective tissue, with infiltration of polymorphonuclear, lymphoid and plasma cells about the blood vessels between the strands of connective tissues. As the infection progressed, the synovial lining was destroyed and completely replaced by granulomatous tissue. Later the cartilage and bone were involved in the process and destroyed. When the bone was involved primarily, the outstanding lesions were a destruction of bone and overlying cartilage. The inflammation of the synovium showed a progression from the superficial to the deeper layers. The changes were characteristic of an inflammatory process that could be readily distinguished from degeneration.

Related references **(1)** Parker F, Keefer CS, Myers WK, Irwin C. Histologic changes in the knee joint with advancing age. Relation to degenerative arthritis. *Archives of Pathology* 1934; **17**: 516–532.

(2) Keefer CS, Parker F, Myers WK, Irwin C. Relationship between anatomic changes in knee joints with advancing age and degenerative arthritis. *Archives of Internal Medicine* 1934; **53**:325–336.

Key message

Infections get into joints by one of three routes: the blood, bone infections or from the overlying skin. Once the joint becomes infected it is quickly destroyed.

Why it's important

This paper is one of a series of contributions on joint pathology that came from the Boston City Hospital Department of Pathology in the 1930s. At that time there was little knowledge of joint pathology, and it was not easy to distinguish between the different causes of joint destruction.

This was one of the first comprehensive descriptions of what happens to joints in septic arthritis. The excellent descriptions of both gross pathology (Figure 16.1) and microscopic changes clearly show the extensive destruction of joints that can result from these infections. In addition to illustrating the degree of joint damage, and distinguishing it from the types of damage done by ageing and osteoarthritis (1, 2), the other main contribution was to document the three main causes of septic arthritis, and to illustrate that in many cases it was due to haematogenous spread from other sites.

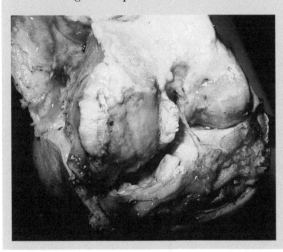

Figure 16.1 Post-mortem knee joint showing severe joint destruction due to septic arthritis, with deep ulceration through the bone and cartilage of the lateral femoral condyle. This contemporary specimen shows changes very similar to those described by Keefer, *et al.* in this paper. (From: *Slide Atlas of Rheumatology* (Dieppe P, Bacon P, Bamji A, Watt I. eds.). London: Gower Medical Publishing, 1984.)

Strengths

1. Excellent clinical and pathological descriptions of the eight cases.
2. Clear evidence of the serious destruction of joints that can result from a septic arthritis.
3. Differentiation of the three main sources of infections in joints.

Weaknesses

1. Only eight cases are described, in seven of which the infection was in the knee joint, and seven of whom died as a result of the sepsis (in one case the leg was amputated, so that a specimen was obtained without autopsy).
2. There was only one case of local spread from overlying skin and one of spread from a bone focus; so six of the eight were haematogenous in origin. In spite of this they try to differentiate pathology in the three types.
3. They infer the time course of the disease in spite of there only being pathological evidence at one time point in a small number of cases.

Relevance

Distinguished septic arthritis as a serious cause of rapid joint damage, usually resulting from haematological spread from another site.

Paper 2

Gonococcic arthritis: pathogenesis, mechanism of recovery and treatment

Authors

Keefer CS, Spink WW

Reference

Journal of the American Medical Association 1937; **109**:1448–1453

Summary

One hundred and forty cases of gonococcal arthritis seen over 5 years are documented. The diagnosis was based on a history of recent gonorrhoea, evidence of specific gonococcal genital-tract infection, a positive gonococcal complement fixation test in blood or synovial fluid, the presence of gonococci in synovial fluid. The course and clinical features of this condition were described. Particular attention was drawn to the polyarticular nature of the disease, the common involvement of tendon sheaths, the danger of exacerbating the disease by 'vigorous' prostatic massage and the presence of maculopapular or haemorrhagic skin lesions in patients with bacteraemia. Three patients were treated with sulphanilamide with dramatic fever resolution and sterilization of the joints. Seven of the 140 patients died.

Related reference   **(1)**   Keefer CS, Parker F, Myers WK. Histological changes in the knee joint in various infections. *Archives of Pathology* 1934; **18**:199–215.

Key message

This was a common form of arthritis which needed to be distinguished from other forms of polyarthritis including rheumatic fever. The demonstration of gonococci in synovial fluid was an important diagnostic finding, heralding rapid articular cartilage destruction. Treatment with sulphanilamide appeared dramatically effective.

Why it's important

Since the very first descriptions of septic gonococcal arthritis 50 years earlier, this condition has been recognized as a common destructive condition. In laying down clear diagnostic criteria, Keefer and Spink helped to establish more clearly one more distinct rheumatic disease. They still did not differentiate fully between septic gonococcal arthritis and reactive arthritis and the use of the gonococcal complement fixation test has not stood the test of time. Nonetheless, through meticulous scientific method and analysis, in this and an earlier paper (1), they demonstrated synovial changes and the importance of early articular cartilage destruction.

Most importantly, however, they demonstrated that treatment with the anti-microbial agent, sulphanilamide, induced rapid sterilization of the joint and defervescence of fever. By so doing, they enabled both the specialist and the generalist to make an accurate diagnosis of gonococcal arthritis and ushered in the era of cure of the condition through effective anti-microbial chemotherapy.

Strengths

1. Clinical descriptions of arthritis are clear with data based on a large sample.
2. The effects of treatment with sulphanilamide are demonstrated, albeit on a very small number of patients, with dramatic clarity.

Weaknesses

1. No differentiation is made between septic gonococcal arthritis and reactive arthritis.
2. The value of the gonococcal complement fixation test is over-estimated.
3. Anti-microbial treatment was only used in three patients.

Relevance

Scientific analysis of both the clinical and immunological features of gonococcal arthritis allowed ready diagnosis for both the generalist and the specialist. Anti-microbial chemotherapy was shown to be rapidly curative.

Paper 3

Suppurative arthritis complicating rheumatoid arthritis

Authors

Kellgren, JH, Ball J, Fairbrother RW, Barnes KL

Reference

British Medical Journal 1958; 1:1193-1200

Summary

Thirteen patients (one was added as a post-script) were described in which severe bacterial infection complicated pre-existing RA. Most patients had severe disease of up to 20 years' duration with much joint destruction. In 10 of the patients, septic arthritis occurred though in the remainder abscess formation at other sites, including osteomyelitis, was described. A pre-disposing source of infection was identified in a few patients but not in most. Six patients died, sepsis being discovered in most only at necropsy. Radiological investigation was in the main unhelpful and some patients did not have classical features of infection, particularly fever and leucocytosis. Diagnosis was complicated by the pre-existing features of active RA. In earlier patients in the series, the diagnosis of sepsis was unsuspected and joint aspiration and blood cultures were not carried out. Several of the later patients underwent aspiration of suspicious joints with early diagnosis and successful treatment.

Key message

Patients with severe rheumatoid joint destruction are especially susceptible to bacterial sepsis though the clinical features of infection may be atypical.

Why it's important

Although several earlier authors had described patients with RA complicated by septic arthritis, Kellgren, *et al.* demonstrated that 50% of cases of joint sepsis seen at their hospitals over the period of study were in patients with RA. Although an uncommon complication, this paper raised awareness of this lethal but potentially treatable complication. Having raised the index of suspicion, this paper also pointed out for the first time that the diagnosis is especially difficult for two reasons. Firstly, the features of active RA closely mimic those of infection. Secondly, several patients even with widespread sepsis failed to respond with either fever or leucocytosis. The paper indicated for the first time that the absence of classical indicators of sepsis does not exclude the possibility of joint sepsis.

The authors also pointed out the importance of aspirating potentially infected joints. Their statement 'in the light of our experience with these patients, aspiration and culture of fluid from the more painful joints are indicated in every patient with RA in whom there is a sudden deterioration ....' has become one of the central tenets of good clinical rheumatological practice. Moreover, they were able to show that diligent search for infection and rigorous energetic treatment, even with the limited antibiotic repertoire of the day, was able to produce remarkable recoveries. Four of the patients had received either steroid or adrenocorticotropic hormone (ACTH). It is not clear whether this predisposed the patients to sepsis though Kellgren and others cite evidence that this is likely with the implication that this complication should be particularly sought in patients receiving steroid therapy.

Strengths

1. The key points are clearly and powerfully made.
2. The index of suspicion of septic arthritis in this group of patients was clearly raised.
3. The value of joint aspiration in cases where any doubt occurred was emphasized unequivocally.

Weaknesses

1. This is a small series of patients.
2. The death of earlier patients and the survival of later patients could have occurred by chance.

Relevance

The detection of joint sepsis in patients with pre-existing rheumatoid disease remains difficult though a high index of suspicion and routine joint aspiration to search for sepsis has become normal good clinical practice.

Paper 4

Post-operative infection after total hip replacement with special reference to air contamination in the operating room

Author

Charnley J

Reference

Clinical Orthopaedics and Related Research 1972; **87**:167–187

Summary

Reviewing deep infections in 5800 total hip replacements performed between 1960 and 1970, the incidence of infection fell from 7% to 0.5%. This was attributed to stringent measures to prevent exogenous infection in the operating theatre. The performance of surgery within a field of ultra-clean filtered air was the major factor in reducing infection rates. The use of impermeable surgeons' gowns to prevent transmission of bacteria from those within the operating enclosure and improved wound closure techniques, also contributed to the reduced infection rate.

Key message

Most deep post-operative prosthetic hip infections are acquired in the operating theatre. The risk can be minimized by exposing the patient to ultra-clean filtered air and by preventing shedding of bacteria from surgeons and nurses in the operating theatre by use of impermeable theatre clothing.

Why it's important

When joint replacement surgery was in its infancy, it became clear that the risk of prosthetic joint infection was substantial with significant morbidity (Figure 16.2) and mortality. Several factors were incriminated including use of acrylic cement and subsequent blood-borne infection from superficial sites of sepsis.

By a series of painstaking studies using operating enclosures within conventional operating theatres, air filtration systems capable of changing the air 130–300 times and bacteriological assessment using settle plates, the exposure of the wound to bacteria was carefully assessed. Over a decade, Charnley was able to show that exposing the wound to carefully directed ultra-clean air could reduce deep infection rates from around 7% at the outset to 1.4%. Further improvements in the infection rate could then be made by the use of impermeable theatre clothing and newer wound closure techniques.

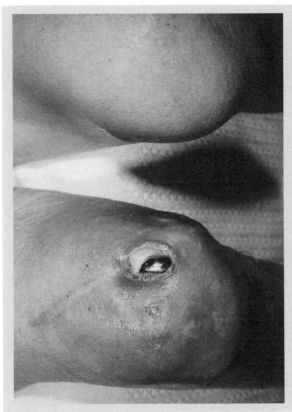

Charnley did note that patients with RA were constitutionally subject to slightly higher infection risk than others, and he concluded that it is unlikely that clean air alone can reduce the infection rate below 1.5%. Subsequently, the introduction of antibiotic-impregnated cement and prophylactic antibiotic therapy also made its contribution, but in these days of multiresistant micro-organisms, the basic tenet of protecting the patient from per-operative infection remains of crucial importance.

Figure 16.2 An infected prosthesis of the knee joint resulting in ulceration through the skin. (From *Slide Atlas of Rheumatology* (Dieppe P, Bamji A, Watt I. eds.). London: Gower Medical Publishing, 1984.)

Strengths

1. Data are drawn from very large numbers of patients operated on at a single centre.
2. Clear end-points are used in terms of measured bacterial colony counts in filtered and unfiltered air and infection rates.

Weakness

The use of operating enclosures was not widely taken up elsewhere due to practical considerations.

Relevance

Systematic and painstaking methods to prevent exposure to infection at the time of surgery is of paramount importance particularly in implant surgery. The clear demonstration of this by an acknowledged pioneer of implant surgery has influenced the practice of joint replacement surgery world-wide.

Paper 5

Allergic complications of meningococcal disease. II. Immunological investigations

Authors

Greenwood BM, Whittle HC, Bryceson ADM

Reference

British Medical Journal 1973; **2**:737–740

Summary

Four patients (of 47 described in a related paper (1)) with arthritis-complicating meningococcal infection were investigated immunologically. Complement-depletion in serum and deposits of meningococcal antigen, together with immunoglobulin and C3, were demonstrated in synovial fluid white cells of the two patients investigated and in one skin biopsy. These findings indicate that arthritis and skin lesions associated with a meningococcal infection are due to immune complex formation rather to actual sepsis.

Related references **(1)** Whittle HC, Abdullahi MT, Fakunle FA, Greenwood BM, Bryceson ADM, Parry EHO, Turk JL. Allergic complications of meningococcal disease. I. Clinical aspects. *British Medical Journal* 1973; **2**:733–737.

(2) Henrick WW, Parkhurst GM Meningococcus arthritis. *American Journal of the Medical Sciences* 1919; **158**:473.

(3) Rolleston H. Lumleian lecture on cerebrospinal fever. *The Lancet* 1919; **1**:645.

Key message

This is the first clear description of arthritis caused by microbial infection but mediated by an immune complex disease.

Why it's important

Arthritis as a complication of meningococcal infection had been well described more than 50 years before this report (2, 3) and allusion had been made to the possibility that arthritis occurring late during convalescence from the acute infection might be due to serum sickness or a related process. These authors were able to demonstrate, via conceptually simple and clear means, that arthritis in this circumstance is likely to be due to immune complex formation rather than direct tissue invasion by viable micro-organisms.

By this means the authors were able to demonstrate that acute infection may lead to synovitis by mechanisms other than persistence of viable micro-organisms. Thus, a half-way house was built between overtly septic disease and disorders such as RA in which no direct evidence of an infective cause is apparent.

Strengths

1. Clear and thorough methodology.
2. This work occurs in the context of other clinical and immunological investigations of a large population of patients with meningococcal disease.

Weakness

Actual immunological data are available for a very small number of patients.

Relevance

The demonstration of an immune mechanism for arthritis in this group of patients has stimulated searches for other micro-organism-driven mechanisms in other forms of inflammatory arthritis.

Paper 6

Human parvovirus-associated arthritis: a clinical and laboratory description

Authors

Reid DM, Brown T, Reid TMS, Rennie JAM, Eastmond CJ

Reference

The Lancet 1985; **1**:422–425

Summary

During an outbreak of human parvovirus (HPV) infection in Scotland, 42 patients were identified with both serological evidence of infection and joint pain. Details were available on 30 patients (27 adults and three children). Each of the three children had a typical rash but seven of the 27 adults had no prodromata nor rash. The intervals between the onset of the rash and the onset of joint pain ranged from 1–16 days. Affected adults were predominantly young women (mean age 30.3 years).

Arthritis consisted mainly of symmetrical small joint involvement of the proximal interphalangeal and metacarpophalangeal joints, though less commonly knees, wrists and ankles were involved. All patients had immunoglobulin (Ig) M and IgG human parvovirus antibodies at presentation. IgM antibodies reached a peak at 8 days and declined to near zero at 60 days. IgG antibodies reached a peak at 40 days and declined more slowly thereafter. In 17 of 24 patients, arthritis resolved within 2 weeks. All but two resolved within 4 weeks though arthralgia persisted in two patients.

Related reference (1)

White DG, Mortimer PP, Blake DR, Woolf AD, Cohen BJ, Bacon PA. Human parvovirus arthropathy. *The Lancet* 1985; **1**:419–421.

Key message

This paper, published simultaneously with (1) clearly describes a clinical arthritis syndrome associated with a common viral infection. Children develop a trivial exanthem but young adults, usually women, develop transient polyarthritis, often without features of the exanthem.

Why it's important

Since the discovery of HPV in 1975, several groups had noted the presence of joint pain amongst a range of other more prominent disease features. For the first time, Reid and colleagues, along with White, *et al.*, clearly delineated one of the most common forms of inflammatory arthritis in the western world. They provided a clear picture of its natural history and likely epidemiology. White and colleagues also made the same observations but under rather different circumstances. By identifying HPV-infected patients attending an early synovitis clinic, they described a more selected population, incidentally demonstrating the value of the relatively new innovation, the 'early synovitis clinic'. Reid's description of a short-lived, spontaneously-resolving disease has been borne out by subsequent observation. White, however, described a more persistent illness in several patients, symptoms persisting for more than 4 years in three of the 19 patients described. In spite of several tantalizing subsequent reports, a clear link between HPV and RA has not been revealed although the possibility that some cases may persist and lead to joint damage remains unresolved.

Strengths

1. Simple classic description of a common disease.
2. Diagnostic serology is clearly described for clinical usage.
3. This description provides a clear basis for diagnosis and treatment by both specialists and generalists.

Weaknesses

1. Epidemiology of this condition is hinted at rather than assessed.
2. Small numbers of patients were documented, not all of these after direct clinical examination by the authors.

Relevance

This and other subsequent papers allowed a common disorder to be diagnosed readily, especially by primary care physicians. Rapid diagnosis thus prevents unnecessary suffering by the patients and inappropriate use of resources.

Paper 7

Lyme arthritis: An epidemic of oligoarticular arthritis in children and adults in three Connecticut communities

Authors

Steere AC, Malawista SE, Snydman DR, Shope RE, Andiman WA, Ross MR, Steele FM

Reference

Arthritis and Rheumatism 1977; **20**:7–17

Summary

An epidemic form of arthritis has been occurring in eastern Connecticut at least since 1972, with the peak incidence of new cases in the summer and early autumn. Its identification has been possible because of tight geographical clustering in some areas, and because of a characteristic preceding skin lesion in some patients. The authors studied 51 residents of three contiguous Connecticut communities (39 children and 12 adults) who developed an illness characterized by recurrent attacks of asymmetric swelling and pain in a few large joints, especially in the knee. Attacks were usually short (median 1 week) with much longer intervening periods of complete remission (median 2.5 months), but some attacks lasted for months. To date the typical patient has had three recurrences, but 16 patients have had none. A median of 4 weeks (range 1–24) before the onset of arthritis, 13 patients (25%) noted an erythematous papule that developed into an expanding, red annular lesion, as much as 50 cm (19.5 in) in diameter. Only two of 159 family members of patients had such a lesion and did not develop arthritis (p<0.000001). The overall prevalence of the arthritis was 4.3 cases per 1000 residents, but the prevalence among children living in four roads was 1 in 10. Six families had more than one affected member. Nine of 20 symptomatic patients had low serum C3 levels, compared to none of 31 asymptomatic patients (p<0.005); no patient had iridocyclitis or a positive test for antinuclear antibodies (ANA). Neither cultures of synovium and synovial fluid nor serological tests were positive for agents known to cause arthritis. 'Lyme arthritis' is thought to be a previously unrecognized clinical entity, the epidemiology of which suggests transmission by an arthropod vector.

Related references (1) Putkonen T, Muslakallo KK, Salminen P. Erythema chronicum migrans with meningitis: a rare coincidence of two tick-born diseases. *Dermatologica* 1962; **125**: 184–188.

(2) Steere AC, Malawista SE, Hardin JA, Ruddy S, Askenease PW, Andiman WA. Erythema chronicum migrans and Lyme arthritis. The enlarging clinical spectrum. *Annals of Internal Medicine* 1977; **86**:685–698.

(3) Steere AC, Malawista SE. Cases of Lyme disease in the United States; locations correlated with distribution of *Ixodes dammini*. *Annals of Internal Medicine* 1979; **91**:730–733.

(4) Steere AC, Malawista SE, Newman JH, Spieler PN, Bartenhagen NH. Antibiotic therapy in Lyme disease. *Annals of Internal Medicine* 1980; **93**:1–8.

Key message

A new and distinctive form of arthritis has been discovered in Connecticut; it is probably caused by an arthropod-born infection.

Why it's important

The opening paragraph of this paper is a true 'classic': 'In November 1975 a mother from Old Lyme, Connecticut, informed the State Health Department that 12 children from that small community of 5000, four of whom lived close together on the same road, had a disease diagnosed as JRA'. The authors thereby paid tribute to the observations and actions of the community right at the beginning of this first paper on Lyme disease. The Yale group, led by Alan Steere and Steven Malawista went on to investigate the phenomenon fully, leading to a comprehensive description of the disease, the vector, the causative organism and the treatment (see related references).

The importance of the discovery of Lyme disease is hard to overestimate. Not only is this an important disease, which can be treated effectively, but it has also given us great insights into infections and arthritis. This first paper provided many of these insights and is a model of combined clinical and epidemiological work to sort out a clinical syndrome. In this paper, the authors fully describe their efforts to make sure that the condition is distinctive, and that it is not a previously recognized form of juvenile arthritis or infectious arthritis.

Strengths

1. Superb clinical and epidemiological investigation of a phenomenon that lay people in the community discovered.
2. Clear evidence that Lyme arthritis is a new, distinctive disease.
3. Pre-empts the subsequent association with *Ixodes dammini*, the spirochaete and antibiotic treatment.

Weakness

It would be churlish to criticize this excellent first paper on Lyme arthritis, although it should perhaps be noted that the authors did, at this early stage, call it Lyme 'arthritis' rather than Lyme 'disease'.

Relevance

The original, ground-breaking description of an important, treatable disease and of an important model for the pathogenesis of other forms of arthritis.

Paper 8a

Immunologic relation of streptococcal and tissue antigens. I. Properties of an antigen in certain strains of Group A streptococci exhibiting an immunologic cross-reaction with human heart tissue

Author

Kaplan MH

Reference

Journal of Immunology 1963; **90**:595–606

Paper 8b

A immunological relationship between the Group A streptococcus and mammalian muscle

Authors

Zabriskie JB, Freimer EH

Reference

Journal of Experimental Medicine 1966; **124**:661–678

Summary

The two reports by Kaplan and later by Zabriskie and Freimer first established that there was indeed immunological cross-reactivity or molecular mimicry between Group A streptococcal bacterial antigens and human heart tissues. The evidence for this cross reactivity included production of rabbit antisera against streptococcal cell wall antigens which reacted in immunofluorescence with human cardiac muscle, and complete abolition of immunofluorescence staining of heart muscle tissues after absorption of rabbit antisera to Group A streptococcal antigens by streptococcal cell wall extracts. Moreover, the cross-reactive properties of Group A streptococci were found to be most prominent in streptococcal strains most often associated with acute rheumatic fever. Initially Kaplan's work seemed to implicate cross-reactivity with human heart muscle and streptococcal M proteins, whereas the report by Zabriskie and Freimer localized the cross-reactive antigens to streptococcal cell membranes. Later work by both groups of authors demonstrated that patients with acute rheumatic fever produced antibodies which reacted with heart muscle antigens. These observations set the stage for many other workers who expanded this concept as a probable mechanism of disease pathogenesis.

Related references **(1)** Kaplan MH, Svec KH. Immunologic relation of streptococcal and tissue antigens. III. Presence in human sera of streptococcal antibody cross-reactive with heart tissue. Association with streptococcal infection, rheumatic fever, and glomerulonephritis. *Journal of Experimental Medicine* 1964: 119–151.

(2) Van de Rijn I, Zabriskie JR, McCarty M. Group A streptococcal antigens cross-reactive with myocardium. Purification of heart-reactive antibody and isolation and characterization of the streptococcal antigen. *Journal of Experimental Medicine* 1977; **146**:579–599.

(3) Dale JR, Beachey EH. Epitopes of streptococcal M Proteins shared with cardiac myosin. *Journal of Experimental Medicine* 1985; **162**:583–591.

Key message

The observations by Kaplan and shortly thereafter by Zabriskie and Freimer were the first to establish a clear antigenic cross-reactivity between common bacterial antigenic moieties and human tissues–particularly heart muscle and membranes of heart muscle cells. These findings seemed of particular importance since it was already known that Group A streptococcal pharyngeal infection always preceded the clinical onset of acute rheumatic fever by 2–3 weeks, and that marked elevations of serum antibodies to Group A streptococcal antigens were a reliable sign of rheumatic fever. The clear demonstration that Group A streptococcal throat infection might therefore induce a cross-reacting natural immune response to self or autologous heart muscle tissue was the first example of how such molecular mimicry might be implicated in an acute and subsequent chronic debilitating human disease, namely, rheumatic fever and rheumatic heart disease. This concept of molecular mimicry was subsequently expanded by many other investigators to attempt to explain other manifestations of rheumatic fever as well as other entirely different disease states.

Why it's important

These initial observations by two independent groups were the first clear-cut scientific demonstrations that an organism which caused serious infections in humans, namely the Group A beta-haemolytic streptococcus, could also induce serious illness and consequent lifelong disability and impairment by another mechanism not previously recognized or described. This mechanism was molecular mimicry, causing cross-reactivity between antigens present in the infecting organism and vulnerable human tissues such as human heart muscle cells, heart valves, endocardium lining heart chambers and heart valves, and virtually all heart structures including pericardium, myocardium and cardiac conduction system. Subsequent investigations by these two groups as well as a large number of other investigators demonstrated that initial exposure to Group A streptococcal antigens during the early acute pharyngeal infection could initiate a broad anti-streptococcal immune response which could then damage autologous heart muscle, heart valve structures, and endocardium, as well as probably being responsible for the acute arthritis and even the strange central nervous system disturbance of Sydenham's chorea and athetoid movement disoders, known to be sometimes the only clinical manifestation of acute rheumatic fever. These observations completely changed some of the mechanics of thinking about how diseases happen and what actually activates the vast linkage of physiological messages and communications within the living human organism that could initiate and then perpetuate a self-damaging disease process such as chronic rheumatic heart disease. This disease, with its slow evolution of heart valve inflammation, scarring and deformity or its progressive weakening of left ventricular muscle contraction and disability which we now refer to as cardiomyopathy, starts with an initial Group A streptococcal infection in the throat of the subject who then mounts an immune response to a wide variety of Group A streptococcal antigens which then cross-reacts with autologous tissues and induces first an acute and later a chronic inflammatory response.

Strengths

1. Straightforward scientific evidence presented.
2. First to suggest that bacterial or other external antigens in our environment could start a pathological injurious process in the human host which would by molecular mimicry initiate an acute and then a chronic inflammatory process.

Weakness

Most of the early observations by both groups were directly supported by demonstrations of various cross-reacting humoral antibodies,with little mention of cell-mediated or T cell involved immune response. This is understandable since in the early 1960's not much was understood about cell-mediated or T cell induced immune responsiveness. It was only much later that attention to cell-mediated immunity was directed to acute rheumatic fever and consequent tissue damage in rheumatic fever or chronic rheumatic heart disease.

Relevance

The whole concept of molecular mimicry and its basic influence as an important mechanism of human disease has had its ups and downs in being accepted by the medical and scientific community at large. Perhaps the strongest set of facts that such a mechanism is really of major importance is the whole scenario of acute rheumatic fever and the Group A streptococcus.

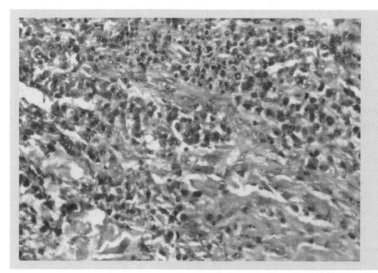

Figure 16.3 Photomicrograph of chronic inflammatory cell infiltrate within a mitral valve of a patient with chronic rheumatic heart disease. Most of the inflammatory cells are small lymphocytes and plasma cells indicating principal involvement of the immune system in this inflammatory process. Haematoxylin and eosin (×380).

CHAPTER 17

Osteoarthritis

Paul Dieppe

Introduction

The story of our developing understanding of osteoarthritis (OA) is far from complete. The papers selected in this section take us through some of the major landmarks of the 20th century, at which point we are still left with much to understand, and a somewhat enigmatic disorder to grapple with.

The different forms of arthritis could only be distinguished when pathology and radiology could be combined with clinical pattern recognition. This process began in the early part of the 20th century with the differentiation of hypertrophic and atrophic forms of arthritis by Goldthwaite (Related reference 1, Paper 1), followed by the superb contribution of Nichols and Richardson (Paper 1), who provided us with the first clear descriptions of OA, but also saddled us with concepts of cartilage degeneration as the basic cause. The 19th century had seen superb clinical descriptions of OA of the finger joints by Heberden and Haygarth. In the 1930s and 40s this form of OA was studied extensively by Stecher, who showed that it had two forms, one idiopathic (and genetic), the other post-traumatic (Paper 2). Until the 1950s, Heberden's nodes had been considered as a separate entity, but this was changed by Kellgren and Moore, who showed the association with large joint OA, and provided us with the definitive description of generalized OA (Paper 3). One of the main and continuing problems in studying OA is the difficulty that we have with definitions, grading and measurement. Jonas Kellgren and John Lawrence, whose contributions to the field were immense, provided us with an x-ray grading system in the 1950s, which remains the gold standard in the 21st century. The application of this system to population studies was pioneered by Lawrence, and led to the seminal observation of the discordance between x-ray changes and symptoms, which changed thinking about this disease for all time (Paper 4). The application of radiographs as an epidemiological tool for the study of OA also allowed this group to make the first associations between occupation and OA (1).

There was only been one major development in the treatment of OA throughout the 20th century, namely the introduction of effective, long lasting prostheses for the hip and knee joints. John Charnley is rightly credited with leading the way here, and his crucial papers of 1960 and of 1961 (Paper 5) would rate as all time classic medical contributions of the last century.

The final three chosen contributions concern more recent attempts to try to understand the aetiopathogenesis of this condition. Only here is the choice difficult and potentially contentious. I could have chosen the work of Henry Mankin on cartilage (2), the work of Eric Radin on biomechanics (3), Paul Byers' contributions to progression (4), or the much more recent innovations in genetics (5). However, it seems to me that biochemistry, pathology and imaging, when combined with clinical observations, remain the key techniques able to help us understand clinical aspects of OA. I have therefore chosen one contribution from the pathologist Peter Bullough who in my view has made the most important contribution to the field (Paper 6), and one paper from Helen Muir and colleagues (Paper 7), in recognition of the huge contribution that Dr Muir made to the investigation of cartilage biochemistry as a window on the pathogenesis of OA, and in the understanding that animal models are an important tool with which to investigate the disease. Finally, I have chosen one paper from my own group, which, with Iain Watt's help, has pioneered the application of new imaging techniques (scintigraphy and MRI) in OA (Paper 8). A further justification for this choice is that its message seems to fit well with the ideas put forward by the four earlier quoted classic contributions, and provides us with a neat circle–from correlations of pathology and radiology with clinical findings in 65 patient studied cross-sectionally in 1909 (Paper 1) to correlations of imaging with clinical findings in 94 patients studied prospectively in the 1990s (Paper 8).

References

1. Kellgren JH, Lawrence JS. Rheumatism in Miners. *British Journal of Industrial Medicine* 1952; **9**:197–207.
2. Mankin HJ. The reaction of articular cartilage to injury and osteoarthritis. *New England Journal of Medicine* 1974; **291**:1335–1340.
3. Radin EL, Paul IL. Response of joints to impact loading. *Arthritis and Rheumatism* 1971; **14**:356–362.
4. Byers P, Contepomi C, Farkas T. A post mortem study of the hip joint. *Annals of Rheumatic Diseases* 1970; **29**;15–31. Prevalence of cartilage lesions in foot joints: a test of the concept of limited and progressive lesions. *Annals of Rheumatic Diseases*, 1970; **29**:15–31.
5. Alo-Kokko L, Baldwin CT, Moskowitz RW, *et al.* Single base mutation in the type II procollagen gene (COL2A1) as a cause of primary osteoarthritis associated with a mild chondrodysplasia. *Proceedings of the National Academy of Sciences USA* 1990;**87**:6565–6568.

Paper 1

'Arthritis deformans'

Authors

Nichols EH, Richardson FL

Reference

Journal of Medical Research 1909; **21**:149–221

Summary

In non-tubercular deforming arthritis there are two pathological types of joint change: (a) the proliferative type, which tends to destroy joint cartilage and lead to ankylosis of the adjacent joint surfaces, and (b) the degenerative type, which tends to destroy the joint cartilage, and produce deformity without ankylosis. These two types do not correspond to two definite diseases, but each type represents reaction of the joint tissues to a considerable variety of causes. In neither type if the original injury is sufficiently severe, or if the causative factor continues to act, is there likelihood of the regeneration of a perfect joint. The nomenclature used in this article is suggested because it describes the pathological process, without any assumption that the aetiology is known in any given case.

Related references　**(1)**　Goldthwaite JE. The treatment of disabled joints resulting from the so-called rheumatoid diseases. *Boston Med Surg J* 1897; **136**:79–84.

(2)　Collins DH. Osteoarthritis. *Journal of Bone and Joint Surgery* 1953; **358**:518–520.

Key message

That there are two main types of arthritis, each of which represents the reaction of a synovial joint to certain types of injury. The proliferative type is characterized by synovial inflammation, the degenerative type by focal areas of loss of articular cartilage.

Why it's important

This article represents the definitive classification of arthritis into the two main types still recognized today, inflammatory and degenerative. This was made possible by a combination of clinical, radiological and pathological expertise; one of the remarkable things about this article, is that its two authors were able to provide clear descriptions of the findings of what would be regarded as three quite different disciplines today: clinical medicine, radiology and pathology. The article is also important for its thesis that each of these two forms of arthritis represent the reaction of joint tissues to a variety of different types of injury, rather than being disease entities.

Subsequently the inflammatory form of arthritis has been split into several diseases, and in some cases the cause is known (gout and septic arthritis for example). In the case of the degenerative type (i.e. OA) it remains appropriate and topical to regard it as the response of a joint to injury. The article is particularly important in the history of OA as it describes and illustrates several patients with different types of this condition, including a woman with

Heberden's nodes, and a man with hip disease ('malum coxae senelis'). This pre-empts the subsequent descriptions of different expressions of OA, featured in other papers in this chapter. In addition, Paper 8, in one sense, brings us full circle to this paper.

Strengths

1. Beautiful, full descriptions of clinical, radiographic and pathological findings.
2. Classical deductive reasoning based on sound observation.
3. Extensively illustrated with line drawings, clinical photographs, photomicrographs and radiographs.

Weaknesses

1. Based on 65 selected cases from one Boston Hospital, only 26 of which came to autopsy.
2. Anchored in the medical science of 1909, which includes several concepts that have been discredited subsequently.
3. Introduction of the term degenerative arthritis, which is one that may have held back research into this form of joint disease.

Relevance

The first clear, comprehensive description of OA, the introduction of the concept of two forms of arthritis, each of which was a reaction of the joints to different forms of insult, and the introduction of the nomenclature 'degenerative arthritis'.

Paper 2

Heberden's nodes: heredity in hypertrophic arthritis of the finger joints

Author

Stecher RM

Reference

American Journal of Medical Science 1941: **201**:801–809

Summary

Heberden's nodes or hypertrophic arthritis of the finger joints may be regarded as a distinct clinical entity. Two types are recognized and distinguishable, one arising as a result of trauma, the other arising spontaneously or idiopathically.

The occurrence of this disease has been shown to be profoundly influenced by race, sex and age differences. A previous study has revealed accurately the incidences of these various classifications. A study of 68 families of patients with idiopathic Heberden's nodes showed that the mothers of such subjects are affected twice as frequently and the sisters three times as frequently as the population in general. These figures, if in error at all, are more likely to be low rather than high. A control series of 43 families selected and studied in the same way showed the sisters of unaffected women to have Heberden's nodes as frequently as the population in general.

The occurrence of multiple cases in the same family cannot be accounted for on the basis of chance alone.

Heredity factors seem best to explain the recorded observations, although the exact mechanism of transmission has not been determined. The conclusions concerning Heberden's nodes are not directly applicable to other forms of hypertrophic arthritis at the present time.

Related references (1) Heberden W. *Commentaries on the history and causes of disease.* London: Payne, 1802.

(2) Haygarth J. *A clinical history of diseases. II. Nodosity of the joints.* London: Gadell and Davies, 1805.

Key message

There are two forms of finger joint OA: one caused by trauma, and the other inherited (Table 17.1).

Table 17.1 Expected-versus-reported prevalence of Heberden's nodes in the sisters and mothers of 68 cases and 43 controls.

	Cases (68)		Controls (43)	
	Mothers (67)	Sisters (129)	Mothers (43)	Sisters (109)
Expected	11	11.4	7	6.3
Observed	21	33	0	5

Why it's important

The early descriptions of OA, such as that of Nichols and Richardson (Paper 1), called the condition a degenerative one, and concentrated on trauma and age as the main causes. Robert Stecher spent a long time studying OA of the finger joints, and studied all the previous literature. He wrote extensively on the subject, and was rewarded with recognition, awards and invitations to speak at prestigious meetings, including (fittingly) giving the 'Heberden Oration'. His particular contributions include the recognition that there are at least two separate forms of finger joint OA: a post-traumatic type and an idiopathic form, and the outcome of this particular paper–the suggestion that the idiopathic form is largely caused by inherited traits. Stecher also uses the nomenclature hypertrophic arthritis, rather than degenerative arthritis, and did much to rekindle interest in OA, and this and his related articles had a high impact at the time and subsequently. Stecher's conclusion that the mechanism of transmission cannot be determined, and that conclusions made from observations of finger joint OA should not be applied to other forms of the disease were very perceptive and remain true today.

Strengths

1. Well illustrated descriptions and illustrations of family trees of three large families with Heberden's nodes.
2. Excellent clinical epidemiology for the time, with a study of 68 index case families and 43 controls, resulting in the clean data, and well calculated ratios of expected-versus-observed rates of Heberden's nodes (see Table 17.1).

Weaknesses

1. His expected rates were based on observations made previously from a different population base, and therefore represent historical controls.
2. The presence or absence of Heberden's nodes in relatives is based on reported history, not examination of the subjects, and may therefore, be erroneous. Stecher recognizes this problem and claims that it is more likely to lead to negative rather than positive bias to his data. He may have been right.

Relevance

Recognition that genetic factors are important in OA, and the differentiation of idiopathic (genetic) finger joint OA from post-traumatic OA.

Paper 3

Generalized osteoarthritis and Heberden's nodes

Authors

Kellgren JH, Moore R

Reference

British Medical Journal 1952; **1**:181–187

Summary

From a study of 391 cases of OA attending a rheumatic clinic we have been able to define a distinct clinical entity for which we suggest the name of primary generalized OA. The condition occurs most often in middle-aged women, and is characterized by a distinct pattern of joint involvement, by a course in which each affected joint passes through an initial painful phase and a more or less acute arthritic phase, and by other distinctive clinical and radiological features.

Generalized OA is a constitutional disorder affecting the diarthrodial joints and probably represents a severe form of idiopathic Heberden's nodes. A therapeutic trial of oestrogen therapy gave negative results, but patients suffering from this disease may be helped considerably by the proper management of their complaints.

Related references (1) Cecil RL, Archer BH. Classification and treatment of chronic arthritis. *Journal of the American Medical Association* 1926; **87**:741–746.

(2) Ehrlich GE. Inflammatory osteoarthritis. *Journal of Chronic Diseases* 1972; **25**:317–328.

Key message

There is a special form of OA (mainly affecting women) that affects several different joint sites in the same individual.

Why it's important

This is one of the most widely quoted papers on OA, being regarded as the original and definitive clinical description of the now generally recognized entity of generalized OA. Kellgren and Moore begin their article by pointing out that hitherto OA of the large joints had been believed to be an age-related degenerative disorder (the legacy of the work of Nichols and Richardson and others). However, they also recognized that the disease called Heberden's nodes (as described by Stecher and others) also seemed to have something to do with OA. So they posed the question 'are Heberden's nodes associated with OA of the large joints?'.

In order to address the question they examined their records from 1,813 cases of all types of arthritis seen in their Department of Rheumatology in Manchester over the last 3 years, and found 120 cases of a generalized form of OA, 110 of which were women. They provide us with a full clinical description of the group, including the joints affected; 103 had Heberden's nodes (most of whom also had thumb base disease), the knees were involved in 64, spine in 57 and hips in 36. Three individual illustrative cases are described in detail, with radiographs and clinical photographs included (Figure 17.1). They describe, for the first time, the tendency of the joints to go through different stages in the evolution of the disease. Because of the high prevalence of this condition in middle-aged women they speculated that it had something to do with the menopause, and took the next, bold step of trying a placebo-controlled trial of oestrogen therapy, which they describe as ineffective. This was one of the first clinical trials of drug therapy for OA.

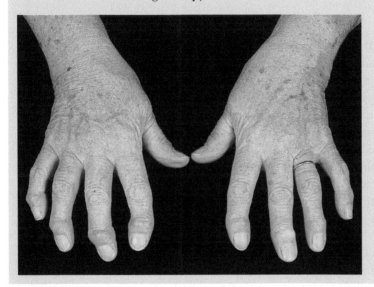

Figure 17.1 The hands of a patient with nodal generalized osteoarthritis, of the sort described in this paper.

Strengths

1. The testing of two hypotheses through clinical research; that Heberden's nodes might be associated with large joint OA, and that oestrogen deficiency might be a factor.
2. Excellent descriptions of the condition, that have never been bettered.
3. The first time that anyone had suggested that there are different stages and phases of activity in the evolution of OA.
4. One of the first clinical trials of drug therapy in OA.

Weaknesses

1. The case selection is not described and is a potential source of bias.
2. No statistical analysis of the expected-versus-observed frequency of the association, or of the clinical trial results.
3. The clinical trial was not randomized and only involved 10 patients in each group, so did not have the power to show whether oestrogens were effective.

Relevance

The definitive description of generalized OA.

Paper 4

Osteo-arthrosis: prevalence in the population and relationships between symptoms and x-ray changes

Authors

Lawrence JS, Bremner JM, Bier F

Reference

Annals of Rheumatic Diseases 1966; **25**:1–24

Summary

A combined urban-rural population in the North of England was questioned about musculo-skeletal pain and loss of work, and was submitted to a clinical examination of the joints and to a routine series of joint x-rays. A sample of blood was tested for rheumatoid factor by the sheep-cell agglutination test. The x-rays were read without knowledge of the history or clinical state.

After standardization of the adult population for age and sex by the unweighted mean, the prevalence of osteo-arthrosis was found to be 52% in males and 51% in females. Five or more joint groups were affected in 9% of males and 12% of females, the proportion increasing rapidly with age to a maximum of 37% in males and 49% in females aged 65 years and over. When minimal disease was excluded, the prevalence of osteo-arthrosis was 19% in males and 22% in females, and five or more joint groups were affected in 0.5% of males and 1.8% of females. Standardization to the 1961 population of England and Wales gave slightly lower prevalences in males.

On the basis of the clinical, radiological and serological findings, the population was divided into a rheumatoid and a non-rheumatoid group. In the non-rheumatoid group there was a significant correlation between x-ray changes of osteo-arthrosis and the frequency of symptoms in the corresponding distribution. This was present in all joints except those of the lumbar spine and was only marginal in the cervical spine. In the rheumatoid groups there was a higher rate of symptoms, but the increase of complaints with the severity of osteo-arthrosis was no greater than that in the non-rheumatoid group. Morning stiffness was associated with an increase in symptoms in the hands and knees in the non-rheumatoid group regardless of whether osteo-arthrosis was present or not.

Obesity was associated with an increase of pain in the knees in persons with osteo-arthrosis but had little influence on those without. Persons with osteo-arthrosis who had been classified as neurotic did not have a higher complaint compared with those not so classified, nor did those with a history of injury. Persons with osteo-arthrosis living in damp houses did not have significantly more than the expected proportion of symptoms, but the numbers in very damp houses were small. Symptoms were only slightly more when bone cysts were present in the metacarpophalangeal joints, but showed no relationship to symptoms in the hip joints.

Related reference   **(1)**   Kellgren J, Lawrence JS. Radiological assessment of osteoarthritis. *Annals of Rheumatic Diseases* 1957; **16**:494–501.

Key message

Radiographic changes of OA are very common in the community, and predispose to joint pain. However, severe radiographic OA is often asymptomatic (Table 17.2).

Table 17.2 Data on the association between x-ray grades and symptoms in people without rheumatoid arthritis, taken from the data in this paper (% of people with symptoms).

Joint	Sex	Radiographic grading 0–1	2	3–4
DIP	M	1.4	8.1	9.4
	F	1.3	6.2	25.0
Hip	M	5.8	0	56.3
	F	9.6	0	100
Knee	M	22.9	41.7	55.5
	F	20.1	43.3	79.5

Why it's important

This paper reports the prevalence of symptoms and x-ray changes of OA of the spine, hips, knees, hands and feet in a large community-based cohort of people in the North of England (1098 men and 1198 women). It illustrates that radiographic changes of OA are extremely common. It also showed up the discrepancy between x-ray changes, which are graded on the Kellgren and Lawrence 0–4 system, and the presence of symptoms, such that many of those with the most severe changes of OA on x-ray are asymptomatic. It is clear that in the spine radiographic changes are practically meaningless and that the discrepancy between pain and x-ray changes in peripheral joints is more obvious in the hand, and least marked in the first metatarsophalangeal joint.

Although the authors are most concerned with prevalence rates, the seminal observation made to our understanding of OA was this discordance between pathology and clinical features. They show clearly that the radiographic surrogate for joint pathology cannot be equated with the clinical syndrome. The observation, which has since been confirmed by many other surveys, has been seen as a problem by many, undermining their concept of a disease. It certainly makes us have to think differently about the nature of OA, but it provided the freedom to ask questions about the causes of pain, which still remain unanswered today. Many of their other observations about associations and features of radiographic OA are unparalleled, and this is a huge paper with a mass of good data.

Strengths

1. Comprehensive clinical and radiographic data on large numbers from a community.
2. A huge amount of data, carefully analysed and reported.
3. Definitive data on the prevalence of radiographic OA in the population.

Weaknesses

1. No concern for potential errors in x-ray readings.
2. Dependence on the Kellgren and Lawrence grading system, which, while useful, has a number of inherent problems, such as the assumptions of linearity and the assumption that bone and cartilage changes occur together.
3. A very complicated paper, muddled in places.
4. No hypothesis testing.

Relevance

The baseline data for prevalence of radiographic OA in the community, and the first and major contribution to show that x-ray changes, while predisposing to symptoms, cannot be equated with them or seen as their cause.

Paper 5

Arthroplasty of the hip: a new operation

Author

Charnley J

Reference

The Lancet 1961; **1**:1129–1132

Summary

There is no summary or abstract to this paper, which reports Charnley's early work on and experience with his new design of hip replacement. In the introduction to this key piece of work he writes:

'In considering how arthroplasty of the hip can be improved, two facts stand out:
(1) After replacement of the head of the femur by a spherical surface of inert material, the failures are essentially long-term. At first the patient may notice no difference between the artificial head and the living one which preceded it. Our problem is to make this temporary success permanent.
(2) Objectives must be reasonable. Neither surgeons nor engineers will ever make an artificial hip joint which will last 30 years and at the same time in this period enable the patient to play football.'

This remains as true in 2001 as it was in 1961.

He then describes the principles and laboratory research which led to the design of his revolutionary low friction arthroplasty, through the use of a polytetrafluorethylene socket and a metallic femoral head, and the cementing of the prosthesis into the femur. He notes that only 97 of his new designed hips have been inserted, and long-term results are awaited, there had only been one death (due to a post-operative myocardial infarction) and the early results were good.

Related references (1) Charnley J. Anchorage of the femoral head prosthesis to the shaft of the femur. *Journal of Bone and Joint Surgery* 1960; **42**(B):28–30.

(2) Charnley J. The long term results of low-friction arthroplasty of the hip performed as a primary intervention. *Journal of Bone and Joint Surgery* 1972; **54**(B):61–76.

(3) Wroblewski BM. Fifteen to 21-year results of the Charnley low-friction arthroplasty. *Clinical Orthopaedics and Related Research* 1986; **211**:30–35.

Key message

A low friction arthroplasty of the hip, with a cemented femoral component, provides a good prosthesis in bioengineering terms, and early clinical results are encouraging.

Why it's important

John Charnely is rightly regarded as the father of modern joint replacement. Of all the papers quoted in this section, this is the only one which heralded a breakthrough of major importance to those who suffer from OA. The introduction and subsequent wide usage of Charnley's hip prosthesis (and subsequent designs and developments in the hip and knee) has brought relief to literally millions of people with OA resulting in severe pain and disability.

Prior to Charnley's work, there had been a number of attempts at replacing the hip with artificial materials, but they had been largely unsuccessful (Charnley describes the problems with the Smith Peterson and Judet hips in the first part of this article). The innovation reported in this paper was the design of a low friction prosthesis through the use of new materials, and the design, which included a small femoral head, cemented into the femur. This design has proved as good as any of those subsequently developed, most of which have used the same principles as Charnely. For example, the related paper of Wrobeleski (3) demonstrates excellent long-term outcomes.

Strengths

1. Charnley was ahead of his time, his insight into the need for a low friction bearing, and the use of long-lasting high molecular weight plastics and bone cement revolutionized the outcome of joint replacement, and changed this from a poor option to the preferred option for severe joint disease.
2. A wonderful, concise description of the scientific rationale for his innovations.

Weaknesses

1. Relatively small numbers of cases studied over a short period of time, and no convincing outcome measures reported.
2. This is Charnley saying 'trust me, I'm a surgeon', but, he was right.

Relevance

An innovation that changed medicine, surgery and the prospects for those with severe OA for ever and for the better. One of the great contributions of all time.

Paper 6

The geometry of diarthrodial joints, its physiological maintenance and the possible signficicance of age-related changes in geometry to load distribution and the development of osteoarthritis

Author

Bullough PG

Reference

Clinical Orthopaedics and Related Research 1981; **156**:61–7

Summary

Diarthrodial joints are governed by physiological mechanisms that maintain stability and an equitable distribution of load. Modelling continues throughout life to maintain the necessary physiological incongruity. However, in old age the system seems to go awry, and the result is an increasing congruity yielding possibly increased stability but interfering with cartilage nutrition and altering the distribution of load. The increasing maldistribution of load with age, it is proposed, mechanically overtaxes the previously underloaded and, presumably, atrophic cartilage. Overtaxing the cartilage in turn leads to further depletion of proteoglycans, collagen fraying and eventually OA. Thus arthritis, at least in one of its forms, appear to be inevitable because of the maldistribution of load that results from age-related changes in joint shape, possibly dictated by the joint's requirement for stability.

Related references **(1)** Bullough PG, Goodfellow J, O'Connor J. The relationship between degenerative changes and load bearing in the human hip. *Journal of Bone and Joint Surgery* 1973; **55**(B):746.

(2) Lane LB, Bullough PG. Age-related changes in the thickness of the calcified zone and the number of tidemarks in adult human articular cartilage. *Journal of Bone and Joint Surgery* 1980; **62**(B):372.

Key message

Age-related changes in the congruity of joints leads to OA, through alterations in the load-bearing surface.

Why it's important

Fittingly, this paper is reported in an edition of the journal dedicated to Truetta, who was one of the first observers to stress the importance of vascularity and bone turnover in the aetiopathogenesis of OA. This essay summarizes much of the very important work done by Peter Bullough and his colleagues in the 1970s (see also related references). He (re)-described the changes in bone vascularity and in the tidemark seen in normal joints with age-ing and in OA, suggesting that bone turnover and changes in bone shape are crucial, and he also showed that cartilage damage develops at sights of maximal loading of joints. He put these observations together with his very extensive experience of the morbid anatomy and pathology of osteoarthritic joints to produce a clear story as to how OA develops.

Strengths

1. A clear, concise, plausible story on the aetiopathogenesis of OA.
2. Paper based on a combination of careful pathological observations and descriptions and laboratory-based tests of hypotheses on joint congruity and loading.
3. Well illustrated.

Weaknesses

1. This is an essay, it contains very little data.
2. Bullough asks you to believe him, but, like Charnley, he is probably right.

Relevance

This work emphasized the dynamic nature of the response of the joint to injury, and was therefore the forerunner of much of the recent work on turnover of cartilage and bone.

Paper 7

An experimental model of osteoarthritis: early morphological and biochemical changes

Authors

McDevitt C, Gilbertson E, Muir H

Reference

Journal of Bone and Joint Surgery 1977; **59**:24–35

Summary

An experimental model of OA resulting from laxity of the joint was induced in 18 mature dogs (at least 2 years old) by sectioning the anterior cruciate ligament of the right knee (stifle) with a stab incision, the left knee providing a control. A sham operation was also performed in three other dogs, in which a stab incision was made but the ligament left intact. The dogs were killed at various intervals from 1 to 48 weeks later. Morphological changes in bone, cartilage, synovial membrane and joint capsule were examined in all joints and biochemical changes in the cartilage of three dogs killed after 2, 8, and 16 weeks. All the changes resulting from the operation progressed with time and became indistinguishable from those found in three dogs with natural OA of the knee. There were no changes in the joints which had had the sham operations. As the time of onset is known, this experimental model in a larger species enables a study to be made of the biochemical as well as the morphological changes in the early stages of OA.

Related references

(1) Pond N, Nuki G. Experimentally induced osteoarthritis in the dog. *Annals of Rheumatic Diseases* 1973; **32**:387–8 (Abstract).

(2) McDevitt C, Muir H, Pond N. Canine articular cartilage in natural and experimentally induced osteoarthritis. *Biochemical Society Transactions* 1973; **1**: 287–8 (Abstract).

(3) McDevitt C, Muir H. Biochemical changes in the cartilage of the knee in experimental and natural osteoarthritis in the dog. *Journal of Bone and Joint Surgery* 1976; **58**(B): 94–101.

(4) Brandt KD, Braunstein EM, Visco DM. Anterior cruciate ligament transection in the dog: a bona fide model of canine osteoarthritis, not merely of cartilage injury and repair. *Journal of Rheumatology* 1991; **18**:436–446.

Key message

An experimental model of OA in a large animal results in changes that are indistinguishable from those of the naturally occurring disease, and the model can be used to study the early biochemical changes of OA.

Why it's important

One of the many serious problems in studying OA in humans is the fact that one never knows how, why or when it started. The onset of the clinical disease is insidious, and often appears to have been triggered by an event (such as a serious joint injury) that occurred many years previously.

In this paper, McDevitt and colleagues provide a full, definitive description of what became known as the 'Pond-Nuki model' of OA, OA in the dog induced by a stab incision to divide the cruciate ligament. This was the first good animal model of OA which allowed investigators to document early changes at any stage after the initiating event, in a species of sufficient size to allow good tissue samples to be available, and one in which the disease occurs naturally. This model, and others like it, have been used extensively to study OA over the last two decades.

This paper describes elegant studies of the phenomenon. The authors used some controls in which a stab incision was made but the ligament not divided, to show that the OA resulted from the ligament transection, and was not just the result of a surgical assault on the joint. They also compared the artificial arthritis with the naturally occurring disease in the same species. Finally, they showed how biochemical changes could be correlated with histological ones, heralding a new era in the investigation of OA. One of the key findings in this paper was the demonstration of increased hydration of the articular cartilage in the early phases of the disease.

Strengths

1. Careful experimental design, with good controls.
2. Correlation of histology with biochemical changes in the cartilage.
3. Analysis of the outcome at various time points after the insult.

Weaknesses

1. Relatively small numbers of animals described.
2. Lack of clarity on the exact site of the sections taken for biochemical analysis.
3. Biochemical changes only studied after a relatively short time period (16 weeks maximum).

Relevance

Introduction of a new, relevant model of human OA, in which early changes could be described and in which morphological changes can be correlated with biochemical ones.

Paper 8

The prediction of the progression of joint space narrowing in osteoarthritis of the knee by bone scintigraphy

Authors

Dieppe P, Cushnaghan J, Young P, Kirwan J

Reference

Annals of Rheumatic Diseases 1993; **52**:557–563

Summary

Objectives: To test the hypothesis that bone scintigraphy will predict the outcome of OA of the knee joint.

Methods: 94 patients (65 women, 29 men, mean age 64.2 years) with established OA of one or both knee joints were examined in 1986, when radiographs and bone scan images (early and late phase) were obtained. The patients were recalled, re-examined, and had further radiographs taken in 1991. Paired entry and outcome radiographs were read by a single observer, blind to date order and other data. Scan findings and other entry variables were related to outcome. Progression of OA of the knee was defined as an operation on the knee or a decrease in the tibiofemoral joint space of 2 mm (0.08 in) or more.

Results: Over the 5 year study period 10 patients died and nine were lost to follow-up. Fifteen had an operation on one or both knees (22 knees). Of the remaining 120 knees (60 patients) analysed radiographically, 14 (12%) had progressed in the manner defined. Of 32 knees with severe scan abnormalities, 28 (88%) showed progression, whereas none of the 55 knees with no scan abnormality at entry had progressed. The strong negative predictive power of scintigraphy could not be accounted for by disease severity or any combination of entry variables. Pain severity predicted a subsequent operation, but age, sex, symptom duration, and obesity had no predictive value.

Conclusions: Scintigraphy predicts subsequent loss of joint space in patients with established OA of the knee joint. This is the first description of a powerful predictor of change in this disease. The finding suggests that the activity of the subchondral bone may determine loss of cartilage.

Related references **(1)** McAlindon TE, Watt I, McCrae F, Goddard P, Dieppe P. Magnetic resonance imaging in osteoarthritis of the knee: correlation with radiographic and scintigraphic findings. *Annals of Rheumatic Diseases* 1991; **50**:14–19.

(2) McCrae F, Shouls J, Dieppe P, Watt I. Scintigraphic assessment of osteoarthritis of the knee joint. *Annals of Rheumatic Diseases* 1992; **51**:938–942.

(3) McCarthy C, Cushnaghan J, Dieppe P. The predictive role of scintigraphy in radiographic osteoarthritis of the hand. *Osteoarthritis and Cartilage* 1994; **2**:25–28.

Key message

If a bone scan shows inactive subchondral bone in the knee joint in a patient with OA, that joint will not progress radiographically over the next 5 years.

Why it's important

Bone scintigraphy is a technique generally used to detect bony metastases; it indicates areas of high bone turnover. In a series of papers by this group, scintigraphy was used to show that the subchondral and marginal bone of osteoarthritic joints is active, that this activity turns on and off (substantiating the idea of Kellgren and Moore that the activity of OA was phasic, Figure 17.2), and then by correlating scintigraphic, clinical and radiographic findings with time, showed that scintigraphic activity was predictive of radiographic progression in both the knee and the hand.

Prior to this, fuelled by the early descriptions of OA as a disease of articular cartilage by Nichols and Richardson and others, there had been a general assumption that cartilage is the main tissue affected in this disease, and that cartilage should be the main target for therapeutic interventions. However, this was one of the first pieces of empirical research to implicate bone pathology as one of the major factors in the pathogenesis of progressive OA. It helped the development of a paradigm change in our thinking about OA, which is now regarded as a disease process of the whole joint organ in which bony, synovial and capsular changes are as important as cartilage damage. It has also helped switch attention from cartilage to bone in thinking about therapeutic targets. Subsequently, MRI has shown similar bone changes, as outlined in McAlindon, *et al.* (1).

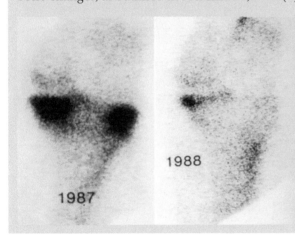

Figure 17.2 Late phase (3 hour) bone scans of the knee of a patient with OA taken 1 year apart. The first scan (1987) shows extensive retention of isotope in the tibial subchondral bone, indicating high turnover. One year later, most of this activity has disappeared and isotope retention is limited to the 'rim pattern' described by McCrae and colleagues, indicating activity in osteophytes only. This illustrates the phasic nature of the activity of OA.

Strengths

1. A relatively large and long-term prospective study.
2. Careful attention to detail in scoring scans and radiographs and in the analysis of variables that might affect progression.

Weaknesses

1. The definition of radiographic progression and non-progression is somewhat arbitrary.
2. The use of knee replacement as a surrogate for progression may be erroneous.
3. The patients were a highly selected group, coming from a hospital practice.

Relevance

Empirical research to show that bone pathology is important in the progression of OA. The first, and to date the strongest predictor of OA outcome.

CHAPTER 18

Crystal deposition diseases

Daniel J McCarty

Introduction

Progress in any field proceeds by a series of modest steps forward. Each step is influenced by steps preceding it and influences those that follow. Although I have been involved in research into arthritic diseases that involve deposition of microcrystals in joint tissues for nearly 40 years, I find that choosing six to eight papers out of thousands published in the past century a daunting and somewhat subjective task. My first choice of papers was (immodestly) my paper with JL Hollander reporting the definitive identification of monosodium urate (MSU) crystals in gouty arthritis. The discovery of calcium pyrophosphate dihydrate crystals and 'pseudogout' was a direct result of this work. Both papers have been transferred by our editors to the joint fluid section of this volume leaving me with fresh choices.

The synthesis, characterization and demonstration of a dose-related inflammatory response to MSU crystals fulfilled Koch's postulates in a non-infectious disease (Paper 1). The discovery of the first cell-derived chemotactic factor and the principal mechanism of action of colchicine, perhaps the oldest known effective drug, were derived from this work (Paper 2). Gout is arguably the most treatable disease in all of medicine because MSU crystal deposition is possible only from saturated urate solutions. Saturation is markedly influenced by local temperature. Solubilization of MSU crystals from cooler body parts often requires serum levels of 0.24 mmol/l (4 mg/dl) or less. Effective control of hyperuricemia and MSU crystal deposition followed the introduction of effective, relatively non-toxic, drugs which inhibited renal tubular resorption of uric acid (probenecid, Papers 3a and b) or inhibited the synthesis of uric acid by blocking xanthine oxidase (allopurinol Paper 4).

As MSU crystal formation is driven by a systemic rise in uric acid levels, CPPD crystal deposition requires locally increased inorganic pyrophosphate (PPi) levels in synovial fluid and joint tissues. Plasma PPi levels are normal in patients with this condition. Just as effective control of hyperuricemia and gout was preceded by quantitative studies of uric acid metabolism, effective control of CPPD crystal deposition requires such studies of PPi metabolism. Generation of PPi from extracellular adenosine triphosphate (ATP) by ectonucleoside triphosphate pyrophosphohydrolase in synovial fluid was quantitatively sufficient to account for the PPi production rate *in vivo* as estimated by PPi pool size and turnover rate in human knee joints, and for the PPi quantities elaborated by human cartilage in organ culture extrapolated to the estimated mass of cartilage in human knee joints (Paper 5).

The originators of the term 'chondrocalcinosis' found that most joints with such calcified cartilage became severely degenerative over time (Paper 6). Joints not affected as part of the 'nodal osteoarthritis' pattern such as the wrist, carpus, elbow, shoulder, hip and metacarpal phalangeal often showed such changes. Lastly, it seemed appropriate to recognize the role of the kidney tubules in both the aetiology of hyperuricemia and as targets for drugs used to lower serum uric acid. Our current understanding is based on a four component model (Paper 7).

Paper I

Acute arthritis in man and dog after intrasynovial injection of sodium urate crystals

Authors

Faires JS, McCarty DJ

Reference

The Lancet 1962, **2**:682–685

Summary

Synthetic monosodium urate monohydrate crystals identical by x-ray diffraction powder pattern to crystals purified from a gouty tophus were sterilized and injected into the knees of two normal (non-gouty) subjects and into the stifle joints of 20 healthy dogs. Swelling, tenderness, warmth and redness of overlying skin and finally pain ensued (three-legged gait in dogs). Crystals were identified in synovial fluid neutrophils. Inflammatory intensity and neutrophilic response were directly proportional to the dose of injected crystals.

Characterization of the suspected aetiologic agent, reproduction of the signs and symptoms in subjects not affected with the disease, and recovery of the aetiologic agent from the lesions fulfilled Koch's postulates for proof of aetiology, albeit in a metabolic, rather than an infectious disease.

Related references

(1) Seegmiller JE, Howell RR, Malawista SE. The inflammatory response to injected sodium urate. *Journal of the American Medical Association* 1962; **180**:469–475. (Independent study showing acute inflammation after injection of synthetic monosodium urate crystals into joints of gouty patients.)

(2) Freudweiler M. Studies on the nature of gouty tophi. *Deutches Archiv fir Klin Med* 1899; **63**:266. (Showed that synthetic sodium urate crystals caused inflammation in a normal human and in several animal species.)

(3) McCarty DJ, Brill J. *Annals of Internal Medicine* 1964; **60**: 486–505. (An abridged translation of the work of Freudweiler and His with comments.)

Key message

This paper established that sodium urate crystals cause acute inflammation. The classic work of Freudweiler and his mentor, Wilhelm His Jr, appears to have been lost to posterity, perhaps due to the untimely death of the former at age 31 years. We discovered it during an intensive search of the older literature. The work of Seegmiller, *et al.* confirmed the inflammatory response to urate crystals, but release into the joint space of endogenous tophaceous urates could not be ruled out (1).

Why it's important

It explains why long-term lowering of serum urate results in far fewer acute attacks of gout. Also led to the discovery of the mechanism of action of colchicine.

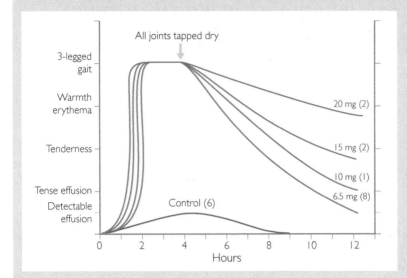

Figure 18.1 Clinical response in dogs to intrasynovial injection of crystalline sodium urate.

Strength

A dose-dependent relationship was established between monosodium urate crystals and an acute inflammatory reaction as seen in acute gouty arthritis. Koch's postulates remain the gold standard for proof of aetiology.

Weakness

The injected material was sterile as it had been autoclaved but no proof that the crystals had not entrapped pyrogen was provided. The limulus assay for pyrogen had not yet been developed. The standard test at that time was development of an elevated rectal temperature in rabbits after intravenous injection of the test material. This was not done either. But even if it had been done, it would not have been sufficiently sensitive to detect amounts of pyrogen sufficient to cause joint inflammation.

Relevance

Demonstration of the phlogistic properties of urate crystals.

Paper 2

Polymorphonuclear leukocyte motility in vitro. IV. Colchicine inhibition of chemotactic activity formation after phagocytosis of urate crystals

Author

Phelps P

Reference

Arthritis and Rheumatism 1970; **12**:1–9

Summary

Colchicine, then regarded as a highly specific treatment, and since the 1930s as a prophylactic agent for acute gout, blocked the release of a cell-derived chemotactic factor in doses as low as 10^{-10}M. Other actions of the drug such as inhibition of phagocytosis or cell adhesiveness require concentrations 10^{-6}M.

Related references (1) Phelps P. Polymorphonuclear leukocyte motility in vitro. III. Possible release of a chemotactic substance following phagocytosis of urate crystals. *Arthritis and Rheumatism* 1969; **12**:197–204.

(2) Wallace SH, Omokoku B, Ertel NH. Colchicine plasma levels – implications as to pharmacology and mechanisms of action. *American Journal of Medicine* 1970; **48**:443–448.

(3) Spilberg I. Colchicine and pseudogout. *Arthritis and Rheumatism* 1980; **23**:1062–1063.

(4) Alvarellos A, Spilberg I. Colchicine prophylaxis in pseudogout. *Journal of Rheumatology* 1986; **13**:804–805.

Key message

Colchicine, at concentrations easily achieved in plasma by usual doses and known to be effective in the suppression of gouty inflammation, almost completely abolished the release of a chemotactic glycopeptide by polymorphonuclear leukocytes that had phagocytosed particulates such as microcrystals. These data explained: (a) why the drug is effective in non-gouty conditions such as pseudogout and calcific periarthritis; (b) why the drug was more effective when given intravenously (10-fold greater plama concentration), and (c) why the drug is not an effective general antiinflammatory agent.

Why it's important

This study showed that colchicine is specific therapy for inflammation induced by the endocytosis of particulate matter by polymorphonuclear leucocytes and not, as long thought, specific for gouty inflammation *per se*. It represented the death knell of the last surviving 'diagnostic' therapeutic trial. It also explained the mechanism of action of the oldest known drug. Herbal colchicine was known in ancient Asia Minor as 'hermodacyl' (the finger of Hermes).

Strengths

1. Very clever experimental design enabling simultaneous measurement of chemotaxis, random cell motility and crystal phagocytosis.
2. The effect of varying drug dose was determined using a crystal dose-response curve for each of these variables.

Weakness

No *in vivo* correlation of suppression of chemotactic factor formation in patients with acute gouty arthritis was attempted. This was partially addressed in subsequent experiments using the canine model.

Relevance

Demonstrated the mode of action of colchicine in crystal-induced arthritis.

Paper 3a

The clinical and metabolic effects of Benemid in patients with gout

Authors

Talbot JH, Bishop C, Norcross BM, Lockie LM

Reference

Transactions of the Association of American Physicians 1951; **64**:372–377

Paper 3b

Benemid (p-di-n-propylsulfamyl)-benzoic acid as uricosuric agent in chronic gouty arthritis

Authors

Gutman AB, Yü TF

Reference

Transactions of the Association of American Physicians 1951; **64**:279–288

Summary

Independent simultaneous reports demonstrating the uricosuric properties of probenecid, the first effective practical treatment for hyperuricemia. Aspirin in large (≥ 5 g/day) doses had been used previously for this purpose but salicylism was frequently severe.

Related references **(1)** Garrod AB. Observations on certain pathological conditions of the blood and urine in gout, rheumatism and Brights' disease. *Transactions of the Medical-Chirogical Society* London 1848; **31**:83–98.

(2) Burns JJ, Yü TF, Ritterband A, Perel JM, Gutman AB, Brodie BB. A potent new uricosuric agent, the sulfoxide metabolite of the phenylbutazone analogue G 25671. *Journal of Pharmacology and Experimental Therapeutics* 1957; **119**:418–426.

(3) Jain AK. Effect of single doses of benzbromarone on serum and urinary uric acid. *Arthritis and Rheumatism* 1974;**21**:456–458.

(4) Gutman AB, Yü TF. Protracted uricosuric therapy in tophaceous gout. *The Lancet* 1957; **2**:1258–1260. (Follow-up study showing control and even resolution of gouty tophi.)

(5) Loeb JN. The influence of temperature on the solubility of monosodium urate. *Arthritis and Rheumatism* 1972; **15**:189–192.

Key message

Both studies measured serum and urinary uric acid in gouty subjects using colorimetric methods. Toxicity to probenecid was dose-related between 500 and 2000 mg/day. The Gutman-Yü study showed that treatment induced acute gouty attacks and uric acid crystalluria, and that the effect of the drug could be reversed by increased protein intake (increased *de novo* purine synthesis) and by aspirin ingestion in the range of 1–3 g/daily (block of probenecid effect on urate tubular reabsorption). The Talbot study noted mobilization of urate from a non-miscible pool, suggesting that tophaceous urates would be reabsorbed by lowering serum uric acid levels sufficiently.

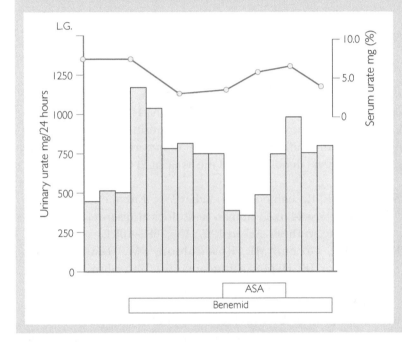

Figure 18.2 Suppressive effect of addition of acetylsalicylic acid (ASA) (2.6 g daily) to Benemid (2.0 g daily) on urinary urate excretion in a case of chronic gout maintained on a low protein, low purine diet. Each column represents 24 hours.

Why it's important

Tophaceous deposits can cause destruction of bone, cartilage and other tissues, producing chronic gouty arthritis. Probenecid represented the first relatively safe drug to rid the body of established tophaceous masses and prevent new masses from forming.

Strength

Almost everything now known about probenecid, it's mechanism, dose, toxicity, drug interactions, and so on was presented in the initial two reports.

Weakness

Until the advent of the specific uricase spectrophotometric method for quantifying uric acid, non-specific colorimetric methods were used. These measured reducing substances generally but were sufficiently accurate for the type of clinical studies described here.

Relevance

The first definitive treatment for gout.

Paper 4

Effects of a xanthine oxidase inhibitor on thiopurine metabolism, hyperuricemia and gout

Authors

Rundles RW, Wyngaarden JB, Hitchings GH, *et al.*

Reference

Transactions of the Association of American Physicians 1963; **76**:126–140.

Summary

First report of the use of the hypoxanthine analogue allopurinol, a competitive inhibitor of xanthine oxidase, to lower serum uric acid levels in gouty patients. Hitchings and Elion shared the Nobel Prize for this and other work on antagonists of purine metabolism. Now widely over-prescribed, allopurinol revolutionized the treatment of hyperuricemia, providing a powerful means of reversing urate crystal deposition and the associated tissue destruction.

Related references **(1)** Seegmiller JE, Rosenbloom FM, Kelley WN. Enzyme deficit associated with a sex-linked human neurological disorder and excessive purine synthesis. *Science* 1967; **155**:1682–1684.

(2) Kelley WN, Greene ML, Rosenbloom FM, Henderson JF, Seegmiller JE. Hypoxanthine-guanine phosphoribosyltransferase deficiency in gout. *Annals of Internal Medicine* 1969; **70**:155–206.

(3) Becker MA, Meyer U, Wood AW, Seegmiller JE. Purine overproduction in man associated with increased phosphoribosylpyrophosphate synthase activity. *Science* 1973; **179**:1123–1126.

(4) Palella TD, Silverman LS, Schroll CT, Homa FH, Levine M, Kelley WN. Herpes simplex virus-mediated human hypoxanthine-guanine phosphoribosyltransferase gene transfer into neuronal cells. *Molecular and Cellular Biology* 1988; **8**:457–460. (Early *in vitro* attempt at gene therapy of Lesch-Nyhan neuronal cells. This syndrome is high on the list of severely incapacitating single gene abnormalities and as such is a strong candidate for attempts at normal gene insertion therapy.)

Key message

Allopurinol blocked conversion of hypoxanthine to xanthine and xanthine to uric acid, causing a rapid fall in serum urate levels.

Why it's important

The use of allopurinol, sometimes in combination with probenecid, achieved plasma urate levels low enough to dissolve tophaceous deposits in nearly all patients. It was also quantitatively converted to its ribonucleotide by hypoxanthine-guanine phosphoribosyl transferase (HGPRTase) thereby depleting the pool of phosphoribosylpyrophosphate (PRPP) a key substrate in the *de novo* synthesis of inosinic acid, the parent purine precursor of uric acid. Lastly, as its ribonucleotide, it acted as a pseudofeedback inhibitor of the enzyme catalyzing the first step of inosinic acid synthesis. Allopurinol can produce serious side-effects but considering its potency and specificity, it is relatively benign.

Strengths

1. The precise mechanism of inhibitors of xanthine oxidase by this hypoxanthine analog was known.
2. The uric acid balance studies were carefully done using specific (uricase) assays.

Weakness

The drop in serum uric acid was accompanied, as expected, by a fall in urinary uric acid excretion that was not matched by an equivalent use in urinary xanthine and hypoxanthine in most patients. This mystery was later solved (1, 2).

Relevance

Demonstration of the efficacy of allopurinol in rapidly lowering serum and urinary uric acid levels.

Paper 5

Inorganic pyrophosphate generation from adenosine triphosphate by cell-free synovial fluid

Authors

Park W, Masuda I, Cardenal-Escarcena A, Palmer DL, McCarty DJ

Reference

Journal of Rheumatology 1996; **23**:665–671

Summary

Quantitative studies of ATP hydrolysis to PPi by synovial fluid nucleoside triphosphate pyrophosphohydrolase showed that this reaction could account for the formation of all extracellular PPi in joint tissues. The limiting factor was the availability of the substrate extracellular ATP. Down regulation of local PPi concentration may prevent or reverse calcium pyrophosphate crystal deposition in cartilage and other articular tissues. By analogy with urate crystals in gout, this may reverse or prevent the associated tissue damage. These data explain why CPPD crystals are commonly found in association with osteoarthritis (OA) but not rheumatoid arthritis (RA). Extracellular ATP is elevated in OA joint fluid and is very low in fluid from inflamed joints. The rate of ATP conversion to PPi in rheumatoid joint fluid may approach zero.

Related references

(1) Camerlaine M, McCarty DJ, Silcox DC, Jung A. Inorganic pyrophosphate pool size and turnover rate in arthritic joints. *Journal of Clinical Investigation* 1975; **55**:1373–1381.

(2) Howell DS, Muniz 0, Pita JC, Enis JE. Extrusion of pyrophosphate into extracellular media by osteoarthritic cartilage incubates. *Journal of Clinical Investigation* 1975; **56**:1473–1480.

(3) Ryan LM, Wortmann RL, Karas B, McCarty DJ. Cartilage nucleoside triphosphate (NTP) pyrophosphohydrolase. I. Identification as an ectoenzyme. *Arthritis and Rheumatism* 1984; **27**:404–409.

(4) Masuda I, Halligan B, Barbieri J, Haas A, Ryan LM, McCarty DJ. Molecular cloning and expression of a porcine chondrocyte nucleotide pyrophosphohydrolase. *Gene* 1997; **197**:277–287.

Key message

Conversion of ATP to PPi by joint fluid ecto-nucleoside triphosphate pyrophosphohydrolase measured *ex vivo* accounts for all PPi production by synovial tissues.

Why it's important

If it is assumed that the biologic activity of CPPD crystals can result in destructive joint changes then attempts should be made to prevent and/or dissolve them. The study cited showed that conversion of ATP, at levels measured *ex vivo*, to PPi by joint fluid ecto-nucleoside triphosphate pyrophosphohydrolase under physiologic conditions was sufficient to account for all PPi production by synovial tissues. Substrate availability, not ecto-enzyme, is the limiting factor in the reaction. Control of joint tissue PPi level and CPPD crystal deposition will probably require control of extracellular ATP levels.

Strengths

1. Studies were quantitative using precise methods to control for PPi hydrolysis and generation of ATP products other than PPi.
2. PPi generated was compared with the results of previous intra-articular PPi pool and turnover studies and with PPi quantities released from articular cartilage incubated in organ culture.

Weaknesses

1. Studies were done *in vitro* using ATP levels measured *ex vivo*, i.e. in fluid obtained from joints afflicted with various forms of arthritis.
2. It is possible that the *ex vivo* measured ATP levels were too high.

Relevance

Demonstration of the enzyme system responsible for extracellular pyrophosphate production using quantitative methods.

Paper 6

Natural course of articular chondrocalcinosis

Authors

Zitnan D, Sitaj S

Reference

Arthritis and Rheumatism 1976; **19**(suppl.):363–390

Summary

Longitudinal radiographic study of familial calcium pyrophosphate crystal deposition in Hungarians living in Slovakia. The trait leading to cartilaginous calcification followed a Mendelian autosomal dominant pattern with complete penetrance by the fourth decade of life. Initially the affected joints appeared normal radiographically, except for the calcification. Degenerative joint disease, sometimes very severe, followed inexorably over time.

Related references (1) Martel W, Champion CK, Thompson GR, *et al.* A roentgenologically distinctive arthropathy in some patients with pseudogout syndrome. *American Journal of Roetgenology, Radiation Therapy and Nuclear Medicine* 1970; **109**:587–605.

(2) Menkes CJ, Simon F, Chourki M. Les arthropathies destruictices de la chondrocalcinose. *Revue Rhumatologie et Maladie Osteoarticulaire* 1973; **40**:115–123.

Key message

The finding that degeneration followed calcification suggests that prevention or reversal of crystal deposition might prevent or reverse destructive tissue changes as has been shown in gout.

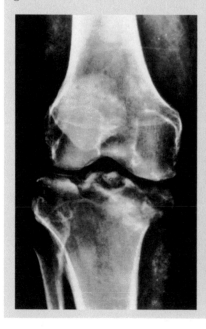 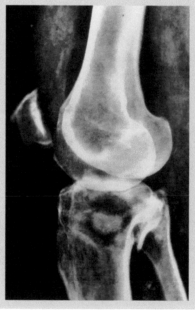

Figure 18.3 Acute Charcot joint in a black man with chondrocalcinosis: left – anteroposterior view; right – lateral view. Acute collapse of the medial tibial plateau with an auto-arthrogram due to powdered bony fragments and joint rupture into the calf. Clinically the process resembled a severe septic arthritis.

Why it's important

Extensive longitudinal studies of the phenotypic effects of a single gene mutation on joint structure and function provides a unique insight into the natural history of a metabolic disease. It provides hope that effective therapy might be developed.

Strength

It is likely that the effects of a single gene mutation were studied as all patients were ethnic Hungarians living in a single Slovak village.

Weakness

It is difficult to extrapolate the findings to sporadic cases of chondrocalcinosis or even affected families of other ethnic groups, e.g. French, Dutch, Japanese, German, English, Swiss.

Relevance

Associated chondrocalcinosis with the onset of a destructive arthropathy in joints but usually affected by classical osteoarthritis.

Paper 7

Evidence for a post-secretory reabsorptive site for uric acid in man

Authors

Diamond HS, Paolino JJ

Reference

Journal of Clinical Investigation 1973; **52**:1491–1499

Summary

Innovative studies on human normal and gouty subjects using pharmacological inhibitors of urate secretion (pyrazinamide or low dose aspirin) and of urate reabsorption (probenecid, sulphinpyrazone, or high dose aspirin) or of both secretion and reabsorption (high dose aspirin) clearly established that uric acid handling by the kidney was a four component system. Pinpointed site of action of probenecid and sulphinpyrazone as inhibition of post-secretory urate absorption.

Related references (1) Sorenson LB, Levinson DJ. Isolated defect in post-secretory reabsorption of uric acid. *Annals of the Rheumatic Diseases* 1980; **39**:180–183.

(2) Simkin PA. Urate excretion in normal and gouty men. *Advances in Experimental Medicine Biology* 1977; **76**:41–45.

(3) Berger L, Yü TF. Renal function in gout. An analysis of 524 gouty subjects including long term follow up studies. *American Journal of Medicine* 1975; **59**:605–613.

Key message

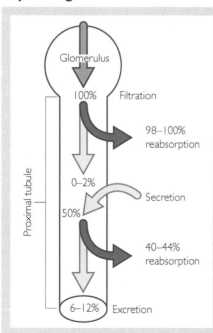

The renal handling of uric acid is complex. Many investigators contributed evidence for complete glomerular filtration, then complete tubular reabsorption followed by active tubular secretion. This three component system became a four component system with the evidence for post-secretory reabsorption. The observation is important because both low and high serum uric acid values can be explained by the effect of organic acids on secretion or on post-secretory absorption. Probenecid, sulphinpyrazone and large (5–6 g/day) doses of salicylates block reabsorption whereas acetoacetic, beta hydroxybutyric, pyrazinoic and lactic acids inhibit secretion.

Figure 18.4 Schematic depiction of handling of uric acid by the kidney showing the four components.

Why it's important

The data led to a model that explains the observed clinical effects of organic acids, including those used as uricosuric drugs.

Strength

Carefully controlled studies were carried out in a clinical research centre using human subjects.

Weakness

Only the uninhibited believe data derived from the use of inhibitors!

Relevance

Demonstration of the complex way in which urate is handled by the kidney.

CHAPTER 19

Osteoporosis

Cyrus Cooper

Introduction

Osteoporosis is defined as a reduction in bone mass and disruption of bone architecture, resulting in reduced bone strength and increased fracture risk. Fragility fractures are the hallmark of osteoporosis, and they are particularly common in the spine, hip and forearm. These fractures show a steep age-related increase and have a major impact on the health of elderly populations in the western world, causing significant morbidity and mortality. They impose huge financial burdens on health services throughout the world. Demographic changes and increasing life expectancy will lead to a dramatic increase in the number of people suffering from fractures over the next few decades (Figure 19.1) unless more effective action is taken to prevent the disorder.

In recent years, there has been significant progress in our understanding of the causes, diagnosis and prevention of osteoporosis (Figure 19.2). Techniques have now been developed which permit prediction of future fracture risk, and the explosion of therapeutic modalities available should significantly reduce fracture risk in future generations. These two themes (assessment of fracture risk, and interventions to retard bone loss with ageing) comprise the major topics in this anthology of classic papers. However, they are by no means the only advances which have been made in our understanding of osteoporosis over the last three decades. The cellular basis of age-related bone loss has now been elucidated, and is known to result from an increase in the rate of bone remodelling and an imbalance between the activity of osteoclasts and osteoblasts. Bone remodelling occurs at discrete sites within the skeleton and proceeds in an orderly fashion, with bone resorption always being followed by bone formation, a phenomenon referred to as coupling. If these two processes are not matched, the resulting remodelling imbalance results in irreversible bone loss. Predisposing factors include oestrogen deficiency in the postmenopausal woman, age-related osteoblast

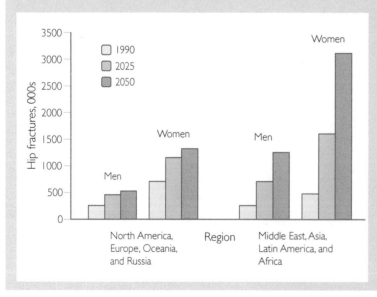

Figure 19.1 Estimated number of hip fractures (in thousands) for men and women in different regions of the world in 1990–2050.

senescence and secondary hyperparathyroidism, as well as a number of diseases and drugs (most notably corticosteroids) which alter the rate of bone turnover. Other determinants of bone strength include bone geometry (for example hip axis length), the accumulation of fatigue damage, and loss of trabecular connectivity.

Over the last 30 years, significant progress has also been made in the development of methods for the non-invasive assessment of bone mass. These include dual energy x-ray absorptiometry, quantitative computed tomography and broadband ultrasound attenuation. Dual energy x-ray absorptiometry is the most widely used technique because of its high reproducibility, low radiation dose and ability to measure bone mineral density at both appendicular and axial sites in the skeleton. Bone density, so measured, is a major determinant of bone strength and fracture risk. The strength of this relationship is comparable to that between blood pressure and stroke, and equates to an 8–12-fold difference in fracture risk across the distribution of bone density in the population. Addition of risk factors to bone mineral density values may lead to enhanced prediction of fracture; the most important of these are a previous history of fragility fracture and, in the elderly, risk factors for falling. Although a useful clinical adjunct in the management of patients with osteoporosis, mass bone density screening of the general population at any age cannot be justified. Clinical indications for bone densitometry have now been clarified, which include important historical risk factors such as previous low trauma fracture, radiological evidence of vertebral deformity, glucocorticoid therapy and oestrogen deficiency.

Preventive strategies against osteoporotic fracture can be applied throughout the life course. They include non-pharmacological interventions to increase peak bone mass (nutrition and exercise), to reduce age-related bone loss, to decrease the risk of falling, and to reduce the impact of falls. In addition, a number of pharmacological interventions have recently been developed which aim to reduce future fracture incidence by altering bone turnover. These include calcium and vitamin D, the bisphosphonates, and the selective oestrogen receptor modulators. Guidelines for the cost-effective use of these agents have now been developed, and their implementation will lead to marked improvement in the morbidity and mortality attributable to osteoporotic fractures.

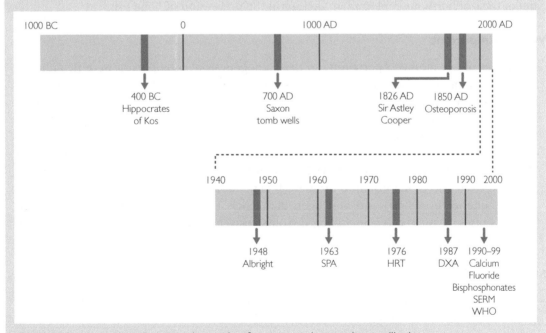

Figure 19.2 Historical evolution in the study of osteoporosis over three millenia.

Paper 1

Postmenopausal osteoporosis: its clinical features

Authors

Albright F, Smith PH, Richardson AM

Reference

Journal of the American Medical Association 1941; **116**:2465–2474

Summary

This manuscript provides the first clinical description of postmenopausal vertebral osteoporosis, and links the disorder directly to oestrogen deficiency. Clinical data are presented for 42 patients with osteoporosis, 40 of whom were postmenopausal women. Ten of these had undergone a premature menopause, and one had primary hyperparathyroidism. The serum calcium biochemistry of these subjects was essentially normal and the profile of fractures encountered was typical, with a preponderance of vertebral deformities.

Related reference   (1)

Riggs BL, Khosla S, Melton U. A unitary model for involutional osteoporosis: estrogen deficiency causes both type I and type II osteoporosis in postmenopausal women and contributes to bone loss in ageing men. *Journal of Bone and Mineral Research* 1998; **13**:763–773.

Key message

This is the first detailed clinical description of postmenopausal vertebral osteoporosis and directly links the disorder to oestrogen deficiency. The manuscript provides a basis for subsequent trials of hormone replacement therapy in the prevention of bone loss.

Why it's important

A number of key messages pertaining to the pathogenesis of osteoporosis were first alluded to in this manuscript. The authors distinguished clearly between osteomalacia (a mineralization abnormality in which calcium hydroxyapatite cannot be incorporated into osteoid matrix) and osteoporosis (in which there is a reduced overall amount of bony tissue, with adequate mineralization of the available matrix). The authors also postulate the importance of oestrogen deficiency in the pathophysiology of postmenopausal bone loss, and propose that hormone replacement therapy (HRT) might have a beneficial effect on calcium retention in the disorder. They go on to distinguish between age-related or involutional bone loss (a consequence of disuse) and oestrogen deficiency. Finally, they outline important secondary causes of osteoporosis including thyrotoxicosis, hypercortisolism, and primary hyperparathyroidism.

Strength

The manuscript constitutes a clear and readable account of the clinical manifestations of postmenopausal osteoporosis.

Weakness

The study is essentially a case series, relying on astute clinical observation and a synthesis of the previous literature.

Relevance

This initial clinical description of the disorder complements the classical descriptions of hip fracture published over a century earlier by Sir Astley Cooper, which documented that: (a) incidence rates of osteoporotic fracture increase steeply with age; (b) that rates are higher among women than among men; and (c) that the disorder has a predilection for skeletal sites containing substantial amounts of trabecular bone. It provides a forerunner of the controlled trials of HRT which convincingly demonstrated that oestrogen replacement following the menopause retards bone loss while it is continued.

Paper 2

The loss of bone with age, osteoporosis, and fractures

Authors

Newton-John HF, Morgan DB

Reference

Clinical Orthopaedics and Related Research 1970; **71**:229–252

Summary

This classical manuscript brings together available literature three decades ago on measurements of bone density between fracture cases and non-fracture controls. The authors realize the implication of a universal loss of bone with age in normal persons, and suggest that osteoporosis is simply an increase in the rate of age-related bone loss. Analysis of the data leads to the conclusion that: (a) all persons lose bone with age, and (b) that the risk of fracture is largely determined by the amount of bone. The authors demonstrate that the increase in frequency of fractures with advancing age is explained by the universal loss of bone with age.

Related references (1) Aaron JE, Gallagher JC, Anderson J, *et al.* Frequency of osteomalacia and osteoporosis in fractures of the proximal femur. *The Lancet* 1974; **1**:229–233.

(2) Nordin BEC, Peacock M, Aaron J, *et al.* Osteoporosis and osteomalacia. *Clinics in Endocrinology and Metabolism* 1980; **9**:177–204.

(3) Riggs BL, Melton LJ. Involutional osteoporosis. *New England Journal of Medicine* 1986; **314**:1676–1686.

Key message

The authors propose that fracture risk is largely accounted for by variation in bone mass in the general population, and that the age-related increase in fracture rate is determined by the normal loss of bone with age.

Why it's important

The authors construct one of the earliest systematic reviews, including the literature on: (a) the age of onset of bone loss; (b) the magnitude of bone loss, and (c) the variance in bone loss with age among men and women. The information is utilized to compare bone loss rates in the peripheral and axial skeletons of each gender, and to explore the association between bone loss and fracture. The findings confirm that all bones lose mineral with advancing age and that bone loss commences at around 40–45 years among women and 50–65 years among men. Greater rates of bone loss were found in women and bone loss continued throughout later life. Estimation of fracture incidence rates from proportions of the population falling below different bone density thresholds generated incidence curves which were almost identical to those derived from epidemiological studies conducted at the time. The authors concluded, for the first time, that osteoporosis is not a discreet disease process which can be easily separated from normality. Rather, it is simply a term used to characterize individuals at the extreme of the distribution of bone density in later life, whose fracture risk is correspondingly increased. The pattern of the age-related increase in hip and wrist fracture was able to be explained entirely on the basis of the pattern of bone loss with age.

Strengths

1. A wonderful review of the literature of its day.
2. Clear elucidation of several problems in the definition of osteoporosis which have remained controversial ever since. These include the continuous distribution of bone density in the general population, the variation in bone loss rates with advancing age, and the absence of a threshold in the relationship between bone density and fracture.

Weakness

The mathematical explanation of the relationship between changing bone density and fracture risk is obscure, but the reasoning behind the relationships is sound.

Relevance

This manuscript is ahead of its time in proposing that osteoporosis might be defined by points on the distribution of bone density at any given age, but that fracture risk is likely to increase smoothly with declining bone density. The clear distinction between osteoporosis and fracture is therefore established; this relationship was enshrined in the World Health Organization (WHO) definition of the disorder.

Paper 3

The diagnosis of osteoporosis

Authors

Kanis JA, Melton LJ, Christiansen C, Johnston CC, Khaltaev N

Reference

Journal of Bone Mineral Research 1994; **9**:1137–1141

Summary

This manuscript provides the basis for the WHO diagnosis of osteoporosis. The article stems from the deliberations of the WHO Study Group on osteoporosis in 1994, which generated the first widely used threshold for osteoporosis definition on the basis of bone mineral measurement (2.5 SD below the young normal mean value at the skeletal site of interest).

Related references **(1)** Consensus Development Conference. Diagnosis, prophylaxis and treatment of osteoporosis. *American Journal of Medicine* 1993; **94**:646–650.

(2) World Health Organization. *Assessment of fracture risk in its application to screening for postmenopausal osteoporosis.* Technical Report Series. Geneva: WHO, 1994.

(3) Melton U, Chrischilles FA, Cooper C, Lane AW, Riggs BL. How many women have osteoporosis? *Journal of Bone and Mineral Research* 1992; **7**:1005–1010.

Key message

Osteoporosis is defined as a bone mineral measurement more than 2.5 SD below the young normal mean value.

Why it's important

With the advent of accurate and precise non-invasive measurement methods of bone mineral, the issue as to whether osteoporosis might be defined exclusively on the basis of such measurements, or whether a fracture was mandated, became highly controversial. This manuscript, summarizing a lengthier WHO report, clearly established the rationale for defining osteoporosis on the basis of bone mineral measurements alone. Prospective studies revealed that the risk of fragility fractures increased progressively and continuously as bone mineral density declined. A fracture threshold, at which the disorder could be defined, was not therefore readily apparent. The WHO study group based their choice of a threshold on the prevalence of clinically relevant associations; the threshold of 2.5 SD below the young normal mean was appropriate to identify approximately 20% of postmenopausal women as having osteoporosis (Figure 19.3). This threshold also had high specificity for prediction of future fracture. Finally, the article provides estimates of the lifetime fracture risk among men and women at age 50 years for the proximal femur (17.5% and 6% respectively), vertebra (15.6% and 5.0% respectively) and wrist (16% and 2.5% respectively).

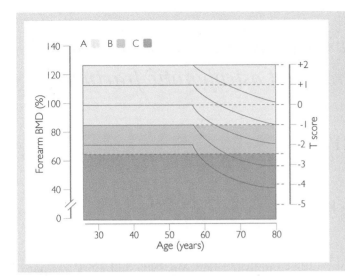

Figure 19.3 WHO definition of osteoporosis: (A) normal bone density, (B) osteopenia, and (C) osteoporosis.

Strengths

1. Provides a succinct description of the WHO definition of osteoporosis.
2. Describes the importance of adopting a bone density threshold relating to the young normal mean.
3. As a decision threshold among younger postmenopausal women (e.g. 50–79 years), the WHO definition remains extremely useful and provides a particularly helpful cost-effective cut-point at which relatively expensive drugs may be prescribed for long periods in patients with the disorder.

Weaknesses

1. More recently, it has become clear that this definition has deficiencies when applied to very elderly samples of the population (e.g. 80 years and over) where prevalence rates rise to high levels.
2. It is also of unproven value in men.

Relevance

The WHO definition of osteoporosis was initially proposed as a tool with which to express the frequency of the disorder in different populations. However, it has subsequently been demonstrated that it also meets the requirements for a therapeutic threshold in women aged 50–79 years. It therefore underpins the clinical management of patients with this disorder, particularly in the prescription of newer antiresorptive agents such as the bisphosphonates and selective oestrogen receptor modulators.

Paper 4

Meta-analysis of how well measures of bone mineral density predict occurrence of osteoporotic fractures

Authors

Marshall D, Johnell O, Wedel H

Reference

British Medical Journal 1996; **312**:1254–1259

Summary

A meta-analysis of prospective cohort studies published between 1985 and 1994 was performed to determine the ability of measurements of bone density in women to predict later fractures. Eleven separate study populations, including 90 000 person-years of observation time and over 2000 fractures, were included. All measurement sites were found to have similar predictive capacity (relative risk 1.5, 95% CI 1.4–1.6) for decrease in bone mineral density, except measurements at the spine for prediction of vertebral fracture (relative risk 2.3, 95% CI 1.9–2.8), and measurements at the proximal femur for hip fracture (relative risk 2.6, 95% CI 2.0–3.5). The predictive ability of decrease in bone mass was similar to that of a 1 SD decrease in blood pressure for stroke, and better than a 1 SD increase in serum cholesterol concentration for cardiovascular disease.

Related references **(1)** Cummings SR, Black DM, Nevitt MC, *et al.* Bone density at various sites for prediction of hip fractures. *The Lancet* 1993; **341**:72–75.

(2) Ross PD, Davis JW, Epstein RS, Wasnich RD. Pre-existing fractures and bone mass predict vertebral fracture incidence in women. *Annals of Internal Medicine* 1991; **114**:919–923.

(3) Seeley DG, Browner WS, Nevitt MC, *et al.* Which fractures are associated with low appendicular bone mass in elderly women? *Annals of Internal Medicine* 1991; **115**:837–842.

Key message

A decrease in bone mineral density by 1 SD is associated with a doubling in the risk of future fracture. This predictive ability is similar to that of blood pressure measurement for stroke, and better than that of serum cholesterol concentration for cardiovascular disease.

Why it's important

Measurement of bone mineral density is a key method for the early identification of individuals at high risk of fracture, although it is only one of a number of risk factors for fracture. Bone density is a continuously distributed variable in the general population, and the issue as to whether screening programmes incorporating this measurement are effective, remains controversial. This study provided a systematic review of 11 prospective studies in which measurements of bone density among women were related to future fracture risk. The results were surprizingly uniform, in suggesting that each standard deviation decrease in bone density results in a doubling of the risk of future fracture (Figure 19.4). There was some evidence for enhanced predictive capacity among measurements made at the site of fracture, but even measurements made at distant sites retained significant positive predictive value. At a lifetime fracture incidence of around 30%, bone mineral measurements had 89% specificity, 34% sensitivity, 58% positive predictive value, and identified approximately 21% of all fractures. The results clearly demonstrated that bone density measurements could predict risk of fracture, but that they were not sufficiently predictive to warrant population-wide screening. The results led to clarification of the precise circumstances in which bone density measurements were justifiable, in the management of individual patients at the highest risk (see Paper 3).

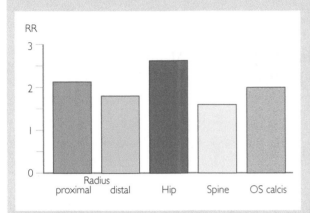

Figure 19.4 Predictive value of bone density at different skeletal sites for future hip fracture.

Strengths

1. This important and timely review clarified the predictive capacity of bone density for future fracture.
2. Clearly demonstrated the lack of effectiveness of a mass screening programme using bone densitometry.
3. Also clearly demonstrated the predictive capacity of bone density measurements in individuals at the highest risk.

Weaknesses

1. The data could not be extrapolated to men or to younger women, in whom further research is needed.
2. Analysis did not include quantitative computed tomography, although ultrasound measurements of the calcaneus were found to be predictive.

Relevance

Clarification of the relationship between baseline bone density measurement and future risk of fracture helped to position this new technology appropriately within clinical guidelines for the evaluation and treatment of osteoporosis. Bone density measurements are now widely used in the management of patients at the highest risk, in whom knowledge of the results alters clinical or therapeutic decision-making. The key clinical indications for densitometry include: (a) prevalent vertebral deformity; (b) previous low trauma fracture; (c) use of corticosteroid therapy, and (d) oestrogen deficiency. When used in this setting, measurements permit the most cost-effective use of therapy over prolonged periods of time with the objective of preventing fractures.

Paper 5

Hormone replacement therapy and risk of hip fracture: population based case-control study

Authors

Michaelsson K, Baron JA, Farahmand BY, Johnell O, Magnusson C, Persson PG, Persson I, Ljunghall S, on behalf of the Swedish Hip Fracture Study Group

Reference

British Medical Journal 1998; **316**:1858–1863

Summary

This population-based case-control study in six Swedish counties compared 1327 women aged 50–81 years with hip fracture, and 3262 randomly selected controls. The objective was to determine the relative risk of hip fracture associated with postmenopausal HRT, including the effect of duration and recency of treatment, the addition of progestogen, the route of administration, and the dose of oestrogen. Compared with women who had never used HRT, current users had a marked reduction in risk of hip fracture (OR = 0.35, 95% CI 0.24–0.53). The protective effect was markedly attenuated, and not statistically significant among former users of hormone replacement (OR = 0.76, 95% CI 0.57–1.01). For every year of therapy, the overall risk decreased by around 6%. Last use 1–5 years previously, with a duration of use more than 5 years, was associated with protection; cessation of therapy for longer than 5 years results in removal of the protective effect of HRT. Transdermal hormone replacement gave similar risk estimates to that from oral regimens.

Related references (1) Grady D, Rubin SM, Petitti DB, Fox CS, Black D, Ettinger B, *et al.* Hormone therapy to prevent disease and prolong life in postmenopausal women. *Annals of Internal Medicine* 1992; **117**:1016–1037.

(2) Cauley JA, Seeley DG, Ensrud K, Ettinger B, Black D, Cummings SR. Estrogen replacement therapy and fractures in older women. Study of Osteoporotic Fractures Research Group. *Annals of Internal Medicine* 1995; **122**:9–16.

(3) Kiel DP, Felson DT, Anderson JJ, Wilson PWF, Moskowitz MA. Hip fracture and the use of estrogens in postmenopausal women. *New England Journal of Medicine* 1987; **317**:1169–1174.

Why it's important

Many studies have shown that HRT can reduce bone loss over relatively short periods of time (3–5 years). Case-control and cohort studies performed two decades ago also suggested that HRT was associated with a reduced risk of hip fracture. However, closer scrutiny of these data suggested that anti-fracture efficacy might be concentrated among current users of HRT. Risk estimates for older women, in whom longer periods had elapsed since cessation of HRT, were found to be closer to unity. This case-control study, coupled with data from the United States, confirmed that HRT was associated with a reduced risk of hip fracture among current users, but clearly demonstrated an attenuation of this protective effect after cessation of use. In particular, women who had ceased use more than 5 years previously were found to have no significant residual protection. The results have great importance for the use of HRT in the prevention of osteoporotic fracture. They suggest that treatment might be commenced several years after the menopause without loss of efficiency in reducing fracture risk. They also suggest that continuation of treatment, to the ages at which fractures occur, is necessary for the intervention to have a major public health impact.

These findings countered the prevailing view at the time, that a decade of HRT immediately following the menopause would suffice to retard bone loss and prevent hip fractures over the subsequent 20–30 years. They have led to substantial efforts to improve compliance with long-term HRT, and to develop other oestrogen-like interventions for use in osteoporosis and cardiovascular prevention.

Strengths

1. The study was of large size, population-based, and had a high response rate.
2. The validity of oestrogen replacement was of the highest quality and cross-checked against various hospital registers.

Weaknesses

1. The principal limitations of the study were possible confounding and non-response bias.
2. There was also relatively low statistical power to explore the association between hip fracture and different types of HRT.

Relevance

This paper confirmed that HRT should be continued for long periods of time in order to obtain optimal protection against hip fracture. No overall hip fracture protection remained after 5 years without HRT, although therapy could be initiated several years after the menopause without loss of fracture protection. Oral and transdermal therapy were equally effective in reducing the risk of hip fracture, and the addition of progestogen permitted a lower dose of oestrogen.

Paper 6

Vitamin D_3 and calcium to prevent hip fractures in elderly women

Authors

Chapuy MC, Arlot ME, Duboeuf F, Brun J, Crouzet B, Arnaud S, Delmas PD, Meunier PJ

Reference

New England Journal of Medicine 1992; **327**:1637–1642

Summary

This manuscript reports a randomized controlled trial of the effects of supplementation with vitamin D_3 and calcium on the frequency of hip and other non-vertebral fractures. Three thousand two hundred and seventy healthy ambulatory women, mean age 84 years, were included in the 18 month study. They were randomized to receive a supplement of calcium 1.2 g, and vitamin D_3 800 IU, or double placebo. The results confirmed a 43% lower (p = 0.04) incidence of hip fracture and 32% lower (p = 0.02) incidence of non-vertebral fractures among the women treated with calcium and vitamin D_3. In this group, the mean serum parathyroid hormone concentration decreased by 44% from baseline and the serum 25–hydroxyvitamin D concentration increased by over 50%.

Related references	(1)	Chapuy MC, Arlot ME, Duboeuf F, *et al.* Effect of calcium and cholecalciferol treatment for three years on hip fractures in elderly women. *British Medical Journal* 1994; **308**:1081–1082.
	(2)	Lips P, Graafmans WC, Ooms ME, Bezemer PD, Bouter LM. Vitamin D supplementation and fracture incidence in elderly persons – a randomized placebo controlled trial. *Annals of Internal Medicine* 1996; **124**:400–406.
	(3)	Dawson-Hughes B, Harris SS, Kraw EA, Dallal GE. Effect of calcium and vitamin D supplementation on bone density in men and women 65 years of age or older. *New England Journal of Medicine* 1997; **337**:670–676.

Key message

This large randomized controlled trial established that calcium and vitamin D were effective in the primary prevention of hip fracture among elderly women resident in French nursing homes.

Why it's important

The key contributors to fractures among elderly women are a reduction in bone mass and an increased frequency of falls. Part of the decrease in bone density with advancing age can be explained by increased parathyroid hormone secretion, resulting from vitamin D deficiency and low calcium intake that are not compensated for by an increase in 1,25-dihydroxyvitamin D production. This trial was the first study to demonstrate convincingly that supplementation with calcium and vitamin D was able to normalize serum parathyroid hormone, retard bone loss and reduce the rate of fractures among elderly women.

The study was followed by attempts to demonstrate whether similar anti-fracture efficacy might be obtained from the use of vitamin D alone, as the addition of calcium reduces compliance, and adds to expenses. Unfortunately, a follow-up study in The Netherlands, which evaluated a supplement of 400 IU cholecalciferol daily among elderly men and women failed to demonstrate effectiveness against hip fracture. The results of further studies are awaited before the best modality for treatment of secondary hyperparathyroidism in the elderly can be established. However, this manuscript led to the introduction of calcium and vitamin D as the basal therapy for patients with osteoporosis in the placebo arms of subsequent randomized controlled trials, and confirmed the effectiveness of this intervention in patients at high risk of future fracture.

Strengths

1. This was a pragmatic randomized controlled trial performed in the general population with a clear result.
2. It has led to an important change in health policy, and confirms that pharmacological intervention, even in the elderly, can lead to a reduction in fracture incidence.

Weakness

The extent to which the intervention acted on hip fracture incidence through an influence on falling was less well studied.

Relevance

Calcium and vitamin D supplementation are now established as first-line treatment for osteoporosis. Although the magnitude of their effect is less than that observed for more potent inhibitors of resorption such as the bisphosphonates, this trial clearly established that suppression of secondary hyperparathyroidism can translate into a reduction in hip fracture incidence. Whether similar effects can be obtained by delivery of vitamin D alone, or whether combined calcium and vitamin D supplementation is required, remain the subject of current trials.

Paper 7

Randomized trial of effect of alendronate on risk of fracture in women with existing vertebral fracture

Authors

Black DM, Cumming SR, Karpf DB, Cauley JA, Thompson DE, Nevitt MC, Bauer DC, Genant HK, Haskell WL, Marcus R, Ott SM, Torner JC, Quandt SA, Reiss TF, Ensrud KE, for the Fracture Intervention Trial Research Group

Reference

The Lancet 1996; **348**:1535–1541

Summary

Two thousand and twenty-seven women aged 55–81 years with low femoral neck BMD and with at least one vertebral deformity on thoracolumbar radiographs, were enrolled in this 3 year placebo- controlled trial of alendronate. Women were followed up to identify incident vertebral and non-vertebral fractures. The incidence of new morphometric vertebral fractures among women in the alendronate group was markedly lower than that in the placebo group (relative risk 0.53, 95% CI 0.41–0.68). The relative risk of hip fracture (0.49, 95% CI 0.23–0.99) and of wrist fracture (0.42, 95% CI 0.31–0.87), was also markedly lower among women given alendronate.

Related references **(1)** Watts NB, Harris ST, Genant HK, *et al.* Intermittent cyclical etidronate treatment of postmenopausal osteoporosis. *New England Journal of Medicine* 1990; **323**:73–79.

(2) Liberman UA, Weiss SR, Broll J, *et al.* Effect of oral alendronate on bone mineral density and the incidence of fractures in post-menopausal osteoporosis. *New England Journal of Medicine* 1995; **333**:1437–1443.

(3) Harris ST, Watts NB, Genant HK, *et al.* Effects of risedronate treatment on vertebral and non-vertebral fractures in women with postmenopausal osteoporosis: a randomized controlled trial. *Journal of the American Medical Association* 1999; **282**:1344–1352.

Key message

This large randomized controlled trial confirmed that alendronate reduces vertebral and hip fracture among women with low bone mass and pre-existing vertebral deformities.

Why it's important

Although randomized trials have shown increases in bone mass associated with several therapies including oestrogens, calcitonin, calcitriol, sodium fluoride, and the bisphosphonates, few have reported reductions in the incidence of vertebral fracture, and only one a reduction in the incidence of hip fracture (see Paper 6). The aminobisphosphonate alendronate, has been shown to increase bone mineral density at the spine and hip, and to reduce the risk of radiographically-defined vertebral fracture among women with low BMD. The Fracture Intervention Trial established that three years of alendronate therapy among post-menopausal women with low bone mass and pre-existing vertebral fractures not only reduced incident vertebral fracture, but also the incidence of hip and wrist fracture. The bisphosphonates (etidronate, alendronate and risedronate) have now been widely evaluated in the prevention and treatment of osteoporosis, and have been shown to reduce the rate of bone loss among healthy postmenopausal women; to reduce the incidence of fractures among elderly patients with osteoporosis, and to be effective in the management of corticosteroid-induced osteoporosis. The more potent bisphosphonates have marked effects on bone resorption, and may improve bone microarchitecture and mineralization, as well as reducing bone turnover. They have an established role in the prevention and treatment of postmenopausal osteoporosis, as well as in the management of corticosteroid-induced osteoporosis.

Strengths

1. Established the necessary design for evaluation of treatments in osteoporosis.
2. Sufficiently large to establish clearly effectiveness of alendronate on the incidence of vertebral fracture, and also provide some evidence on the risk of limb fractures.

Weakness

The stringent recruitment criteria to the study did not permit adequate evaluation of adverse effects. It was only after release of the agent that the association with oesophageal discomfort and ulceration were recognized, and strict guidance was issued as to the means whereby the agents should be administered.

Relevance

The bisphosphonates are now routinely used in the management of osteoporosis. This trial was among the first studies to establish their role in management. It also remains one of the only studies to demonstrate that an anti-resorptive drug reduces the incidence of hip fracture.

Section 3

Regional and Miscellaneous Disorders

CHAPTER 20

Back pain

Malcolm IV Jayson

Introduction

Back problems are extremely common. Epidemiological studies in the general population have show a lifetime prevalence of significant episodes of back pain of 70–80% and experience of back pain within the month previous to the survery of 30–40%.

The back is an extremely complex structure with numerous potential sources of back pain. This includes not only the nerves but also the thecal sheaths, blood vessels, ligaments, periostium, muscles and other tissues.

Commonly it is difficult and often impossible to define the specific source of a patient's symptoms. Much pathology can be demonstrated but this frequently bears only a very poor relationship to the development of back pain. Modern medical technology, including MRI and CT scanning, technetium scans and neurophysiology, have frequently served to heighten the confusion rather than provide specific answers in any individual case. Moreover we now know that the perception of pain commonly depends upon central amplification so that patients with trivial organic damage have an enhanced perception of the severity of their pain and disability. This phenomenon of central amplification probably accounts for the enormous increase in back disability seen in recent years.

With this background it is hardly surprising that our knowledge and understanding of the pathogenesis of many back pain syndromes has evolved very slowly and it is only in recent years that we have learned to distinguish the concepts of nociception, pain experience, distress and illness behaviour.

Although much original work on the pathology of disease on the spine was undertaken by pathologists such as Schmorl and Junghanns (1932, see Related reference, Paper 1), there was no clear identification of the disc as being responsible for back problems until the classic studies of Mixter and Barr (1934, Paper 1). There has been one or two previous descriptions of disc prolapse causing nerve root damage but in general it was thought that protrusions from the back of the disc were chondromas. Mixter and Barr re-examined pathological specimens in the museum and showed that they were disc herniations and that they could damage the nerve root. They described a series of patients treated successfully with surgery.

This paper led to an explosion of interest in the intervertebral disc and for many years thereafter orthopaedic surgeons uncritically operated on virtually every back pain patient whether or not there was a defined protrusion and sciatica. There were some successes but also many disasters. In part the problem was lack of appropriate diagnostic tools. Myelography is an invasive procedure and often correlated poorly with symptoms. Many surgeons operated without previous specific indentification of disc protrusion and nerve root damage. Surgery for sciatica with an appropriately defined disc prolapse has become a very successful operation.

The principal function of the spine is to support the trunk and at the same time allow flexibility of movements. The relationship between the structure and function of the intervertebral disc is all important. Nachemson and Morris (1964, Paper 2) initiated physiological research into the biomechanics of the disc showing that it was possible to measure the pressures within the disc in life and during a wide variety of physical activity. In a long series of papers they established the effects of posture and exercise in both healthy and degenerate discs. This work proved to be the foundation of modern ergonomics. Modern advice used in industry on the correct ways to lift directly stems from these studies. This approach led to an improved design of seating. The Volvo Car Company invested heavily in this research and used it to produce their ergonomic car seats. These principles are now adopted by virtually all car manufacturers.

A more general approach to biomechanics has included a long series of studies of muscle function and strength in various postures. Extensive research has been conducted on the biomechanics of the human spine and machines developed in efforts to improve quantification of spine function. The results of these studies however, have been relatively disappointing. Despite considerable investment in technology, the results of attempts to quantify spine function have only correlated very poorly with back pain. We now know that there are other important pathogenic mechanisms apart from disc prolapse. Kellgren (1938, see Chapter 21, Paper 8) showed that nociceptive stimulation of soft tissues could lead to referred pain experienced in the lower limbs. Far too often it is assumed that pain in the leg must mean nerve root damage. This study was the first to identify pain in the lower limb referred from the soft tissues and to appreciate that this is different from radicular pain. The actual mechanism of nerve root damage was originally thought to be due to direct trauma by the disc herniation pressing on the nerve. Hoyland, *et al.* (1989, Paper 3) identified the significance of vascular damage and in particular venous obstruction leading to nerve root swelling, fibrosis and neural atrophy. More recent studies have shown two level compression within the spine causing isolated segments of poor perfusion. Increasingly it is apparent that vascular damage plays an important part of the pathogenic process and occurs as a consequence of both disc herniation and degenerative disease.

The disc itself may be a source of pain. There is a correlation between the severity of disc degeneration and back pain, albeit rather poor. It is known that in the healthy disc innervation is restricted to the outer layers of the annulus fibrosus. One difficulty has been to identify why disc degeneration may lead to pain in some patients but not in others. The study by Freemont, *et al.* (1997, Paper 4) identified the ingrowth of nociceptive fibres into the inner annulus and the nucleus of painful degenerate disc, and indicates an important pathogenic mechanism in the production of back pain.

Nevertheless, our understanding of the pathogenesis of many back pain problems has been poor. Waddell (1987, Paper 5) drew attention to the distinction between back disability and back pain. He pointed out that back pain is an extremely common and world-wide phenomenon, yet the severity of disability associated with back pain appears very much a disorder of Western civilization and has developed as a recent epidemic. He identified the role of psychosocial factors in exacerbating patients' perception of the severity of the back pain problem, and leading to the degrees of distress and disability which we commonly see. In this context, Bigos, *et al.* (1991, Paper 6) undertook a prospective study in which he examined baseline data and followed-up workers in order to identify pre-back pain factors predictive of future back episodes. As would be expected, workers with a previous history of backache developed future back episodes. In addition, they also showed that job dissatisfaction was a major predictive factor for future backache. Again this emphasizes the role of psychological distress and other psychosocial factors in the back pain scenario.

The traditional management of back pain has been long periods of rest often with bed rest, lying flat, and cautious and careful remobilization. This approach was challenged by Deyo, *et al.* (1986, Paper 7). They showed that this advice is wrong and indeed may promote disability. They introduced the concept of only a short period of bed rest and early mobilization and activation. Since then others have shown that the best results are obtained by minimizing the period of rest and restriction of activity, and returning to normal function as soon as possible. The benefits may be due to a combination of physical effects on the spine and psychological effects in avoiding the reinforcement of the concept of disability. This philosophy has been extended into the management of chronic back pain. For patients for whom there is no specific solution, intensive rehabilitation programmes including physical rehabilitation and psychological counselling seem to offer the best way forward. Programmes incorporating this approach are now available in many centres.

Paper 1

Rupture of the intervertebral disc with involvement of the spinal canal

Authors

Mixter WJ, Barr JS

Reference

New England Journal of Medicine 1934; **211**:210–215

Summary

This study reported a series of 19 cases of herniation or rupture of the intervertebral discs in the cervical, dorsal and lumbo-sacral spine with the development of both spine pain and neurological damage. Previously it was thought that the swellings from discs were neoplasms but the authors identified that rupture of the disc is much more common and recommended that the treatment of this condition is essentially surgical.

Related reference   **(1)**   Schmorl G and Junghanns H. *Archiv und Atlas der normalen und pathologischen Anatomie in typischen Röntgenbildern.* 1932. Georg Thiem, Liepzig.

Key message

Prolapse of nucleus pulposus and fracture of the annulus is a common cause of back problems.

Why it's important

In a pathological study Schmorl and Junghanns (1) had demonstrated disc prolapse but had not considered the clinical significance of these findings. Other authors had identified disc lesions leading to both spinal cord and nerve root pressure but generally it was thought they were due to chondromas, and apart from one or two individual case reports the phenomenon of disc prolapse was not recognized. This study indicated the importance of disc herniation as a specific cause of spine problems and that operative removal of the prolapse could be a successful form of treatment. It was this paper which led to an explosion of interest in the surgical management of back problems. Following this publication there was a dramatic increase in the amount of lumbar spine surgery. This was frequently undertaken uncritically and for back pain rather than for sciatic pain. Much of this was performed in North American private practice. For many patients surgical intervention was inappropriate. We now know that surgery can be very effective for patients with clearly defined nerve root compression and sciatic pain. However, the place of surgery for patients with back pain without significant nerve root compression is still to be defined.

Strengths

1. This study first drew attention to disc herniation as a diagnostic entity.
2. It was the first to provide specific diagnoses for some of our back problems and for some patients provided an important therapeutic advance.

Weaknesses

1. We now know that there is a mass of disc pathology which correlates very poorly with back symptoms.
2. The enthusiasm of the authors for the surgical approach led to many unnecessary operations.

Relevance

This paper was an important milestone in the modern development of our understanding of back pain problems. Although it provided an important advance it also led to much unnecessary and inappropriate surgery.

Paper 2

In vivo *measurements of intra-discal pressure*

Authors

Nachemson A, Morris JM

Reference

Journal of Bone and Joint Surgery 1964; **46**(A):1077–1092

Summary

Following pilot studies on cadaveric discs, the authors inserted a specially constructed needle with a pressure-sensitive polyethylene membrane at the tip into normal lumbar discs (Figure 20.1) in a series of 16 patients with long-standing back problems at other levels, many of whom had undergone previous spine surgery. They obtained basic data on the intra-discal pressures at rest, and demonstrated increases on sitting, standing and during various physical activities. They also were able to analyse the effects of the Valsalva manoeuvre, the application of an inflatable corset and the changes associated with spinal fusion at adjacent levels. They were able to determine the stresses on the disc in different positions and under different conditions of rest. They also undertook discography and determined the size of the nucleus, using this to develop equations calculating the total load on the disc in various postures and activities.

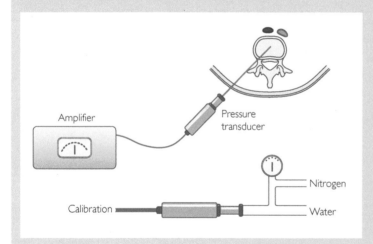

Figure 20.1 Experimental design for measuring intradiscal pressure *in vivo*.

Key message

Measurement of intradiscal pressure in living subjects at rest and in a variety of postures and physical activities is a practical procedure of value for understanding the physiology of the human spine.

Why it's important

This was the first study of the physiology and biomechanics of the human spine in life. The authors measured the intra-discal pressure during a variety of physical activities and showed that this technique was safe. They were able to record the variations in pressure in various postures, and in particular showed the increase associated with sitting, with lower values on reclining.This study and a long series of subsequent papers analysed much more clearly the effects of posture, weightlifting and so on. They led to a proper understanding of the ergonomics of the back. Much of the current advice on posture, the provision of lumbar supports, particularly in car seats, and advice on the right and wrong ways to lift and carry have been derived from this work.

Strength

For the first time *in vivo* measurements were made of intra-discal pressures and the changes associated with various physical activities and postures.

Weakness

This particular study was restricted to patients who already had back problems elsewhere. Although the study was restricted to the normal discs in these subjects, previous autopsy studies had shown radical effects on disc mechanics when there was evidence of disc degeneration. In subsequent papers they addressed this issue measuring disc pressures in normal subjects.

Relevance

This study was the stimulus for much research in ergonomics and in particular the effects of posture and weightlifting, and in providing appropriate advice and support for patients with back problems. This research provided a fundamental stimulus to the scientific understanding of the function of the human spine.

Paper 3

Intervertebral foramen venous obstruction. A cause of periradicular fibrosis

Authors

Hoyland JA, Freemont AJ, Jayson MIV

Reference

Spine 1989; **14**:558–568

Summary

The authors undertook a cadaveric study of 160 lumbar foramina. They demonstrated that disc herniation and osteophytic outgrowths into the intervertebral foramen may compress the neural structure. but much more commonly were associated with compression and distortion of the large venous plexus within the intervertebral foramen. In the absence of direct nerve compression the most severe neural changes were associated with venous compression, congestion and resultant dilatation. Pathological changes within and around the nerve root complex included oedema of the nerve roots, peri and intraneural fibrosis and focal demyelination. Inflammatory cells were notably absent. The vascular changes within the thickened fibrous sheath around damaged nerves included basement membrane thickening suggestive of endothelial cell injury. There was an association between venous compression tissue fibrosis, endothelial injury distant from the compression, and neuronal atrophy. It was thought that this was probably due to ischaemia as a result of reduced venous outflow. These observations led the authors to propose that venous obstruction may be an important pathogenic mechanism in the development of peri- and intraneural fibrosis and subsequent nerve damage.

Key message

Degenerative disease of the spine and disc herniation are associated with nerve root damage. This paper draws attention to venous obstruction with impaired nutrition as an important pathogenic mechanism in addition to the direct effects of pressure.

Why it's important

The study drew attention to the importance of vascular damage in the pathogenesis of nerve root symptoms. Previously the focus had been on the direct effects of pressure by an osteophyte or a herniated disc on the nerve root. However, it is well recognized that the direct evidence of pressure may not be obvious. At surgery engorged veins around the nerve roots are often described. This particular study brought together these different observations and indicated an important pathogenic mechanism. It has led onto much more detailed studies on the role of vascular damage in back pain problems. It also provided an explanation for the association of spinal problems with cardiovascular disease and with smoking. Both may be associated with vascular damage and impairment of blood supply within the vertebral canal and thus play important roles in mediating back pain problems. Further work from this group together with others analysed the cellular content in proliferating tissue associated with mechanical herniation. In particular there is cellular infiltration which does not include polymorphs but which appears to be a reaction to nucleus pulposus and other tissues, again contributing towards the pathogenic process.

Strength

This is a systematic study carefully quantifying the degrees of obstruction of the interverte-bral foramen and statistically relating these to evidence of venous obstruction and in turn to fibrosis and neural damage.

Weakness

In a cadaveric study it is not possible to relate the venous obstruction and nerve root damage to pain syndromes in life. Subsequently other workers have critically examined the role impaired blood flow *in vivo* and demonstrated its importance.

Relevance

This study indicated important mechanisms of nerve root damage associated with mechani-cal problems of the spine which are not a direct result of mechanical pressure on the nerves. It led to consideration of alternative approaches to treatment based upon the evidence of vascular damage.

Paper 4

Nerve ingrowth into diseased intervertebral disc in chronic back pain

Authors

Freemont AJ, Peacock TE, Goupille P, Hoyland JA, O'Brien J, Jayson MIV

Reference

The Lancet 1997; **350**:178–181

Summary

The authors examined samples of intervertebral discs obtained at spine fusion examining specimens from both painful degenerate discs and adjacent normal discs. Cadaveric controls were also obtained. Immunohistochemical techniques were also used to test for general nerve markers, Substance P and a protein expressed during axonogenesis (Growth associated protein 43 (GAP 43)). In healthy control discs, the nerve fibres were restricted to the outer and middle thirds of the annulus fibrosus. However, in the subjects with chronic low back pain the nerves commonly extended into the inner third of the annulus and into the nucleus pulposus. The nerves were usually accompanied by blood vessels although sometimes isolated nerve fibres were seen at disc matrix. Non-associated fibres expressed GAP 43 but both vessel and non-vessel associated fibres expressed Substance P. When comparing pain and non-pain levels in the spine, again nerve ingrowth was more frequent at the painful levels.

Key message

The finding of isolated nerve fibres that expressed Substance P deep within diseased intervertebral discs and their association with pain, suggests an important role for nerve growth into the intervertebral disc in the pathogenesis of chronic low back pain.

Why it's important

There is a correlation between the presence of imaging evidence of disc degeneration and back pain. However, this relationship is relatively poor. There are patients who may show advanced damage in the spine and no pain and *vice versa*. Previous neurophysiological studies have concentrated on healthy discs and it was demonstrated that innervation is restricted to the outer part of the disc. This study has shown that there is variable ingrowth of nociceptive fibres into the inner annulus and the substance of the nucleus pulposus and that this development correlates with the presence of pain. Differences in the growth of nerve fibres within the disc may well explain why the development of pain varies so considerably between different people.

Strength

This is the first systematic study using modern immunohistochemical techniques to examine the distribution of nerve fibres within the disc and to relate these findings to clinical symptoms.

Weaknesses

1. It is difficult to obtain control discs for a study such as this. An adjacent unaffected disc exposed at the time of spinal fusion for a damaged disc was used, but clearly the adjacent disc may have pathology not easily identifiable.
2. Another set of controls were cadaveric spines. In these circumstances it is not possible to determine accurately whether back pain has been present in life.
3. There is also a possibility the immunohistochemical appearances have changed following death, although experimental work suggests that this is unlikely.

Relevance

This study has provided important data on the neurophysiological structure of the healthy and damaged intervertebral disc.

Paper 5

A new clinical model for the treatment of low back pain

Author

Waddell G

Reference

Spine 1987; **12**:632–644

Summary

The author has produced a theoretical framework to understand the natural history of low back pain. Most episodes of pain should be benign self-limiting conditions. Low back disability as opposed to pain is a relatively recent Western epidemic. He critically examined the role of medicine in that epidemic, and constrasted the traditional medical model of the disease with a bio-psycho-social model(Figure 20.2) and used this to explain many clinical observations. Although rest is the commonest treatment prescribed after analgesics, there is a little evidence of long lasting benefit. There is little doubt about the harmful effects of prolonged bed rest. Conversely, there is no evidence that activity is harmful. It does not necessarily make the pain worse. Experimental studies have shown that controlled exercises not only restore function, reduce distress and illness behaviour and promote apparent return to work, but actually reduce pain. Clinical studies confirm the value of active rehabilitation in practice.

To achieve the goal of treating patients rather than spines we must approach low back disability as an illness rather than low back pain as a physical disease. As a result we must distinguish pain from disability and the symptoms and signs of distress and illness behaviour from those of physical disease. Management should change from the negative recipe of rest for pain to more active restoration of function.

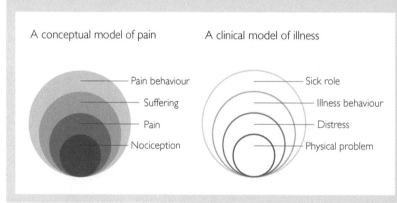

A conceptual model of pain

A clinical model of illness

- Pain behaviour
- Suffering
- Pain
- Nociception

- Sick role
- Illness behaviour
- Distress
- Physical problem

Figure 20.2 An illustration of the bio-psycho-social concept of illness. On the left is the model devised by Loeser, and on the right the Glasgow Illness Model, with an adaptation by Waddell to the problems of chronic back pain.

Related reference (1) Melzack R, Wall PD. Pain mechanisms: a new theory. *Science* 1956; **150**:971–999.

Key message

Low back disability is not the same as low back pain. The development of disability is a relatively recent Western epidemic, and it is necessary to distinguish the symptoms and signs of psychological distress and pain behaviour from those of physical disease. When assessing patients one should not only consider the specific syndromes but also the need to treat the whole person. In particular one should alter the philosophy of management so that the patient takes an active role sharing responsibility for his or her own progress, and that there is a change from rest to rehabilitation and restoration of function.

Why it's important

This was a fundamental publication drawing together a vast range of studies and provided a reasoning for a holistic approach to back pain problems. He reviewed the epidemiology of low back pain pointing out that over the years there has been a dramatic increase in the numbers of working days lost due to back incapacities. In contrast in less developed countries, although back pain is almost universal, there was very little disability before the introduction of Western medicine.

He identified the need to distinguish the physical problem from the resulting distress and this in turn from illness behaviour and from the adoption of a sick role. This required a bio-psycho-social analysis and indicates the importance of psychological and social influences in modifying individual perception of and response to disease. The gate control theory by Melzack and Wall (1) may provide a neurophysiological mechanism for this concept. On this basis he described a series of symptoms and signs which may be used to identify magnified or inappropriate illness behaviour, and which help to distinguish these factors from those specifically related to physical disease. With this understanding he looked at the evidence regarding the use of bed rest. He identified that protracted rest is harmful due to a wide variety of mechanisms and proposed a much more active approach in which patients' participation in the rehabilitative process is fundamental.

Strengths

1. This study drew together a mass of evidence on the epidemiology of back pain and of back disability.
2. It provided a theoretical construct enabling improved understanding of back disability and indicating appropriate ways forward.

Weaknesses

1. Although providing an important framework for understanding disability associated with back problems it has been used to explain virtually all back disability, with a result that specific diagnoses may be missed.
2. In many patients there is a specific nociceptive problem but the psycho-social factors have led to a greatly amplified response.
3. The study is useful in avoiding inappropriate intervention procedures when the psycho-social factors are paramount, but equally it may lead to failure to identify specific underlying problems which are capable of being remedied.

Relevance

This study provided the conceptual framework for much of our current understanding of the persistence of back distress and disability.

Paper 6

A prospective study of work perceptions and psychosocial factors affecting the report of back injury

Authors

Bigos SJ, Battie M, Spengler DM, Fisher LD, Fordyce WD, Hanson TH, Nachemson AN, Wortley MD

Reference

Spine 1991; **16**:1–6

Summary

A longitudinal prospective study of 3020 aircraft employees to identify risk factors for reporting acute back pain at work. Pre-morbid data including individual physical, psychosocial and work place factors were recorded over slightly more than 4 years of follow-up. Two hundred and seventy-nine subjects reported back problems. Other than a history of recurrent or recent back problems, the factors found to be most predictive of subsequent reports of back pain in a multivariate model were work perceptions and certain psychosocial responses. In particular subjects who 'hardly ever' enjoyed their jobs were 2.5 times more likely to report their injury (Figure 20.3). The subjects scoring highest on the Scale 3 (HY) of the Minnesota Multiphasic Personality Inventory (MMPI) were 2.0 times more likely to report back pain than subjects with the lowest scores. A history of lack of job task enjoyment, high MMPI Scale-3 score, and a history of back treatment showed that subjects in the highest risk group had 3.3 times the numbers of reports compared with the lowest risk group.

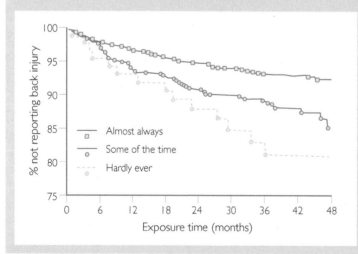

Figure 20.3 A diagram relating to the work APGAR (job enjoyment) versus subsequent job injury. The graph compares the percentage of subjects reporting subsequent back problems to their responses to the statement 'I enjoy the tasks involved in my job'. Those who 'hardly ever' enjoyed their job tasks were at highest risk.

Key message

Psychological factors and in particular job dissatisfaction are important predictors of the future development of back problems.

Why it's important

Back pain is one of the commonest causes of loss of work. The numbers of working days lost has rapidly escalated in recent years. Until this study was produced it was thought that the development of back pain was principally related to mechanical problems associated with work. Much effort went into ergonomic analyses of the workplace situation and magnitudes of weights lifted and so on. Despite this the incidence of work loss continues to increase. This study challenged that view in emphasizing the role of the psychosocial factors. It was well established that a history of a previous back problem is an important risk factor. It has been known for some time that patients with back pain may become distressed. Here for the first time it was shown that job dissatisfaction by itself will predict future back pain.

With this knowledge, epidemiological surveys of back pain and in particular prospective studies are recognized as incomplete if they do not assess the psychosocial background. Failure to get on with one's supervizing officer, the compensation system and medico-legal claims, operant conditioning, and the role of family and friends play important roles in encouraging disability. This study emphasized the multifaceted nature of back problems in industry and has helped explain why previous prevention efforts which focussed purely on physical factors have been unsuccessful. Jobs that are perceived to be a burden, unenjoyable, unfulfilling and providing few assests strongly influence the development of future back problems. People who enjoy their jobs or who are in less emotional distress tend to under-report back injury.

Strengths

1. This was a prospective study in which the baseline data was recorded prior to the development of back pain.
2. It was then possible to relate the development of back problems back to the pre-morbid data.

Weaknesses

1. This study analysed the report of back injury rather than the development of back pain. There is an important difference between the two and it would have been valuable to determine the development of back problems and analyse this data separately from those who actually report and took time off as a result.
2. The subjects all worked in the Boeing Aircraft factory. It was stated that the study was performed in a diverse, highly sophisticated manufacturing industry with the job tasks tending not to be extremely stressful for the back. The data with regard to this particular point is not provided, and the back injury claim rate was found to be similar in fact to other American industries where back stresses are considered to be higher.
3. The study analysed the reports of back injury. Intuitively one would think that psychosomatic factors would be more important in the development of chronicity of back problems. This has not been analysed.

Relevance

This study has indicated the importance of psychosocial factors in predicting the future occurrence of reports of back injury.

Paper 7

How many days of bed rest for acute low back pain?

Authors

Deyo RA, Diehl AK, Rosenthal M

Reference

New England Journal of Medicine 1986; **315**:1064–1070

Summary

Two hundred and three patients with mechanical low back pain were randomly asigned to treatment of either 2 day's bed rest (Group I) or 7 day's bed rest (Group II). Although compliance with the recommendation of bed rest was variable, patients assigned to group I missed 45% fewer days off work than those assigned to group II (3.1 versus 5.6 days, p = 0.01). No differences were observed in other functional, physiological or perceived outcomes. For many patients without neuromotor defects, shorter periods of 2 day's bed rest may be appropriate. If widely applied, this policy may substantially reduce absenteeism from work and the resulting indirect costs of low back pain for both patients and employers.

Key message

For patients with acute low back pain, shorter periods of bed rest promoted more rapid and better recovery than prolonged periods of bed rest.

Why it's important

The traditional management of acute episodes of back pain required prolonged periods of recumbency with the patient lying flat, usually on a firm bed, and only allowed up for toilet or washing. At the same time analgesics were provided to provide pain relief. The patient remained on bed rest until the acute back episode resolved. Mobilization was then undertaken very cautiously with great care being taken to protect the back. This was the first study to challenge this approach to management, and indicated that prolonged periods of immobility promoted the perpetuation of symptoms and disability. It has led to a rethink about the management of back pain.

It has been followed by a succession of studies confirming these findings and indicating the importance of maintaining physical activity and remaining at work. The more recent studies show that patients with acute back pain should remain at work if at all possible. If they need to be off work it should be for the shortest period, and if they need rest in bed it should be for a limited period of time, generally 2 days or less. Prolonged periods of bed rest are now recognized as promoting the perpetuation of disability. A number of different mechanisms are thought to play a part. These include the importance of motion in healing injured soft tissues and joints; the development of stiffness in relation to immobility; improvement of the arterial blood supply and venous drainage in association with spine movement; the development of muscle weakness with prolonged inability, and the psychological effects of prolonged rest including a fear of injuring the back.

Strengths

1. A controlled study comparing two regimes of bed rest for patients with acute back pain.
2. The assessors were blinded to the treatment assignment.

Weaknesses

1. This study included patients with acute and chronic pain, some had previous acute episodes, many had evidence of nerve root irritation.
2. This type of research requires a much larger study examining separately the effects of acute and chronic back pain, and patients without and with sciatica.
3. Although treatment with 2 and 7 day's bed rest was recommended, compliance was limited particularly in the latter group. In terms of practical application, a specific prescription of 2 or 7 day's bed rest is very difficult as many patients modulate their activities in relation to their symptoms.

Relevance

This paper led to a fundamental shift in the approach to management of back pain. In particular it was responsible for the change from recommending prolonged periods of bed rest and protection of the back to maintaining normal activity if at all possible. Failing that, limited periods of inactivity and return to normal function as soon as possible are now recommended.

CHAPTER 21

Soft tissue disorders

Cathy Speed and Brian Hazleman

Introduction

Soft tissue rheumatic complaints encompass disorders of tendon, ligament, bursa, fascia, joint capsule and isolated lesions of muscle. Some chronic pain syndromes such as fibromyalgia are also included. Although they represent a significant proportion of new patient consultations in rheumatology, they remain poorly understood with respect to their pathologies, epidemiology and management. The diverse spectrum of these often complex disorders is frequently underestimated.

Some earlier observations on specific disorders have, until recently, been overlooked. It is only now, with the use of sensitive imaging techniques such as magnetic resonance imaging that the importance of these early observations has been highlighted. This is illustrated in those papers by Smith (Paper 1) and Rathbun and McNab (Paper 2), relating to rotator cuff pathologies, which are a spectrum of commonly encountered complaints. In contrast, there have been clinical papers which have had a significant influence upon opinions relating to soft tissue complaints. Such is the case with the papers presented here by Neer (Paper 3), Steinbrocker (Paper 5) and Brain, *et al.* (Paper 6).

Other more scientifically-based papers have helped vastly to improve our understanding of some soft tissue complaints and were an early recognition of the complexity of the regions that are affected in soft tissue complaints. These include those papers by Kellgren (Paper 8), Upton and McComas (Paper 7) and by Lucas (Paper 4). Soft tissue disorders represent a significant socio-economic burden as a result of lost productivity and costs of health care. However the emphasis upon the relevance of soft tissue complaints in the workplace has shifted from true industrial injury as described in 1945 by Hunter, *et al.* (Paper 9), to less specific complaints with major legal and financial implications for the employer, as emphasized by Hadler in 1986 (Paper 10).

These classic papers help to emphasize not only the complexities of a wide range of complaints, but also of the many challenges which remain to be met in their understanding. Soft tissue rheumatology, as Dixon described over 20 years ago, remains 'the great outback of rheumatology' and truly is a vast and exciting frontier.

Paper I

Pathological appearances of seven cases of injury of the shoulder joint; with remarks

Author

Smith JG

Reference

London Medical Gazette 1834; **14**: 280

Summary

Smith was credited with the first report on rotator cuff tears, which he published in 1834. This paper consisted of a report of five post-mortem cases in which rotator cuff pathology was found in seven shoulders. In each case a tear of subscapularis was demonstrated and in two of these this was the sole rotator cuff pathology. One of these latter two cases involved a full thickness tear, the other partial thickness. The age in some cases was not stated, but included patients in the range of 30–56 years of age.

Smith's findings were as follows:

- In one case global tear of the cuff was described.
- In one case a partial isolated tear of the subscapularis tendon was described and in another an isolated full thickness tear of this tendon was noted.
- In one case full thickness tears of the tendons of supraspinatus, infraspinatus and teres minor was demonstrated, with a partial thickness tear of subscapularis.
- In three shoulders, tears of subscapularis and supraspinatus were noted.
- In all seven shoulders, pathology of the tendon of the long head of the biceps was noted, involving either subluxation or rupture, with or without scarring and reattachment.
- Laxity of the capsule and ligaments of the shoulder and stretching of the cuff tendons or excessive movement of the humeral head was reported in two cases.
- Subdeltoid bursal thickening or open communication with the glenohumeral joint was described in four shoulders.
- Exostoses, covered with an 'enamel like' substance on the undersurface of the acromion was described in two cases and similar findings also noted on the humeral head in one case.
- A 'fracture' of the acromion, forming an 'artificial joint' with fibrocartilage and fibroligamentous capsule was described in three cases.

Related references

(1) Hauser EDW. Avulsion of the tendon of the subscapularis muscle. *Journal of Bone and Joint Surgery* 1954; **X**(A):139–141.

(2) Nevasier RJ, Nevasier TJ, Nevasier JS. Concurrent rupture of the rotator cuff and anterior dislocation of the shoulder in the older patient. *Journal of Bone and Joint Surgery* 1988; **70**(A):1308–1311.

(3) Gerber C, Krushell RJ. Isolated rupture of the tendon of the subscapularis muscle: clinical features in 16 cases. *Journal of Bone and Joint Surgery* 1991; **76**(B);371–380.

(4) Ticker JB, Warner JJP. Single tears of the rotator cuff. *Orth Clin N Amer* 1997; **1**(28):99–116.

Key message

First description of rotator cuff tears (alone or in combination) and associated lesions. Rotator cuff pathology can involve one or more of the tendons of the rotator cuff. Isolated tears of subscapularis can occur. Involvement of the tendon of the long head of the biceps is common. Laxity of the glenohumeral joint should always be considered in patients with rotator cuff pathology.

Why it's important

This paper is considered to be the first to describe tears of the rotator cuff and contains a description of many of the important features of rotator cuff pathology, ranging from global cuff rupture to partial thickness tears and involving multiple portions of the cuff or tendons in isolation.

Whilst isolated tears of the other components of the rotator cuff (supraspinatus, infraspinatus and teres minor) have received much attention, it was not until 1954 that isolated tears of subscapularis were reported (1) and subsequently only rarely did further case reports appear (2). It was not until the last decade that series of such tears have been reported (3). Such series have assisted in elucidating indicators of subscapularis tears, such as the age of the patient (with a non-degenerate cuff), a history of trauma involving hyperextension or external rotation of the adducted arm and pain with the arm in positions below shoulder level as well as during overhead activities (4). Specific features on examination include an increased range of passive external rotation, weakness of internal rotation and a positive lift off test (3, 4).

Involvement of the tendon of the long head of the biceps in rotator cuff disorders is now noted to be common and is related to the intimate association between the cuff and the biceps tendon as the latter runs to insert onto the supraglenoid tubercle of the scapula. Pathology of the rotator cuff should be expected in cases of rupture of this tendon. Capsular and ligamentous laxity of the glenohumeral joint is now well recognized and may result in instability of the shoulder joint and subsequent cuff pathology. It may be related to trauma (unilateral instability) or congenital laxity (multidirectional instability). Subdeltoid bursal changes are now looked for routinely during ultrasonography in the evaluation of the patient with rotator cuff pathology.

Smith's findings of the 'enamel' covered exostoses on the undersurface of the acromion presumably represented osteoarthritic changes and/or impingement, the latter also being the likely aetiology to such findings on the head of the humerus. Lastly, was the 'fracture' of the acromion described by Smith simply the acromioclavicular joint?

Strengths

1. Alerted medical community to a wide range of rotator cuff pathologies.
2. Noted some of the associated pathological changes that can occur in rotator cuff lesions.

Weaknesses

1. No background to the cases was available.
2. Macroscopic pathology only.
3. Interpretation of associated pathological changes was limited.

Relevance

Credited as the first published report of rotator cuff tears. Noted associated factors. Identified isolated tears of subscapularis.

Paper 2

The microvascular pattern of the rotator cuff

Authors

Rathbun JB, Macnab I

Reference

Journal of Bone and Joint Surgery 1970; **52**(B):540–553

Summary

Rathbun and Macnab performed cadaveric studies to examine the vascular supply of the supraspinatus tendon and to compare this with that of other tendons of the rotator cuff. A histological examination of each tendon was also performed. The rotator cuff vascular bed was filled with radio opaque dye and the dye was allowed to harden. The rotator cuff was dissected and soft tissue radiography with a beryllium window allowed the microvasculature to be demonstrated. This technique was performed with the arm of the cadaver at the side and then repeated for the opposite arm with the shoulder abducted.

With the arm adducted, an area of relative avascularity was seen in the supraspinatus tendon near its point of insertion and in the superior portion of the infraspinatus tendon, but not in the other tendons of the rotator cuff. Avascularity was also noted in the tendon of the long head of the biceps. Histological studies showed degenerative changes, calcification and rupture in these areas of avascularity, while healthy tendons were seen where blood supply was good. With the arm in abduction, the vessels within the supraspinatus tendon filled almost completely, but an avascular zone appeared in the subscapularis tendon. The authors suggested that with the arm in the adducted and neutrally rotated position, the zones of avascularity were secondary to a 'wringing out' phenomenon. The authors also postulated that the areas of tendon degeneration were preceded by avascularity.

Related references **(1)** Riley GP, Harrall RL, Constant CR, *et al.* Tendon degeneration and chronic shoulder pain: changes in the collagen composition of the human rotator cuff tendons in rotator cuff tendinitis. *Annals of Rheumatic Diseases* 1994; **53**:359–366.

(2) Mosley HF, Goldie I. The arterial pattern of the rotator cuff of the shoulder. *Journal of Bone and Joint Surgery* 1963; **45**(B):780.

(3) Swiontkowski M, Iannotti JP, Boulas JH, *et al. Intraoperative Assessment of Rotator Cuff Vascularity Using Laser Doppler Flowmetry.* St Louis: Mosby, Year Book, 1990:208–212.

(4) Sigholm G, Styf J, Korner L, Herberts P. Pressure recording in the subacromial bursa. *Journal of Orthopaedic Research* 1988; **6**:123–128.

Why it's important

The 'critical zone' of the supraspinatus tendon is the anterior portion near its point of insertion that appears to be particularly prone to ruptures and calcification. Many of these lesions are degenerative in nature (tendinosis), with underlying pathological changes including alteration of collagen fibre type distribution, with a relative increase in type III collagen, fibrovascular proliferation and microtears (1). The pathogenesis of such lesions is unclear, but vascularity was long considered to play a central role. Other factors may include age, genetics and mechanical impingement.

Prior to the publication of this paper in 1970, the critical zone had been described as a zone of relative avascularity. Although Moseley and Goldie noted in 1963 that the vascular supply to the cuff was rich in anastamoses between tendinous and osseous vessels, many continued to consider avascularity to be the primary cause of rotator cuff tendinopathies (2). Rathbun and Macnab were the first to postulate that these findings may have been an artifact of positioning. Subsequent studies by others using laser doppler demonstrated substantial flow and increased flow in the area of cuff tears (3). It is therefore apparent that other factors play a significant role in the development of rotator cuff tendinopathies. These may include raised subacromial pressure has been demonstrated with flexion of the shoulder (4).

Strengths

1. Elegant demonstration of vascular supply of the rotator cuff.
2. Rational theory to explain findings.
3. Had an important impact upon theories of the pathogenesis of rotator cuff tendinopathy.

Weaknesses

1. Cadaveric studies.
2. Number of cadavers in the study is not stated.
3. No quantitation of blood supply possible.

Relevance

Avascularity is not the sole factor in the development of rotator cuff tendinopathies. Poor vascular supply to portions of the cuff may occur with the arm in specific positions.

Paper 3

Anterior acromioplasty for the chronic impingement syndrome in the shoulder. A preliminary report

Author

Neer CS

Reference

Journal of Bone and Joint Surgery 1972; **54**(A) [1]:41–50

Summary

Neer described the importance of the anterior third and undersurface of the acromion in the impingement syndrome. He based these findings on cadaveric studies and surgical observations. In cadaveric studies he noted that, with elevation of the arm in internal or external rotation, the critical area of the tendons of the rotator cuff (supraspinatus, occasionally in association with the infraspinatus and tendon of the long head of the biceps) pass under the coraco-acromial ligament or the anterior process (but not the posterior two-thirds) of the acromion. Neer extrapolated these findings to develop a surgical approach to the management of 50 patients with partial or complete tears of the rotator cuff or persisting impingement after lateral acromioplasty, which at that time was the standard surgical approach to treatment.

He followed up 47 of these patients for a mean of 2.5 years. A satisfactory outcome was defined as full use of the shoulder, less than 20 degrees of limitation in full overhead extension and at least 75% of normal strength. This was noted in 15 of 16 partial thickness tears, 19 of 20 full thickness tears and four of 11 patients who had previously had lateral acromionectomies.

Key message

Description of importance of anterior subacromial impingement in rotator cuff pathologies, associated radiological findings, and surgical approach to management.

Why it's important

In this paper, Neer popularized the concept of impingement in rotator cuff lesions. He described three different stages of the impingement syndrome:

1. Reversible oedema and haemorrhage, usually in the younger patient.
2. Fibrosis and tendinitis, particularly in 25–40 year old patient.
3. Bone spurs and tendon rupture, particularly in the patient >40 years of age.

From his cadaveric and operative studies, Neer recognized the importance of the anterior third and undersurface of the acromion in the impingement syndrome. He noted that, with elevation of the arm in internal or external rotation, the 'critical area' of the tendons of the rotator cuff (see below) pass under the coraco-acromial ligament and/or the anterior process, but not the posterior 2/3, of the acromion.

Neer also made several other points in this paper:

- He emphasized the importance of non-surgical management of rotator cuff tendinitis.
- It is extremely difficult to distinguish clinically between partial and full thickness rotator cuff tears.
- He described what has come to be recognized as Neer's test: subacromial injection of xylocaine in partial thickness tears to evaluate the effects of impingement.
- Neer emphasized the importance of recognizing that, in pathologies of the tendon of the long head of the biceps, operative intervention should also address subacromial impingement.
- Radiological findings of cysts and/or sclerosis of the greater tuberosity and anterior acromial osteophytes were noted.

Since Neer's initial description of anterior acromioplasty, several workers have reported their favourable results using this technique and it remains popular. Arthroscopic acromioplasty is also now popular but whether it is superior to open surgery is still unclear.

Strengths

1. Clear rational interpretation of a major mechanism in the development of rotator cuff lesions.
2. Extrapolation of hypothesis to the development of an operative approach to management of these conditions.
3. Had a significant impact upon the understanding and management of rotator cuff tears secondary to impingement.

Weaknesses

1. Based on the author's observations from cadaveric studies and a cohort of patients with impingement syndrome, most with rotator cuff tears.
2. The details of these patients are not given.
3. Post-operative follow-up was limited.
4. Outcome based on a subjective scale of 'satisfactory' versus 'unsatisfactory'.
5. No randomized controlled trial was performed.

Relevance

Had a significant impact upon the understanding and management of rotator cuff tears secondary to impingement. Impingement occurs primarily at the anterior third of the acromion and its related undersurface. This area must be focussed upon if surgical intervention is considered.

Paper 4

Biomechanics of the shoulder joint

Author

Lucas DB

Reference

Archives of Surgery 1973; **107**:425–432

Summary

Reviewed the functional anatomy and biomechanics of the glenohumeral joint, basing their review on the work of Inman, *et al.* (1944) (1) and Codman (1934) (2). This review emphasized the importance of the 'force couple' in abduction of the shoulder. This is the mechanism whereby two muscle groups act to abduct the arm, the deltoid acting to elevate the arm whilst the rotator cuff and long head of the biceps act to stabilize the humeral head. This review also emphasized the concept of scapulohumeral rhythm, whereby rotation of the scapula occurs with glenohumeral abduction in order to permit the deltoid to maintain an optimum length-tension ratio during most of the abduction range.

Related references
(1) Inman VT, Saunders J bde CM. Observations on the function of the clavicle. *Clin Med* 1946; **65**:158–166.
(2) Codman EA. *The Shoulder: Rupture of the Supraspinatus Tendon and Other Lesions In or About the Subacromial Bursa.* Boston: Thomas Todd, 1934.
(3) Poppen NK, Walker PS. Forces at the glenohumeral joint in abduction. *Clinical Orthopaedics* 1978; **58**:165.

Key message

Combined action of the deltoid and rotator cuff and biceps allows abduction of the arm by the formation of a force-couple. The deltoid elevates the arm whilst the rotator cuff stabilizes the humeral head in the glenoid.

Why it's important

The glenohumeral joint is not an inherently stable joint. It is the most mobile joint in the body, potentially sacrificing stability for this wide range of movement. This review highlighted the fact that abduction by deltoid requires the head of the humerus to be stabilized in the glenoid fossa by contraction of the muscles of the rotator cuff. It was not until 5 years after the publication of this review that Poppen and Walker demonstrated the importance of the combined action of both supraspinatus and deltoid in the initiation and the first 30 degrees of abduction of the arm (3). If the cuff is insufficient (for example torn or weak), then the humeral head migrates superiorly and impinges upon the cuff and undersurface of the acromion. In addition the glenohumeral joint will be unstable, emphasizing the importance of the rotator cuff as a dynamic stabilizer. This concept allows some insight into the cause of many rotator cuff tendinopathies. Repetitive tasks involving use of the shoulder can result in fatigue of the musculature of the cuff and loss of the stabilizing effect. This in turn can lead to impingement, with repetitive microtrauma leading to tendon lesions.

The relationship between the movement at the glenohumeral joint and rotation of the scapula during abduction is an important component of normal shoulder function and is described as scapulohumeral rhythm. Normal scapulohumeral rhythm involves abduction of the arm to 90 degrees prior to any scapular rotation taking place. Loss of scapulohumeral rhythm is an important clinical sign in many shoulder disorders and re-establishing this rhythm a major goal in shoulder rehabilitation.

Strengths

1. Clarification of previous workers' research.
2. Emphasized the importance of the force couple in elevation of the arm and the role of the rotator cuff as dynamic stabilizers.
3. Emphasized the importance of scapular rotation and scapulohumeral rhythm.

Weaknesses

1. This was not original work but summarized the findings of others.
2. The biomechanics of the shoulder complex is complicated and many aspects remain unclear.

Relevance

Stabilization of the humeral head in the glenoid by the rotator cuff is of paramount importance in normal shoulder function. Rotator cuff tendinopathies can result from, or be the cause of, loss of this stabilizing action.

Paper 5

The shoulder hand syndrome

Author

Steinbrocker O

Reference

American Journal of Medicine 1947; **3**:402–407

Summary

Steinbrocker presented and discussed six cases (five females, one male) of shoulder pain with ipsilateral swelling of the hand, followed by trophic changes in five of these six. Prior diagnoses had been made in these cases, including rheumatoid arthritis (RA), connective tissue disease, periarthritis and septic arthritis. He postulated that these findings were due to a vascular and/or neurological disturbance or to sympathetic dysfunction.

He also listed three stages of evolution. Firstly, an acute or chronic onset of shoulder pain and generalized swelling and stiffness of hand and fingers, appearing simultaneously or sequentially. Vascular disturbance was reported in an unspecified number. A history of possible minor trauma was reported in only one of the six patients in this group. Secondly, over 3–6 months resolution of pain and dysfunction of shoulder and resolution of swelling of hand, but more pronounced stiffness and flexion deformity of the fingers and notable osteopenia of the hand and shoulder on plain x-ray. The third stage involves trophic changes of the hand and flexion contractures of the fingers which may persist for years.

Recovery in this series ranged from 10 months to 7 years, the latter case being only partially recovered when Steinbrocker published this report. Although he noted that Sudeks atrophy, causalgia, reflex sympathetic dystrophy and post-traumatic osteoporosis are all suggested by this clinical picture, he considered these cases to present more acutely than Sudek's and a history of trauma was generally lacking.

Key message

Shoulder hand syndrome is a syndrome of pain, tenderness, and swelling of the hand in association with a painful stiff shoulder. This is now considered to be a form of algodystrophy. Early diagnosis and intervention are important to prevent progression.

Why it's important

Steinbrocker was the first to recognize the shoulder hand syndrome, the clinical picture of tenderness, pain, and swelling of the hand in association with shoulder pain and/or adhesive capsulitis. The onset may be insidious or acute and many cases are related to a medical event such as a myocardial infarction or cerebrovascular accident or to (often minor) trauma. As Steinbrocker noted, diagnostic confusion may occur. Shoulder hand syndrome is now considered to be a form of algodystrophy. The stages that Steinbrocker described are still considered relevant. Stage I may begin with shoulder pain and stiffness or this may be noted after the peripheral symptoms. Swelling, pain, tenderness, hyperpathia, allodynia, vasomotor and sudomotor changes are noted and may persist for up to 6 months. Trophic changes appear in Stage II and soft tissue atrophy, contractures and osteopenia occur in Stage III. Early diagnosis and intervention are important to prevent progression from Stage I. The diagnosis is often a clinical one, but thermography will show asymmetry of cutaneous temperature, while radionuclide studies will show an increased uptake in the blood flow and pool phases and a delay in soft tissue uptake in most early cases. Osteopenia on plain radiography and localized reductions in bone mineral density on DEXA scanning are seen in chronic cases. Treatment includes education, reassurance and encouragement to mobilize actively the affected limb. Pain relief by the use of analgesics, non-steroidal anti-inflammatory drugs (NSAIDs), oral corticosteroids, tricyclic agents, propanalol, dimethyl sulphoxide, sympathetic nerve blocks and calcium channel blockers have all been advocated.

Strength

Described a clinical syndrome with cases as illustrations.

Weaknesses

1. No confirmatory investigations.
2. No discussion of treatment.

Relevance

First description of shoulder hand syndrome.

Paper 6

Spontaneous compression of both median nerves in the carpal tunnel. Six cases treated surgically

Authors

Brain WR, Wright AD, Wilkinson M

Reference

The Lancet 1947; **1**:277–282

Summary

This paper described non-traumatic bilateral carpal tunnel syndrome and had a significant impact on the understanding of hand pain. Prior to this paper, median nerve compression at the wrist had been described almost uniquely in association with trauma. In addition, the classical symptomatology had not been clarified, with some confusion existing as to the reasons for the relative lack of sensory findings. Brain, *et al.* described six cases involving middle aged or elderly women presenting with pain and tingling in the hand in the distribution of the median nerve. In some cases there was a history of increased use of the hand. Wasting and weakness of the thenar muscles was noted, with diminished light touch and two-point discrimination in the median nerve distribution in some. At operation the median nerve was swollen and pink, with surrounding oedema. Surgical release of the carpal tunnel improved the symptoms in all cases although there remained some sensory and/or motor symptoms/impairment in all.

Related references (1) Stopford JSB. *British Medical Journal* 1926; **1**:1028.
  (2) Repaci M, Torrieri F, Di-Blasio F, Uncini A. Exclusive electrophysiological motor unit involvement in carpal tunnel syndrome. *Clinical Neurophysiology* 1999; **110**(8):1471–1474.

Key message

This paper described non-traumatic bilateral carpal tunnel syndrome that led to a significant improvement in the understanding of hand pain. The clinical picture of pain and tingling in the distribution of the median nerve with thenar wasting and weakness but only minor sensory findings was emphasized. Operative findings of a swollen, thickened median nerve below the carpal ligament indicated a 'neuritis'. Carpal tunnel release was highlighted as an effective approach to management of this condition.

Why it's important

Prior to this paper median nerve compression at the wrist, though recognized, was poorly understood. It was considered that such complaint was associated with significant local trauma and was therefore usually unilateral. The symptomatology associated with median nerve compression, particularly the relative lack of sensory symptoms, led to confusion and it had been previously postulated that only the motor branch was involved. In this paper the classical symptoms and signs of bilateral carpal tunnel syndrome were described in a typical group of patients. Impairment of light touch, pinprick and two-point discrimination was noted and subsequently these sensory findings, particularly the latter, have been relied on clinically to gauge the severity of the problem, although correlation with median nerve sensory conduction findings has not been consistently demonstrated. The authors pointed out that their findings were in keeping with previously described stages of compression of a mixed nerve (1). Subsequent studies have confirmed that pure motor fibre involvement is rare (2).

The role of repetitive use of the hand in carpal tunnel syndrome has been confirmed in some epidemiological and experimental studies (1, 2). However, in reviewing epidemiological studies mainly from Finland, Hadler suggested that there was no increased incidence of carpal tunnel syndrome in shop assistants, assembly line workers nor in light mechanical industry. Carpal tunnel syndrome is a prescribed disease. That is, the disease is considered to be a risk of specific occupations (work involving the use of hand-held vibration tools in the case of carpal tunnel syndrome), providing no other predisposing factors are present in that individual. Other disorders can be associated with carpal tunnel syndrome. These include inflammatory arthritides including those induced by crystals, connective tissue diseases, local space occupying lesions, infections and metabolic and endocrine disorders. Pregnancy and renal dialysis may also be associated with the complaint.

The authors discuss the differential diagnosis of carpal tunnel syndrome and its distinguishing features. Differentiation from progressive muscular atrophy, syringomyelia, cervical spine and costoclavicular syndromes and brachial plexus lesions are all discussed. They point out that flexion of the wrist does not always increase compression on the nerve, perhaps explaining the lack of consistency of Phalen's test. Surgical management, involving carpal tunnel release, in such patients is described and remains popular today. This technique had been described earlier by others, but to release the nerve after compression relating to trauma.

Strengths

1. Presented a review of literature and some of the sources of confusion on the subject of hand pain.
2. Presented classical cases and provided a clear rationale to explain the clinical pictures.
3. Discussed the differential diagnosis and distinguishing features.
4. Provided information on each case including investigations, operative findings and follow-up.

Weaknesses

1. Electrodiagnostics were performed only on one case.
2. Observational study of only six cases.

Relevance

Significantly contributed to the understanding of carpal tunnel syndrome. Described typical cases of idiopathic cases and treatment by carpal tunnel release.

Paper 7

The double crush in nerve entrapment syndromes

Authors

Upton AR, McComas AJ

Reference

The Lancet 1973; **II**:359–361

Summary

This paper discussed the anomalies which exist in some cases of carpal tunnel syndrome, specifically that there may be no apparent precipitant, that proximal symptoms or a coexisting ulnar nerve syndrome may be present, obvious nerve pathology at surgery may be lacking, poor correlation between surgical findings and the extent of the symptoms, failure of some cases to respond to carpal tunnel release and the finding of slowing of impulse conduction proximal to the site of compression.

The authors studied this further in 220 patients presenting with numbness or tingling in the hand, some with weakness of intrinsic hand muscles. All had motor unit population studies in the thenar and hypothenar muscles, motor and sensory conduction studies and concentric needle EMG of muscles innervated by C4-T1 nerve roots. These investigations indicated that 85/220 patients had carpal tunnel syndromes, 24 had ulnar neuropathies and six had both. Seventy percent of these had evidence of a cervical root lesion, on the basis of radiological evidence of a cervical vertebral abnormality, neck symptoms, a history of whiplash, clinical evidence of a dermatomal sensory abnormality or EMG evidence of denervation. The authors postulated that single axons, having been compressed (or excessively stretched) in one region, become susceptible to damage at another site, due to serial impairment of axoplasmic flow.

Related references **(1)** Narakas AO. The role of thoracic outlet syndrome in the double crush syndrome. *Ann Chir Main Memb Super* 1990;**9**(5):331–340.

(2) Cassavan A, Rosenberg A, Rivera LF. Ulnar nerve involvement in carpal tunnel syndrome. *Arch Phys Med Rehabil* 1986; **67**(5):290–292.

(3) Dellon AL. Musculotendinous variations about the medial humeral epicondyle. *J Hand Surg Br* 1986; **11**(2):175–181.

(4) Golovchinsky V. Double crush syndrome in lower extremities. *Electryogr Clin Neurophysiol* 1998; **38**(2):115–120.

(5) Richardson JK, Forman GM, Riley B. An electrophysiological exploration of the double crush hypothesis. *Muscle Nerve* 1999; **22**(1):71–77.

(6) Dahlm LB, Archer DR, McLean WG. Axonal transport and morphological changes following nerve compression. An experimental study in the rabbit vagus nerve. *J Hand Surg Br* 1993; **18**(1): 106–110.

(7) Lundborg G, Dahlm LB. Anatomy, function and pathophysiology of peripheral nerves and nerve compression. *Hand Clin* 1996; **12**(2):185–193.

Key message

Compression of a nerve root may occur at multiple levels.

Why it's important

The hypothesis helps to explain the anomalies that are seen in the groups of patients described above and emphasizes the importance of looking for additional lesion(s) in patients with peripheral nerve entrapments. Proximal lesions include not only nerve root entrapment but also thoracic outlet syndrome (1). Anatomical variations in the arm such as the presence of fibrous bands and accessory or overdeveloped musculature have been demonstrated (2), which may explain the double crush syndrome. Electrophysiological studies have also supported the existence of such a condition (3).

Double crush syndrome has subsequently been described in the lower extremities, with peripheral entrapment syndromes occurring in conjunction with proximal nerve lesions at the lumbar spine (4).

While the concept of double crush syndrome has achieved wide clinical acceptance, others remain sceptical. Richardson, *et al.* (5) hypothesized that, since median sensory response is of C6/C7 origin and the median motor response is primarily of C8 origin, then C6 and/or C7 cases would demonstrate an increased frequency of median mononeuropathy by sensory criteria and C8 cases by motor criteria. However, neurophysiological studies failed to support this hypothesis.

Strengths

1. Clearly written and provides a concise summary of the anomalies seen in patients with carpal tunnel syndrome.
2. Provides a rational explanation for the clinical picture(s) seen in this group of patients.

Weaknesses

1. The basis for diagnosis of a cervical root lesion is of uncertain validity, as it is unclear as to how many of the stated criteria for a cervical root lesion were required. Many of these criteria are non-specific and insufficient to make the diagnosis. However electrophysiological evidence in 81 patients was provided.
2. As the paper was written before MRI was readily available it is not possible to substantiate the diagnoses of cervical disc lesions with imaging studies.
3. The hypothesis that impaired axoplasmic flow after initial nerve injury results in an increase in the susceptibility at a second site is elegant but unsubstantiated. However, it has been subsequently demonstrated that morphological and biochemical changes can take place in a compressed neurone (6). These may include alterations in intraneural microcirculation and nerve fibre structure, and in vascular permeability with resulting formation of oedema and deterioration in nerve function (7).

Relevance

Provides a rational explanation for the clinical picture(s) seen in this group of patients.

Paper 8

Observations on referred pain arising from muscle

Author

Kellgren JH

Reference

Clinical Science 1938; **3**:176–190

Summary

Kellgren investigated the pain patterns produced by stimulation of deep muscle, fascia and tendon by injection of small quantities of hypertonic saline. Stimulation of muscle bellies gave rise to diffuse pain often at a distance from the point stimulated. He concluded from this part of his study that diffuse pain from a given muscle may be confused with pain arising from deeper structures. Stimulation of muscle fascia and of tendon was found to be more sensitive and with a more localized distribution of pain. Kellgren then investigated whether the distribution of the referred pain followed a spinal segmental pattern and reported this to be the case. This pattern differs from the segmental innervation of the skin. Kellgren investigated areas of the distribution of referred tenderness on muscle stimulation. He found that referred pain from muscle is associated with referred tenderness from deep structures. Kellgren postulated that the mechanism of reference could be due to a common pathway shared by pain arising from muscular and deep somatic structures.

Related references **(1)** Simons DG. Muscle pain syndromes (I). *American Journal of Physical Medicine* 1975a; **54**(6):288–311.

(2) Simons DG. Muscle pain syndromes (I). *American Journal of Physical Medicine* 1975b; **55**(1): 15–42.

(3) Travell J. Myofascial trigger points: a clinical view. *Advances in Pain Research and Therapy* 1976; **1**:919–926.

(4) Fricton JR. Myofascial pain. In: *Bailliere's Clinical Rheumatology* 1994; **8**(4):857–880.

Key message

Pain arising from skeletal muscle can be diffuse and mild to moderate in nature. It follows a spinal segmental pattern. It may be confused by pain arising from deeper somatic structures.

Why it's important

Kellgren's paper opened the chapter on the concept of diffuse pain arising from muscle and the field has since developed significantly. Specific regional non-inflammatory muscle pain syndromes are now recognized under the term myofascial pain. Kellgren described areas of muscle that he stimulated which gave rise to diffuse referred pain as muscle points. Other workers later took the concept described by Kellgren and developed the theme by describing trigger points (1–3). Trigger points are defined as a localized deep tenderness in a taut band of skeletal muscle that is responsible for the pain in the zone of reference and if treated will resolve the resultant pain. The zone of reference is defined as the area of perceived pain referred from the irritable trigger point, and is usually localized over the trigger point and may spread out to a distant site.

Myofascial pain has specific clinical characteristics including the presence of trigger points in a taut band of muscle, pain in a zone of reference, associated factors such as gastrointestinal, visual and otological disturbances, paraesthesiae and dermatographia. Contributing factors to myofascial pain include trauma, whiplash, psychological stress, the performance of repetitive tasks, physical illness and sleep disturbance (4). Investigations are normal and the pathophysiology is not understood, since no specific pathological lesion has been identified. Treatment involves pain control, stretching, muscle conditioning, postural realignment, acupuncture and trigger point injections, tricyclic agents, counselling and addressing underlying factors.

Strengths

1. Important observations in the pattern of pain arising from muscle.
2. Showed that pain distributions identified by the subjects were reproducible.

Weaknesses

1. Observational study on small numbers.
2. Unclear as to the variation in pain distribution between subjects.

Relevance

The paper identified the distribution and nature of pain arising from muscles and led to the development of the concept of myofascial pain.

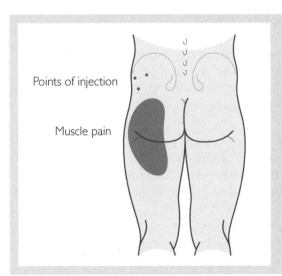

Points of injection

Muscle pain

Figure 21.1 The distribution of pain experienced after stimulation of the gluteus medius muscle.

Paper 9

Clinical effects of the use of pneumatic tools

Authors

Hunter D, McLaughlin AIG, Perry KMA

Reference

British Journal of Industrial Medicine 1945; **2**:10–16

Summary

This paper summarized the literature on the clinical effects of pneumatic tools and presented findings of their own series of cases. Osteoarthritis (OA) in the upper limbs and decalcification of the carpus were discussed but the emphasis and significance of the paper relates to a condition described at that time as 'white finger', now considered part of the hand-arm vibration syndrome (HAVS). Clinical features of numbness, stiffness and pallor of the fingers, in particular the fingers upon which the tool is resting are described. Recurrence on exposure to cold some years after cessation of use of pneumatic tools is noted. Characteristic associations, such as involvement of the non-dominant hand, exacerbation by cold temperatures and increased incidence and severity with tools that vibrate at frequencies between 2000–3500 strokes/minute were reported. Approaches to prevention are suggested, most importantly restricting the use of tools with vibration frequencies in the range of 2000–3500 strokes/minute. Other approaches, including warming the compressed air and shock absorbers are also mentioned, but are noted to have been tried with little success.

Related references (1) International Standards Organization. *Guide for the evaluation of human exposure to whole body vibration.* ISO 2631. Geneva: ISO, 1978.

(2) British Standards Institution. *British Standards guide to measurement and evaluation of human exposure to vibration transmitted to the hand.* BSI 6842. London: BSI, 1987.

(3) International Standards Organization. *Guidelines for the measurement and the assessment of human exposure to hand transmitted vibration.* ISO 5349. Geneva: ISO, 1986.

(4) American National Standards Institute. Guide for the measurement and evaluation of human exposure to vibration transmitted to the hand. ANSI S3–S4. New York: ANSI, 1986.

(5) Gemn G, Pyykko I, Taylor W, Pelmear PL. The Stockholm workshop scale for the classification of cold-induced Raynaud's phenomenon in the hand-arm vibration syndrome (revision of Taylor-Pelmear Scale). *Scandinavian Journal of Work Environmental Health* 1987; **13**:275–278.

(6) Dupuis H, Riedel S. Experience on the reversibility of the vibration induced white finger disease. *Cent Eur J Public Health* 1995; **3** (suppl.):19–21.

(7) Petersen-R, Andersen M, Mikkelsen S, Nielsen SL. Prognosis of vibration induced white finger: a follow up study. *Occup Environ Med* 1995 Feb; **52**(2):110–115.

Key message

The syndrome of vibration white finger, later known as part of the HAVS, is a significant, incapacitating disorder related to the use of vibrating hand-held tools. Other musculoskeletal conditions such as hand and wrist OA can also arise due to the use of such machinery.

Why it's important

The HAVS, consisting of vascular, neurological, and articular disorders (OA) occurring in the upper limbs of vibration-exposed workers as described in this paper, is now well recognized. It became an industrial prescribed disease in 1985. Vibration can be described by its frequency, amplitude, acceleration and direction in addition to the exposure time. The authors reported higher risk with specific frequencies and the medical risks are considered to be directly related to the severity of the vibration and the total vibration exposure time. However, there are too few epidemiological data to enable reliable conclusions to be drawn about precise exposure-response relationships for any of the complaints which form part of the HAVS. As a result, there are four current recommended industry standards for tools: BSI 6842 (1987) (2), ISO 5349 (1986) (3), ANSI S3–34 (1986) (4), ACGIH (1992–93) (4).

In the early literature describing HAVS, dating from the early 1900s, it was given numerous labels, including vibration white finger (VWF), spastic anaemia, dead fingers, traumatic vasospastic disease and occupational Raynaud's phenomenon. In this paper Hunter, *et al.* emphasized the importance of differentiating VWF from primary Raynaud's phenomenon. In VWF, persistent paraesthesia and pain are common in the hands and arms and these occur independently from the 'white attacks'. There are no stages of hyperaemia or cyanosis. Subjective reports can correlate poorly with objective findings. The severity of HAVS can be assessed using numerous scales, including the Stockholm classification (5). However there is currently no simple, reliable objective diagnostic test available.

The aetiology of the disorder remains unclear but appears to be related to blood vessel and nerve (including mechanoreceptor) damage, which occur simultaneously but independently of each other.

The reversibility of HAVS has been studied. A reduction in or cessation of exposure to vibration may have a beneficial effect on finger-blanching symptoms and the cold response of digital vessels but this may not occur for some years (6). Further research has implied that continued work with high vibration hand-held tools, smoking, other circulatory diseases, and low age at the time of diagnosis have an unfavourable influence on the prognosis (7).

Strengths

1. Clearly written, with practical messages.
2. Support their literature review with a large series of their own cases.

Weaknesses

1. Little discussion of pathogenic mechanisms.
2. Literature review and report of a case series rather than randomized controlled trial.

Relevance

Interpretation of the literature, supported by a large case cohort study, on the syndrome now recognized as HAVS, which became an industrial prescribed disease 40 years after the publication of this paper.

Paper 10

Industrial Rheumatology. The Australian and New Zealand experience with arm pain and backache in the workplace

Author

Hadler NM

Reference

Medical Journal of Australia 1986; **144**:191–195

Summary

In a critique of the concept of occupational soft tissue 'disease', Hadler provides an overview of the clinical and socio-political environments that confound the management of soft tissue complaints in the work place. He uses backache and arm pain to illustrate the salient points. From the clinicians' viewpoint, the diagnosis of work incapacity is straightforward and made when the patient states that he/she cannot work. There then follows the period of determination as to whether a specific disorder is present and a management strategy is devised, which may include alteration of factors associated with the workplace.

Socio-political and legal aspects have significantly added to the complexity surrounding work incapacity. These issues address whether the relationship of cause (work) and effect (incapacity) exists and if so what are the specific characteristics of each. Such issues are laden with emotional, social, financial and bureaucratic factors that the clinical care of the patient can become lost in the complexities of the label 'work incapacity'. Hadler points out that there is no evidence that back pain in the workplace is any more common than in the general population (1). He also comments upon the increasing frequency in claims for industrial compensation in Australia, despite significant ergonomic improvements in the workplace and the findings that arm pain in the workplace is less common than in the general population in England and in the USA. Hadler emphasizes the need to consider not only physical activities (static muscle contractions, repetitive activity and direct loading), but also the broader working environment (social, financial, emotional and psychological factors, poor working conditions and insufficient supervision) in the evaluation of musculoskeletal complaints in the work place.

Related reference **(1)** Hadler NM. Industrial rheumatology: clinical investigations into the influence of the pattern of usage on the pattern of regional musculoskeletal disease. *Arthritis and Rheumatism* 1977; **20**:1019–1025.

Key message

Hadler emphasizes the need for the medical profession to focus upon the clinical responsibilities and the search for an explanation for work-related disorders such as arm pain.

Why it's important

In 1977 Hadler coined the term 'industrial rheumatology' in order to highlight the need for the clinician to address discrete musculoskeletal complaints which led to work incapacity. In this paper, written 9 years later, he noted that this field has been profoundly affected by surrounding socio-political issues, in particular financial compensation. The clinician's role in care of the patient with a musculoskeletal complaint which may be related to work, includes diagnosis, identification of the cause(s) if possible, and management strategies. These may include alteration of ergonomic factors and consideration whether cessation of work is necessary and if so, what effects will it have on the patient. However these ideals are often obscured by the issue of 'who is to blame' and financial compensation. Hadler emphasizes the need for the medical profession to focus upon the clinical responsibilities and the search for an explanation for work-related disorders such as arm pain. While use-associated arm pain has been given many labels, the term 'repetitive strain injury' is frequently coined, inferring damage. However, no conclusive pathological findings have been noted. This emotion (and legal) laden term should therefore be avoided.

Strengths

1. Review of the salient clinical and socio-political issues surrounding musculoskeletal complaints and the workplace.
2. Strong reminder to the clinician to focus upon his/her role of care for the patient.

Weaknesses

1. Personal opinion.
2. Unclear in parts.

Relevance

Hadler is one of the few rheumatologists who have been able to consider regional back pain syndromes such as back and arm pain within the biopsychosocial model of disease, as opposed to the purely biomedical model. As a result, he recommended abolition of the term 'repetitive strain injury'.

CHAPTER 22

Fibromyalgia

Hugh Smythe

Introduction

Fibromyalgia is complex but we have learned much about it in the last three decades, especially in the last 10 years. I began with a list of 53 'classic' papers that I thought were essential to cover all relevant aspects of the subject, but have been obliged to reduce these to six main papers. I regret the omission of essential contributions by colleagues whose friendship I value highly. I have limited my selections to a common theme, based around the observations on referred pain of Kellgren and his colleagues (1, 2, 3). It is clear that the pain of fibromyalgia arises neither from the tissues complained of, nor from the unsuspected but characteristic sites of deep pain and tenderness found by the examiner. It is also clear that neural mechanisms are involved in affecting the severity and chronicity of pain, and the presence of associated symptoms. So in dealing with fibromyalgia we must deal with referred pain and tenderness and with amplifying factors.

Beginning their work in 1936, Kellgren and Lewis produced pain by injecting hypertonic saline into their own deep somatic tissues, and those of blindfolded volunteers. The pain experienced was referred, interpreted as arising from structures remote from the stimulus. They later injected interspinous ligaments and found that pain was referred distally in distributions that were different from segmental dermatomes and the term 'sclerotomes' was subsequently used (4). The referred pain was accompanied by referred tenderness. The work of Kellgren was confirmed by others (5, 6), but was subsequently largely forgotten by rheumatology, as well as by medicine in general. But Kellgren recognized the all-important fact that much pain could arise from the spine, saying 'There is little doubt that in many cases obscure pains in the chest and abdomen are due to diseases of the spine. Thus in every case it is well to preserve an open mind at the outset and to examine carefully all the structures which, by virtue of their segmental innervation, could give rise to the pain under consideration'. Kellgren's chapter in Copeman's *Textbook of Rheumatic Diseases* (3) summarizes the early work and thoughtfully develops those aspects of relevance to the clinician and is my first 'classic' reference that I believe should be read by all physicians*.

More recently, the pioneering experimental work of Moldofsky and his colleagues led to the modern definition of fibromyalgia (Paper 1), based on the findings of tender spots and sleep disturbance. This work caused a lot of controversy and discussion about the reality of fibrositis or fibromyalgia, largely laid to rest by the work of the American College of Rheumatology (ACR) who produced robust classification criteria (Paper 2). Such criteria help patient classification for the research studies needed into pathogenesis and treatment. Papers 3 and 4 are experimental studies into the pathogenesis of fibromyalgia, each of which suggest that spinal and other more central mechanisms are important. The final group of papers (Papers 5a–c) bring us back, full circle, to the work of Kellgren, as they indicate that the spine is the likely source of pain in fibromyalgia.

Editors' note: Four different chapter authors selected the pain work of Kellgren as a 'classic' relevant to their area of expertise. One of the original papers is reviewed in the chapter on soft tissue disorders. In the other chapters, to avoid duplication, we have either omitted the reference and/or pointed out its importance through the introduction, as in this case.

References

1. Kellgren JH. Observations on referred pain arising from muscle. *Clinical Science* 1938; **3**:175–190.
2. Kellgren JH. Deep pain sensibility. *The Lancet* 1949; **1**:943–949.
3. Kellgren JH. Pain. In: *Textbook of Rheumatic Diseases* (Copeman W, ed.). 3rd edition. Edinburgh and London: Churchill Livingstone, 1964.
4. Travell J, Bigelow NH. Referred somatic pain does not follow a single segmental pattern. *Federation Proceedings* 1946: **5**:106.
5. Inman VT, Saunders JbdeCM. Referred pain from skeletal structures. *Journal of Nervous and Mental Diseases* 1944; **99**:660–667.
6. Hockaday JM, Whittey CWM. Patterns of referred pain in the normal subject. *Brain* 1967; **90**:485–496.

Paper 1

Two contributions to understanding of the 'fibrositis' syndrome

Authors

Smythe HA, Moldofsky H

Reference

Bulletin of Rheumatic Diseases 1977; **28**:928–931.

Summary

There is a definable entity to which the traditional description of the 'fibrositis syndrome' may be applied. The purpose of this paper is to describe our observations and opinions in order to stimulate others to challenge and possibly modify them.

The patients in our studies showed the invariable association of symptoms of chronic aching, a non-restorative sleep pattern with marked morning stiffness and fatigue, the EEG finding of alpha intrusion in non-REM sleep, and localized tenderness at 12 or more of 14 specific sites. These associations constitute a set of criteria for diagnosis of 'fibrositis' more rigorously defined than those we have previously proposed and used. These criteria were not fulfilled in many subjects with other diffuse soft tissue pain syndromes, such as post-exercise myalgia, and myalgia accompanying viral infections. The 'fibrositis syndrome' is not merely synonymous with chronic widespread soft tissue pain.

Related references

(1) Moldofsky H, Chester WJ. Pain and mood patterns in patients with rheumatoid arthritis. *Psychosomatic Medicine* 1970; **32**:309–318.

(2) Moldofsky H, Scarisbrick P, England R, Smythe H. Musculoskeletal symptoms and non-REM sleep disturbance in patients with 'fibrositis syndrome' and healthy subjects. *Psychosomatic Medicine* 1975; **37**:341–351.

(3) Moldofsky H, Scarisbrick P. Induction of neurasthenic musculoskeletal pain syndrome by selective sleep stage deprivation. *Psychosomatic Medicine* 1976; **36**: 35–44.

(4) Lentz MJ, Landis CA, Rothermill J, Shaver J. Effects of slow wave sleep disruption on musculoskeletal pain and fatigue in middle aged women. *Journal of Rheumatology* 1999; **26**:1586–1592.

Key message

Fibrositis is a distinctive condition characterized by tender spots and disturbed sleep as well as pain and fatigue.

Why it's important

This paper, which was a brief summary of experimental studies published in the related references, brought fibrositis to the attention of modern rheumatologists. There were two critical observations. First the sleep disturbance. The finding of alpha intrusion in non-REM sleep was unexpected and was the first association of a measurable abnormality strongly associated with the pain syndrome. The second was the tender spots. Where did the list come from? Briefly preference was given to points that were generally unknown to patients but commonly found (Figure 22.1). Many of these sites had been attributed to bursitis, tendonitis, costochondritis or other local conditions not confirmed by local pathology. The sharply defined and remarkably predicatable location permitted definitions repeatable by other observers.

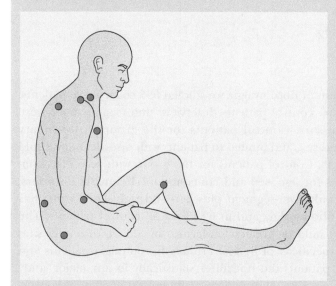

Figure 22.1 A diagram of some of the tender spots found in patients with fibromyalgia and first described in this paper (From Dieppe P, Bacon P, Bamji A, Watt I (eds.), *Slide Atlas of Rheumatology*, London: Gower, 1987.)

Strengths

1. A superb summary of a lot of excellent experimental work.
2. The comparison of 'fibrositis' patients with others with generalized pain.
3. Findings that have stood the test of time.

Weaknesses

1. The studies were small in number.
2. The methods were not all fully validated at this time.
3. The inferences were controversial.

Relevance

The paper that ushered in the modern concept of fibromyalgia.

Paper 2

The American College of Rheumatology 1990 criteria for the classification of fibromyalgia; report of the multicentre trial committee

Authors

Wolfe F, Smythe HA, Yunus MB

Reference

Arthritis and Rheumatism 1990; **33**:160–72

Summary

To develop criteria for the classification of fibromyalgia we studied 558 consecutive patients: 293 patients with fibromyalgia and 265 control patients. Interviews and examinations were performed by trained, blinded assessors. Control patients for the group with primary fibromyalgia were matched for age and sex, and limited to patients with disorders that could be confused with primary fibromyalgia. Control patients for the group with secondary-concomitant fibromyalgia were matched for age, sex and concomitant rheumatic disorders. Widespread pain (axial plus upper and lower-segment plus left- and right-sided pain) was found in 91.6% of all patients with fibromyalgia and in 69.1% of all control patients. The combination of widespread pain and mild or greater tenderness in >11 of 18 tender sites yielded a sensitivity of 88.4% and a specificity of 81.1%. Primary fibromyalgia patients and secondary-concomitant fibromyalgia patients did not differ statistically in any major study variable, and the criteria performed equally well in patients with and those without concurrent rheumatic conditions. The newly proposed criteria for the classification of fibromyalgia are: (1) widespread pain in combination with (2) tenderness at 11 or more of 18 specific tender point sites. No exclusions are made for the presence of concomitant radiographic or laboratory abnormalities. At the diagnostic or classification level the distinction between primary fibromyalgia and secondary-concomitant fibromyalgia (as defined in the text) is abandoned.

Related references

(1) Campbell SM, Clark S, Tindall EA, Forehand ME, Bennett RM. Clinical characteristics of fibrositis. A 'blinded' controlled study of symptoms and tender points. *Arthritis and Rheumatism* 1983; **26**:817–824.

(2) Wolfe F, Allen M, Bennett RM. The fibromyalgia syndrome: a consensus report on fibromyalgia and disability. *Journal of Rheumatology* 1996; **23**:534–539.

Key message

Criteria for the classification of fibromyalgia have been produced from empirical research on carefully selected patient groups.

Why it's important

There was much of clinical value in this study. A history of headache, numbness, irritable bowel or bladder, and dysmenorrhoea was more common in the fibromyalgia group. The best sites were trapezius, lateral elbow, 2nd rib, low cervical, and inner knee. Some earlier criteria had showed high specificity but low sensitivity (1, 2), and were of value in studies requiring a high degree of diagnostic certainty. However, the value of these criteria were in the identification of groups of patients for entry into research studies, uncontaminated with pre-judgments about cause. For these purposes they have served very well, permitting thousands of studies involving many disciplines in many countries.

Strengths

1. Large, well conducted clinical study.
2. Good description of many of the clinical features of fibromyalgia.
3. Excellent classification criteria for research studies.

Weaknesses

1. Relatively poor specificity mean that they are not useful for individual patient diagnosis.
2. Ceiling and floor effects mean that they are of limited value in determining relative severity and associated disability.

Relevance

Prior to this work there had been great debate as to the nature and diagnostic features of fibromyalgia. These criteria are now the accepted ones for classifying the condition.

Paper 3

Elevated levels of substance P and high incidence of Raynaud phenomenon in patients with fibromyalgia: new features for the diagnosis

Authors

Vaeroy H, Helle R, Forre O, Kass E, Terenius L

Reference

Pain 1988; **32**:21–26

Summary

In 30 patients with diagnosed fibromyalgia, the cerebrospinal fluid (CSF) level of immunore-active substance P (SP) was investigated. Compared to normal values (9.6 +/- 3.2 fmol/ml), all patients had elevated levels of SP (36.1 +/- 2.7 fmol/ml, range 16.5–79.1). SP levels were significantly higher in patients who were smokers. We propose elevated CSF levels of SP and Raynaud phenomenon as characteristic features of fibromyalgia with potential as diagnostic markers of the disease, and further that smoking might be an aggravating factor for its pathogenesis and development.

Related references

(1) Russell IJ, Orr MD, Littman B, Vipraio GA, Alboukrek D, Michalek MJ, Lopez Y, MacKillip F. Elevated cerebrospinal fluid levels of substance P in patients with the fibromyalgia syndrome. *Arthritis and Rheumatism* 1994; **37**:1593–1601.

(2) Smythe HA, Gladman A, Mader R, Peloso P, Abu-Shakra M. Strategies for assessing pain and pain exaggeration: controlled studies. *Journal of Rheumatology* 1997; **24**:1622–1629.

(3) Bradley L, Alarcon GS, Sotolongo A, Weigent DA, Alberts KR, Blalock JE, Kersh BC, Domino ML, De Waal D. Cerebrospinal fluid levels of substance P are abnormal in patients with fibromyalgia regardless of traumatic or insidious pain onset. *Arthritis and Rheumatism* 1998; **41**(suppl.9): S256 (abstract).

(4) Welin M, Bragee B, Nyber F, Kritansson M. Elevated substance P levels are contrasted by a decrease in meta-encephalin-arg-phe levels in CSF from fibroymalgia patients. *Journal of Musculoskeletal Pain* 1995; **3**(suppl.1): 4 (abstract).

Key message

Cerebrospinal levels of SP are elevated in patients with fibromyalgia.

Why it's important

This was the first study describing increased levels of a pain neurotransmitter. Subsequent studies (1–4) have confirmed the increase in CSF SP. It is an attractive idea that SP release is due to pain of peripheral origin, but other possibilities exist – either the SP or the release stimulus could come from higher levels. It still remains to be confirmed that the (pain) stimulus for the release of SP originates peripheral to the central nervous system.

Strength

The first description of a subsequently confirmed and interesting observation.

Weaknesses

1. The use of control values from the literature, not their laboratory.
2. Unjustified speculation about cold hands.
3. Technical concerns.

Relevance

The first description of a chemical (neurotransmitter) abnormality in patients with fibromyalgia, suggesting possible new approaches to treatment as well as diagnosis.

Paper 4

Diagnostic epidural opioid blockade in primary fibromyalgia at rest and during exercise

Authors

Bengtsson M, Bengtsson A, Jorfeldt L

Reference

Pain 1989; **39**:170–180

Summary

Nine patients with primary fibromyalgia participated. The patients were studied prior to, and immediately after four identical periods of exercise (bicycle ergometer) each performed 30 minutes after injection with saline, repeated saline, an opioid, and naloxone. All substances were given epidurally, except for naloxone, which was given intravenously. Finally, with the patients resting in bed, lignocaine was injected epidurally. Phsiological variables, general exertion, dyspnoea, lower extremity exhaustion, pain and tender points in the lower half of the body were examined.

Resting pain and tender points diminished slightly after the opioid injection. Lignocaine completely abolished resting pain and tender points. Lower extremity exhaustion was reduced by the opioid. General exertion and dyspnoea were unaffected by the opioid. In conclusion the results support the hypothesis that the pain in fibromyalgia is of peripheral nocioceptive or spinal origin. We raise the hypothesis that the fatiguability is, at least partly, due to inhibition because of pain.

Key message

Epidural injections of lignocaine abolish the pain and tender points of fibromyalgia.

Strength

Well designed experimental study.

Weaknesses

No control patients with generalized pain but without fibromyalgia.

Relevance

The fact that the pain and tender spots can be abolished by epidural lignocaine suggests that the pain may arise from spinal or more peripheral sites.

Paper 5a

Increased rates of fibromyalgia following cervical spine injury

Authors

Buskila D, Neumann L, Vaisberg G, Alkalay D, Wolfe F

Reference

Arthritis and Rheumatism 1997; **40**:446–452

Paper 5b

Function of the hypothalamic-pituitary-adrenal axis in patients with fibromyalgia and low back pain

Authors

Griep EN, Boersma JW, Eef GWM, Lentjes A, de Kloet ER

Reference

Journal of Rheumatology 1998; **25**:1374–1381

Paper 5c

The C6-7 syndrome – clinical features and treatment response

Author

Smythe HA

Reference

Journal of Rheumatology 1994; **21**:1520–1526

Summary

These three papers are grouped together to make a common point. After cervical injury, all of the extra tender points required to meet criteria for fibromyalgia were in the upper body (Buskila, *et al.* 1997). The patients studied by Griep, *et al.* were selected from patients with chronic low back pain. In those meeting criteria for fibromyalgia the extra points were predominantly in the lower body (Griep, *et al.* 1998). The patients in the C6–7 syndrome paper were all previously documented to have tenderness at the upper body sites included in the ACR criteria for fibromyalgia (91 of 151 met all criteria). They had lost the upper body tenderness with support to the lower neck throughout sleep. They remained symptomatic, with a different pattern of upper body tender points; and most responded to adjusted strategies (Smythe 1994). Together these three papers point to specific regions of the spine as the site of origin of the referred pain in fibromyalgia.

Key message

Fibromyalgia may arise from spinal problems, and effective management may depend on treatment of spinal abnormalities.

Why it's important

These papers indicate that the spine is the origin of the pain in fibromyalgia. Rheumatologists are not comfortable with neck and back problems. The literature indicates that our colleagues in other disciplines equally fail to help those with chronic neck and back problems so that referral is not yet a useful option. Failure to identify and address these problems may account for treatment failures; fitness programmes cannot succeed if the patient does not have a safe neck and low back.

Strengths, weaknesses and relevance

These papers are concerned with selected groups of patients, and the findings need to be confirmed by others. The proof of the intriguing concept that spinal problems may underlie fibromyalgia in many patients will come if other groups can show that fibromyalgia can be treated through management strategies aimed at spinal problems.

CHAPTER 23

Geographical disorders

Adewale Adebajo

Introduction

Rheumatic disorders are not the same all over the world. Rheumatology research in the 20th century has been dominated by work from the developed world, resulting in an inevitable emphasis on the diseases as seen in the countries of origin of the researchers. But much can be learnt by examining rheumatic disorders in other parts of the world, where there are some different diseases, as well as a different expression of some of the most common forms of arthritis. These differences can have either genetic or environmental causes.

The first paper in this selection describes a classical epidemiological study carried out in the developing world (the Philippines) by the WHO-ILAR-COPCORD group, a study group formed to aid understanding of the importance of musculoskeletal diseases throughout the world. This model epidemiological study emphasizes the high frequency of rheumatic complaints in the developing world.

The next 3 papers are concerned with the altered expression of common rheumatic diseases in different countries. Paper 2 is concerned with gout, which is particularly common in Polynesians; the importance of this particular contribution is that it suggests that there is a strong genetic component to this susceptibility. Paper 3 is about rheumatoid arthritis (RA) in Africa. This is a fascinating subject, which has been investigated by several groups. The chosen paper is one of the earliest contributions, indicating that RA, along with other 'autoimmune disorders' is relatively uncommon in Africa. Subsequent work has suggested that this is in part related to rural (as opposed to urban) living, and that things might now be changing, with the prevalence of RA currently increasing in some parts of the developing world, whereas it may be decreasing in the developed world. These investigations are of potential importance to our understanding of possible environmental triggers to RA. Paper 4 discusses geographical variations in another common form of arthritis, osteoarthritis (OA). This classic contribution was one of the first to point out that hip OA is relatively uncommon in Hong Kong Chinese, in spite of the fact that Heberden's nodes (sometimes used as a surrogate marker of a genetic predisposition to the disease) are common in this racial group. The authors speculate that squatting may be an important factor in protection of the hip.

The final three papers in this selection concern diseases which are specific to certain regions of the world. There are several such disorders, but we have limited our choice to three; Kashin-Beck disease (Paper 5) and Mseleni disease (Paper 6) are two 'endemic' forms of OA, first thought to be due to dietary toxins, but now thought more likely to be forms of dysplasia or avascular necrosis, and to be more likely to be genetic rather than environmental in origin. Ross River arthritis (Paper 7) is an example of a form of infectious arthritis limited in distribution by the fact that it depends on the presence of a mosquito born virus. However, this classic paper draws attention to the fact that travel and migration mean that we have to be aware of the possibility of such disorders anywhere in the world now.

There are many other forms of arthritis limited to certain regions of the world that might have been included, such as Blount's disease. But this selection includes what we believe to be classic papers, as well as giving a reasonable overview of the spectrum of rheumatic disorder seen in different countries, and the reasons for these differences.

Paper 1

Rheumatic disease in a Philippine village II: WHO-ILAR-APLAR COPCORD Study. Phases II and III

Authors

Wigley R, Manahan L, Muirden KD, Caragay R, Pinfold B, Couchman KG, Valkenburg HA

Reference

Rheumatology International 1991; **11**:157–161

Summary

A survey of rheumatic complaints in a remote village area of the Philippines was carried out. In phase one a screening questionnaire identified 269 adults (comprising 131 males and 138 females) as having rheumatic symptoms out of 950 adults (comprising 482 males and 468 females) studied. In phase two, 234 (87%) of positive respondents were re-questioned using a more detailed proforma. This detailed proforma identified 196 adults with peripheral joint pains, 67 adults with neck pain and 137 adults with back pain. One third of adults attributed their symptoms to work and 127 adults had to stop work because of their complaints. Disability including an inability to carry loads affected 1.8% of the study population. It was observed that 82% of adults with rheumatic complaints still required help for their symptoms. In Phase three of this study, 166 adults with rheumatic symptoms were medically examined. Osteoarthritis of the knee was found in 25 adults and 17 adults had Heberden's nodes. There were 16 adults with epicondylitis, 16 adults with rotator cuff pain and 35 adults were diagnosed as having levator scapulae insertion pain.

Related references (1) Darmawan J, Muirden KD, Wigley R, Valkenburg HA. Arthritis community education by leather puppet shadow play in rural Indonesia. *Rheumatology International* 1992: **12**:97–101.

(2) Wigley R. Primary prevention of rheumatic disease. *Journal of Rheumatology* 1993; **20**:605–606.

Key message

This paper is the landmark study of the WHO/ILAR Community Orientated Programme for the Control of Rheumatic Diseases (COPCORD). This paper has provided the template for further community studies around the world.

Why it's important

The WHO/ILAR (COPCORD) was born out of a recognition by the World Health Organization (WHO) that rheumatic diseases in general are insufficiently appreciated and understood. In particular the social and economic impact of rheumatic diseases, particularly in the developing world, is largely unknown due to an information deficit. In partnership with the International League against Rheumatism (ILAR), the WHO believes that crucial to tackling this issue is a need to overcome the information deficit.

COPCORD surveys have now been conducted in the Asia/Pacific region, South America and similar projects in Africa are scheduled. The main principles behind the COPCORD projects are that such surveys should be applicable to the majority of the world's population, which means rural communities in developing countries. Furthermore, they should also be community-orientated rather than hospital-based. These surveys should emphasize existing resources and have a low cost structure. They should consider disease prevention and avoid ignoring traditional non-western health care methods.

This paper reflects these core COPCORD principles and provides a reference for the design of such COPCORD surveys. The paper describes the three phases involved in the survey, consisting of an initial simple screening questionnaire followed by a more detailed proforma and finally, clinical examination of positive responders together with the use of available investigations. This study also draws attention to the concept of rheumatic disease prevention and control in the community.

Strengths

1. Provides a reference guide for community surveys of rheumatic complaints in developing countries.
2. It describes very clearly the difficulties encountered in carrying out these surveys in developing countries.

Weaknesses

1. A small section makes reference to children which is confusing as the methodology was aimed at adults.
2. No economic data is included.
3. The authors were unable to provide a reliable estimate of population prevalence.

Relevance

This landmark COPCORD study has enabled clinicians in various parts of the world to conduct community surveys to determine the frequency and pattern of rheumatic complaints in their region, and to make comparisons across regions. This study also raised the concept of rheumatic disease prevention and control in the community. Information derived from these studies are crucial for health service planning and the allocation of health resources, particularly in the developing world (1, 2).

Paper 2

Hyperuricaemia, gout and diabetic abnormality in Polynesian people

Authors

Prior IA, Rose BS, Harvey HP, Davidson F

Reference

The Lancet 1966; **1**:333–338

Summary

The prevalence of hyperuricaemia and gout in three groups of Polynesians living in different environmental conditions in the Pacific were studied. The three groups consisted of New Zealand Maoris and two groups of Maoris living in the Cook Islands. One group of Cook Island Maoris lived in Raratonga, an urban population, and the other group lived in Pukapuka, a rural population. Overall, 755 New Zealand Maoris, 471 Raratongans and 379 inhabitants of Pukapuka were studied. More than 40% of both males and females in all three groups were hyperuricaemic. The attack rate for gout amongst the males was 10.2% among the New Zealand Maoris, 2.5% among Raratongans and 5.3% among the Pukapukans. Ten of the 38 gouty males also had diabetes which developed after the onset of gout in all but one patient. Obesity and hypertension were common among the New Zealand Maoris with gout, but not among the Cook Islanders. These findings suggest the influence of important genetic factors among Polynesians contributing to hyperuricaemia, gout, and diabetes.

Related reference   (I)

Zimmet PZ, Whitehouse S, Jackson L, Thomar K. High prevalence of hyperuricaemia and gout in an urbanised Micronesian population. *British Medical Journal* 1978; **1**:1237–1239.

Key message

The high prevalence of gout in Polynesians is probably genetic in origin.

Why it's important

This is the first study of Maoris with the same ethnicity living in three different environmental conditions. Despite their different environmental exposure all three populations had a high prevalence of hyperuricaemia suggesting that genetic factors were largely responsible. This study provided the first firm epidemiological evidence to indicate that genetic factors may be involved in the hyperuricaemia and occurrence of gout observed among the Polynesian people. Prior to this time it was presumed that the remarkably high prevalence of hyperuricaemia and clinical gout among the Polynesians was due solely to environmental factors associated with westernization, including changes in diet such as increased calorie intake, increased fat intake and alcohol. In particular these environmental factors were believed to be responsible for the high level of hyperuricaemia and clinical cases of gout found among the New Zealand Maoris.

The second population group which the authors studied consisted of Maoris (Raratongans) who had lived under town conditions for 10 years or more and had been exposed to a western diet and other environmental features of the western life. The third population group consisted of the entire population of Pukapuka whose inhabitants were very isolated and their way of life had not changed notably over many years. Thus they were on subsistence-type living with a traditional rural diet.

Whilst the highest prevalence of clinical gout was found among the New Zealand Maoris, the observation of a significantly increased level of hyperuricaemia among the Raratongans as well as the Pukapukans, indicates a strong genetic predisposition to hyperuricaemia among Polynesians despite the different living conditions. These observations have led to further studies of hyperuricaemia and gout among this ethnic group (1) with a focus on a reduced renal clearance of uric acid.

Strengths

1. The hypothesis is clear and the message is simple.
2. Comprehensive demographic details are given about the communities studied.

Weaknesses

1. Potential pathophysiological mechanisms involving genetic factors are not adequately discussed.
2. Potential genetic factors are not discussed.

Relevance

This study of the prevalence of hyperuricaemia and gout further emphasizes the value of studying the same ethnic population exposed to different environments as a way of determining the relative importance of genetic and environmental factors in the causation and pathogenesis of diseases. This information is important in the development of public health measures for the prevention of gout.

Paper 3

Autoimmune disease in parasitic infections in Nigerians

Author

Greenwood BM

Reference

The Lancet 1968; **2**:380–382

Summary

In order to determine the prevalence of autoimmune diseases in West Africa, all patients with autoimmune conditions seen at the University College Hospital, Ibadan, Nigeria, over a 10 year period (1957–1966) were reviewed. Forty-two patients were diagnosed as having RA, two patients as having systemic lupus erythematosus (SLE) and one patient with systemic sclerosis. Other non-rheumatological conditions identified during this period were eight patients with ulcerative colitis, six patients with myasthenia gravis, four patients with pernicious anaemia and one patient with Hashimoto's thyroiditis. Overall there were only 104 patients with autoimmune diseases out of the total of 98 454 patients studied. No patient with primary Sjögren's syndrome or polyarteritis nodosa was found. The number of patients with RA observed during this period was compared with expected values based on figures obtained for England and Wales. Based on this comparison, the expected frequency of patients with RA was six times the number actually observed in the West African population.

Related references **(1)** Muller AS, Valkenburg HA, Greenwood BM. Rheumatoid arthritis in three West African populations. *East African Medical Journal* 1972; **49**:73–83.

(2) Adebajo AO, Reid DM. The pattern of rheumatoid arthritis in West Africa and comparison with a cohort of British patients. *Quarterly Journal of Medicine* 1991; **80**:633–640.

Key message

This paper was the first to provide evidence to support anecdotal reports suggesting that autoimmune diseases in general, and RA in particular, was uncommon in West Africa. This paper was also the first to raise the possibility of a protective effect by tropical infections such as malaria, on the occurrence of autoimmune diseases.

Why it's important

Prior to this study, there had been anecdotal reports suggesting that RA was rare in Africa in general, and in West Africa in particular. This study was the first to show in a systematic manner that autoimmune diseases including RA was less common in West Africa than in Europe. This study has provided the foundation for further studies looking at the prevalence of RA in sub-Saharan Africa. These studies have included recent studies in West Africa which confirm that although the prevalence of RA may be on the increase, the disease still remains relatively uncommon. This study is the first to raise the possibility of a protective effect from tropical infections such as malaria. This hypothesis has been put forward as a possible explanation for the lower prevalence of RA in West Africa.

This fascinating hypothesis has recently been revisited in the light of genetic studies showing that certain human leucocyte antigen (HLA) haplotypes such as HLA DRB1* 1302-DQB1* 0501 are associated with protection against malaria. In contrast, HLA-DR4 and HLA-DR1 (both associated with susceptibility to RA in most populations) are relatively uncommon in the region. These observations taken together with Greenwood's findings, suggest that malaria (which is endemic in West Africa), has led to the selection of those HLA haplotypes which protect against the development of malaria with a concomitant decrease in HLA haplotypes associated with the development of autoimmune diseases such as RA. The potential link between RA and tropical infections in West Africa remains the subject of ongoing studies (1, 2).

Strengths

1. Provides strong evidence to support previous anecdotal reports indicating that RA was uncommon in certain populations in sub-Saharan Africa.
2. Provides the first review of the prevalence of autoimmune diseases in Africa.

Weaknesses

1. The methodology was poor and the nature of the catchment population was not adequately described.
2. The study suffered from the methodological problems commonly associated with retrospective hospital-based studies, such as that of patient selection and ascertainment bias.

Relevance

This study provided evidence that RA was uncommon in sub-Saharan Africa when compared with Europe and North America. This study has contributed to other studies world-wide including ongoing studies looking at the complex relationship between genetic and environmental factors in the aetiology of RA. Whilst the possibility of RA being due to an infectious agent has long been a widely considered hypothesis, this study was the first to indicate that directly or indirectly, certain infections may actually protect against the development of RA. This study also provides some evidence for the belief that RA is on the increase in Africa and Asia but on the decrease in Europe and North America. It provides a reference for ongoing longitudinal studies to explore this possibility.

Paper 4

Osteoarthritis of the hip and other joints in Southern Chinese in Hong Kong

Authors

Hoaglund F T, Yau A C, Wong WL

Reference

Journal of Bone Joint Surgery 1973; **55**(A):545–557

Summary

A random study of the finger joints, hips and knees of 500 hospitalized Hong Kong Southern Chinese patients above the age of 54 years was carried out in September 1967. Radiographs of the hands, pelvis and knees were obtained in all patients. The first 211 patients (112 men and 99 women) underwent a history and physical examination. 98% of these patients indicated that they regularly used the squatting position, particularly for toileting purposes which involved maximum hip flexion and 10–30 degrees of hip abduction. Among the 211 patients examined, 30% of the men and 31% of the women had evidence of Heberden's nodes. There was an increase in the presence of Heberden's nodes with increasing age in both men and women. The prevalence of radiological evidence of moderate and severe OA involving the distal interphalangeal joints was comparable to that of previous British studies. Those Chinese patients who had OA involving their finger joints had a much higher incidence of OA involving other joints when compared to those patients whose finger joints were not involved.

Related reference (1) Kellgren JH, Lawrence JS. Osteo-arthrosis and disc degeneration in an urban population. *Annals of Rheumatic Diseases* 1958; **17**:388–397.

Key message

This was the first description of a study in a non-Caucasian population which looked at clinical and radiological features of OA in a systematic fashion using a large cohort of patients. In particular, the study draws attention to potential relationships between ethnic differences and the pattern of joint involvement in OA.

Why it's important

This paper was the first to document in a detailed manner clinical and radiological aspects of OA in a non-Caucasian population. This paper has increased awareness of the potential benefits which could be derived from studying the pattern of OA in different racial groups. The study arose from the observation that hip surgery in the Hong Kong Chinese is rarely performed for conditions other than joint destruction due to sepsis or tuberculosis.

The authors found that the prevalence of Heberden's nodes among their study population was similar to that which had previously been reported for British populations. This contrasted with their finding that OA of the hip was significantly less common in their study population, than had been reported among Caucasian populations. Thus, this paper confirmed using a significant population size and detailed radiological examinations, that OA of the hip was indeed uncommon in the Chinese population.

In this paper, the authors raise interesting hypotheses as to why OA of the hip might be less common in the Chinese. They suggest that squatting, particularly for toilet needs and the extreme range of motion required, might protect the hip joint against the development of OA among the Chinese. In addition they also point out that predisposing factors such as congenital dysplasia of the hip and slipped capital femoral epiphysis appear to be less common among the Chinese and that this might be an additional explanation of the low prevalence of OA of the hip in this population.

These hypotheses have served to stimulate other studies looking at racial differences in OA (1). The majority of these studies have used a combination of clinical assessment as well as the detailed radiological assessments described in this paper.

Strengths

1. An example of astute clinical observations leading to a prospective study.
2. It provides detailed information for the first time on OA in a non-Caucasian population.

Weaknesses

1. This population was hospital-based and consequently subject to possible ascertainment bias. However, the authors felt there was minimal ascertainment bias due to poor health provision or the high cost of hip surgery, as these were not significant problems in their population.
2. It would have been of greater interest if this study had been extended to all adults rather than only adults above the age of 54 years.

Relevance

This paper draws attention to the usefulness of studying racial differences in the pattern of joint involvement in OA. It points out that genetic factors, environmental factors and in particular socio-cultural factors, may all influence the prevalence and pattern of joint involvement in OA. These observations should help to shed further light on our understanding of the aetiopathogenesis of OA

Paper 5

The clinical course of Kashin–Beck disease

Author

Nesterov AI

Reference

Arthritis and Rheumatism 1964; **7**:29–40

Summary

This paper reviews the clinical features and clinical course of Kashin–Beck disease. It describes three grades of Kashin–Beck disease and includes case histories to illustrate each of these subtypes. Overall, the disease is described as a chronic disabling condition characterized by generalized OA involving peripheral joints and the spine, but without systemic manifestations. Kashin–Beck disease occurs principally in childhood and results in growth disturbances. It is endemic in Eastern Siberia, Northern China and Northern Korea. The paper discusses the aetiopathogenesis of this condition and in particular the possibility that it is due to ingestion of cereal grain, grown in the affected regions of the world where the grain has become infected with the fungus *Fusaria sporotrichiella*.

Related reference   (1)   Sokolov L. Endemic forms of osteoarthritis. *Clinics in Rheumatic Diseases* 1985; **11**:187–202.

Key message

This is the first review of Kashin–Beck disease. The review documents the history, clinical features and aetiopathogenesis of the disease.

Why it's important

This first review of Kashin–Beck disease comprehensively covers all aspects of the condition including its clinical and radiological manifestations. The paper documents the history of Kashin–Beck disease from its earliest description in 1861, when features of the disease were first noticed to be prevalent amongst the Cossacks who lived in the eastern area of Russia. The review refers to multiple sources of data collection including the Soviet Health Service and both the Institutes of the Academy of Medical Sciences and the Irkutsk Institute of Orthopaedics. The review also draws heavily from personal observations.

Kashin–Beck disease is described from its insidious and often asymptomatic onset in childhood to its subsequent slow progression. The paper subdivides Kashin–Beck's disease into three subtypes; the mild form of the disease (referred to as the first degree), the moderate form of the disease (referred to as the second degree), and the severe form of the disease (referred to as the third degree). Illustrative case histories for each of these subtypes is given. The mild form of the disease manifests as thickening and slight deformities of the interphalangeal or wrist joints, demonstrable both clinically and radiologically. Crepitus is frequently present in the knees. The moderate form of Kashin–Beck disease is characterized by the complete clinical and radiological picture of a deforming OA. In this phase of the disease, the extremities become shorter as the joints become deformed. The patient experiences significant joint pains and there is accompanying progressive disability. In its most advanced form, Kashin–Beck disease is characterized by a combination of chronic deforming OA together with more general clinical features such as muscular pain and weakness. Spinal involvement may also occur, thereby further limiting mobility.

The paper discusses radiological and histological features of the disease, with radiographs showing irregularity in often premature but focal ossification of the epiphyseal growth plate. The authors draw the inference that the basic problem could reside in the growth plate of articular cartilage due to nonspecific damage. The authors, however, also point out that histological data suggests that articular cartilage shares with the growth plate a focal apparently episodic necrosis of chondrocytes.

The paper discusses Kashin–Beck disease as having a possible environmental causation. Evidence is put forward to support the hypothesis that Kashin–Beck disease is due to toxins resulting from cereal grain grown in the affected areas of the world where the grain has become contaminated with the parasitic fungus, *Fusaria sporotrichiella*. The contamination of cereal grain with this fungus is believed to be due to the climatic conditions in these regions of the world. The author points out that public health measures had already begun to lead to a decrease in incidence of Kashin–Beck disease, and that elimination of new cases of the disease should eventually be possible.

Strengths

1. A comprehensive review describing all aspects of the condition.
2. Appropriate illustrative case reports are given.
3. The postulated cause of the disease is well described.

Weaknesses

1. No specific epidemiological data is given.
2. No data is given to substantiate the paper's claim that the incidence of Kashin–Beck disease is falling.

Relevance

This excellent overview of Kashin–Beck disease brought this disease to the attention of the rheumatology community outside the Soviet Union. Kashin–Beck disease was the first form of endemic OA to be described, and its description has formed the basis for the search for further forms of endemic OA world-wide (1).

Paper 6

Unusual hip disease in remote part of Zululand

Authors

Whittman W, Fellingham SA

Reference

The Lancet 1970; **1**:842–843

Summary

An unusual form of hip disease was identified near the Mseleni Mission Station of Bombo district, Zululand, South Africa. A random sample of households was carried out as part of a community survey. Out of a total population of 236 men studied, 25% of men were affected. Of 636 women studied, 66% of women were affected. Of 551 boys studied, 4% of boys were affected and of 569 girls studied, 7% of girls were affected. The associated disability was measured by the need for a walking stick. Seven percent of men, 35% of women, 0.2% of boys and 0.7% of girls required the use of a walking stick. Thirty-seven x-rays of the pelvis were reviewed. The majority of these (24 radiographs) showed evidence of advanced OA.

Related reference   (1)   Yach D, Botha JL. Mseleni joint disease in 1981; decreased prevalence rates, wider geographical location than before, and socioeconomic impact of an endemic osteoarthrosis in an underdeveloped community in South Africa. *International Journal of Epidemiology* 1985; **14**:276–284.

Key message

This is the first description of Mseleni's disease. This study adds Mseleni's disease to the small group of joint disorders referred to as endemic OA.

Why it's important

This is the first report of Mseleni's disease and is the first form of endemic OA described from the African continent. Prior to this, a similar condition known as Kashin–Beck disease had been described. Kashin–Beck disease is commonly observed in South Eastern Siberia, Manchuria, Northern China, the Shaanxi province of China and North Korea. The disease is characterized by OA affecting both the peripheral joints and the spine. Mseleni's disease resembles dysplasia epiphysealis multiplix, and is found among the Mseleni area of Northern Zululand in South Eastern Africa, near the border with Mozambique (1). It is a painful disorder most commonly affecting the hip joint although other joints, in particular the knees and ankles, may be involved. This report emphasizes the progressive nature of the condition with associated increasing disability leading to the need for walking aids and even an inability to walk at all.

This paper draws attention to the radiological features of this condition. The authors emphasize the radiological features of large osteophytes, protusio acetabuli, the deformity of the femoral head with medial subluxation and the rarity of subarticular cysts. The authors speculate on a nutritional deficiency or toxins similar to that postulated for Kashin–Beck disease, with potential candidates being veld foods, wild vegetables and palm beer.

Strengths

1. Clear and easy to read.
2. The excitement of identifying a new form of endemic OA is conveyed.

Weaknesses

1. The methodology was poor with no description of the overall catchment population.
2. No indication as to whether or not some individuals may have had OA due to other causes.
3. The demographic, clinical and serological features of those individuals with Mseleni's disease was not adequately described.

Relevance

This first report of Mseleni's disease added yet another form of endemic OA to the existing literature. There is the possibility that the study of these conditions will serve to provide further insight into the aetiopathegenesis of OA.

Paper 7

Ross River virus arthritis in Papua New Guinea

Authors

Scrimgeour EM, Aaskov JG, Matz LR

Reference

Transcripts of the Royal Society of Tropical Medicine and Hygiene 1987; **81**:833–834

Summary

Over a 1 year period between 1980 and 1981 a survey was carried out of all patients present-ing with acute polyarthritis at Port Moresby General Hospital located in the capital of Papua New Guinea. Twenty-four Melanesian patients were identified and assessed for possible Ross River virus infection. All of these patients had an acute onset of symmetrical polyarthritis involving both large and small joints. In three patients, a diagnosis of Ross River virus infec-tion was confirmed by appropriate serological tests. In three other cases serological tests were suggestive of Ross River virus infection, but were not diagnostic. Synovial biopsies from the knees of two patients with Ross River virus arthritis and one patient with suspected Ross River virus infection were obtained. The biopsies showed mild chronic synovitis with synovial cell hyperplasia.

Related reference   **(1)**   Nimmo JR. An unusual epidemic. *Medical Journal of Australia* 1928; 1:549–550.

Key message

This study confirms an association between acute polyarthritis and Ross River virus infection. This study also confirmed the presence of Ross River virus among the population group of Papua New Guinea.

Why it's important

This paper draws attention to the prevalence of arthritis caused by mosquito-born viruses in the tropics and sub tropics. The paper also confirmed the association between polyarthritis and Ross River virus infection (1). Synovial biopsy specimens further indicated that Ross River virus infection can cause an inflammatory polyarthritis.The paper highlights the prob-lem of the requirement of a serological service for the precise diagnosis of Ross River virus arthritis. Unfortunately such a service is not available in many parts of the tropics, leading to misdiagnosis and under diagnosis of the condition.

    This paper was the first to identify patients with polyarthritis and Ross River virus infection in Papua New Guinea. The paper describes the characteristic clinical features of Ross River virus comprising sudden onset of fever and a symmetrical polyarthritis. The paper also points out that treatment is essentially symptomatic. This paper draws attention to the potential for the spread of the alpha virus across the region of the Pacific islands and the consequent pub-lic health implications of Ross River virus infection.

Strengths

1. The serological aspects of Ross River virus infection are well described.
2. Good illustrative cases of Ross River virus infection are given.

Weaknesses

1. True prevalence estimates are not given as the study was hospital-based.
2. The demographic features of the hospital catchment population is not given.
3. No relationship to rainfall or other climatic variations is given.

Relevance

This study emphasizes Ross River virus infection as a cause of acute polyarthritis. The study has provided evidence that Ross River virus arthritis occurs across the region of the Pacific islands. With increasing migration and travel, this paper draws attention to the need to be aware of Ross River virus infection as a cause of polyarthritis in anyone living in, or who has visited the tropics or sub tropics.

CHAPTER 24

Associations of other systemic diseases with arthropathies

H Ralph Schumacher, Jr

Introduction

One of the important developments of the 20th century is the recognition and emphasis on the fact that musculoskeletal manifestations can be caused by a wide variety of systemic diseases, many of which are treatable, or as some are familial diseases, preventable in family members. The editors have selected a small number of papers to highlight identification of these associations. There are of course also many other examples. The classifications on the rheumatic diseases as published in textbooks or the *Primer on the Rheumatic Diseases* can be referenced to show the many associations (1, 2). Careful clinical observers can almost certainly help us identify still unrecognized associations and their implications.

Papers featured in this section focus on clinical observation most often with histopathological studies to confirm or support new hypotheses. Do not forget there is still more to be learned by biopsies of unexplained lesions. Application of new molecular and immunohistochemical tools may even increase the value of biopsies. The recognition that clinical syndromes seemed to differ from known diseases was important in identification of amyloid arthropathy in dialysis patients and of the arthropathy in haemochromatosis. In these as well as in sarcoidosis and acromegaly musculoskeletal symptoms had often previously been attributed to rheumatoid arthritis (RA) or osteoarthritis (OA) or left unexplained.

Evaluation of large series confirmed associations. In ochronosis musculoskeletal involvement had long been noted but we elected to highlight the identification of the biochemical defect. In most of these diseases studies now are using genetic and molecular techniques to characterize further mechanisms and improve therapies but challenges remain. Sarcoidosis is treated only symptomatically with corticosteroids. Is it really an infection? Despite identification of the arthropathy of haemochromatosis, the joint disease remains the most resistant aspect often not responding to even early phlebotomy. Results are somewhat more encouraging with at least some aspects of early treatment of acromegaly. Gene or enzyme therapies will eventually be coming for haemochromatosis and alcaptonuria-ochronosis.

References

1. Klippel J, Dieppe P (eds.). *Rheumatology*. 2nd edition. London: Mosby, 1998.
2. Schumacher HR (ed.). *Primer on the Rheumatic Diseases*. 11th edition. Atlanta: Arthritis Foundation, 1999.

Paper I

Clinical and pathological studies of joint involvement in sarcoidosis

Authors

Sokoloff L, Bunim JJ

Reference

New England Journal of Medicine 1959; **260**:841–846

Summary

Five cases of sarcoidosis were presented in which polyarthritis was a conspicuous feature. Each also had other systemic features of sarcoidosis. Synovial biopsies in three patients showed typical non-caseating granulomas. Searches for other causes of granulomatous synovitis were unrevealing. Sarcoidosis was proposed to be a more frequent cause of arthritis than previously recognized and it was proposed that previous cases might have been misdiagnosed as rheumatic fever or RA. An association with erythema nodosum was noted in one case, and the frequent association with erythema nodosum was noted in some previous cases with more transient arthritis.

Related references **(1)** Burman MS, Mayer L. Arthroscopic examination of knee joint: report of cases observed in course of arthroscopic examination including instances of sarcoid and multiple polypoid fibromatosis. *Archives of Surgery* 1936; **32**:846–874. (The report by Sokoloff and Bunim was not the first to document an association of arthritis with sarcoidosis but it most clearly established the association.)

(2) Kaplan H. Sarcoid arthritis. *Archives of Internal Medicine* 1963; **112**:925–935. (This report of arthritis in nine of 23 patients with sarcoidosis in a US military hospital in Germany clearly separated the acute migratory arthritis seen with erythema nodosum as having a good prognosis in contrast to the chronic disease.)

(3) Lofgren S. Primary pulmonary sarcoidosis. II. Clinical course and prognosis. *Acta Medica Scandinavica* 1953; **145**:424–431. (One of the early reports of the transient acute sarcoidosis leading to the commonly used eponymous designation.)

Key message

Sarcoidosis can cause an arthritis that is separate from the bone disease. Only one of these cases had joint erosions despite a chronic course in some. This therefore needed to be distinguished from the other currently recognized diseases.

Why it's important

This paper was important as it reinforced previous isolated observations and established that sarcoid arthritis can occur. This was one of a series of papers occurring around this time emphasizing that many systemic diseases can have specific joint manifestations. Previously there had frequently been a tendency to make two diagnoses such as still calling the arthritis rheumatoid without detailed examination. This has been critical in making what we now call RA a considerably cleaner concept.

Strength

Meticulous histological studies that suggested that mechanisms of arthritis might not be identical in all cases. Some had only non-specific inflammation; similar cases continue to be reported.

Weaknesses

1. This and other early observations were not yet able to separate out the Lofgren's syndrome.
2. The African American patients in this series had very limited follow-ups at the time of the report.
3. Details of their later courses were not reported.
4. Little was discussed about treatments but few alternatives were available at that time.

Relevance

We now recognize some 100 causes of arthritis and this is one that frequently enters diagnostic considerations.

Paper 2

Acromegalic arthropathy

Authors

Bluestone R, Bywaters EGL, Hartog M, Holt PJL, Hyde S

Reference

Annals of Rheumatic Diseases 1971; **30**:243–258.

Summary

A series of 42 consecutive hospitalized patients with acromegaly were studied for the presence of musculoskeletal problems. Peripheral joint abnormalities were found in 26. Carpal tunnel syndrome was seen in 22 and was bilateral in 20. Twenty patients had back pain. Soft tissue swelling was more common than joint effusion. There was no evidence of inflammatory arthritis. Joint spaces were often initially wide on radiographs due to hypertrophied cartilage. Histologically there was active cartilage cell proliferation in the basal and middle layers of cartilage presumably due to excess growth hormone. Four patients had severe arthrosis of hips and/or knees. All had severe long-lasting acromegaly. Osteophytosis of the anterior parts of the thoracic and lumbar vertebrae was often prominent.

Related references **(1)** Waine H, Bennet GA, Bauer W. Joint disease associated with acromegaly. *American Journal of the Medical Sciences* 1945; **209**:671.

(2) Kellgren JH, Ball J, Tutton GK. The articular and other limb changes in acromegaly. *Quarterly Journal of Medicine* 1952; **21**:405.

(3) Trainer PJ, Drake WM, Katznelson L, Freda PU, *et al.* Treatment of acromegaly with the growth hormone-receptor antagonist pegvisomant. *New England Journal of Medicine* 2000; **342**:1171–1177.

Key message

Musculoskeletal problems occur at all stages of acromegaly. Effective treatment reversed the carpal tunnel syndrome only. Despite the frequent back pain, mobility was often well maintained or even greater than normal probably due to thickened discs and lax hypertrophied ligaments.

Why it's important

This and earlier smaller series noted above identified a potentially treatable cause of arthritis. As better treatments now become available early diagnosis may not only resolve the soft tissue problems but also prevent the later secondary OA. These observations also gave important insights into effects of growth hormone on cartilage and bone. Acromegalic ulcers on cartilage described earlier by Kellgren, *et al.* (2) were confirmed in more extensive pathological studies. The dramatic bridging osteophytes illustrated are very similar to lesions later described as DISH (diffuse idiopathic skeletal hyperostosis) that are probably also related to growth hormone-like molecules. Ten patients had symptoms suggestive of mild Raynaud's phenomenon and two had severe morning stiffness causing potential confusion with other rheumatic diseases. Fatigue is now also noted as a prominent symptom of acromegaly further risking confusion.

Strength

X-rays were obtained on most and allowed correlation with extensive and detailed pathological studies on three cases (two necropsies and one surgery).

Weaknesses

1. Disc and capsular calcifications were noted but not studied further. We still are not sure about the relationship of chondrocalcinosis to acromegaly.
2. Soft tissues were described in less detail than bone and cartilage.

Relevance

This valuable resource on early as well as chronic musculoskeletal problems in acromegaly has led to increased attention to joint symptoms and signs as clues to this diagnosis.

Paper 3

The nature of the defect in tyrosine metabolism in alkaptonuria

Authors

LeDu BN, Zannoni VG, Laster L, Seegmiller JE

Reference

Journal of Biological Chemistry 1958; **230**:251–256

Summary

This disease had been identified as a mendelian recessive trait by Garrod in 1902 who coined the term 'inborn error of metabolism' suggesting that an enzyme defect would explain this disease. This report described the definitive biochemical evidence and showed absence of homogentisic acid oxidase in a liver from a patient with alkaptonuria and ochronosis. Liver biopsy was performed during abdominal surgery for an oesophageal hiatus hernia. There was no detectable homogentisic acid oxidase in the liver homogenate but all other enzymes in the tyrosine oxidation pathway were the same as in normal human liver and liver from other mammals.

Related references **(1)** Fernandez-Canon JM, Granadino B, Beltran-Valero de Bernabe D, Renedo M, Fernandez-Ruiz F, Penalva MA, Rodriguez de Cordoba S. The molecular basis of alkaptonuria. *Nature Genetics* 1996; **14**:19–24. (This is one of a series of papers from this group and others describing the cloning of the human homogentisic acid oxidase gene and showed that it is the gene responsible for alkaptonuria. The gene is located on chromosome 3q2. Missense mutations co-segregate with the disease.)

(2) O'Brien WM, Banfield WG, Sokoloff L. Studies on the pathogenesis of ochronotic arthropathy. *Arthritis and Rheumatism* 1961; **4**:137–152. (Affinity of the cartilage for homogentisic acid or its precursors is described.)

(3) Hunter T, Gordon DA, Ogryzlo MA. The ground pepper sign of synovial fluid: A new diagnostic feature of ochronosis. *Journal of Rheumatology* 1974; **1**:45–53. (A clever practical observation that may allow easy detection of this rare syndrome.)

Key points

Normal levels were demonstrated for all enzymes of the tyrosine oxidation system except for homogentisic acid oxidase. There was no evidence that absence of enzyme was due to an inhibitor.

Why it's important

This study set the stage for a series of studies on this autosomal recessive disorder showing that homogentisic acid polymers deposited in cartilage and other tissues causing the disease of ochronosis. This also set the stage for the continued genetic studies and established the still unrealized potential for therapy of this devastating and still poorly managed disease.

Strength

Meticulous biochemical studies identified the single enzyme defect that had been suspected.

Weaknesses

1. Tissues other than the liver were not studied.
2. The exact nature of the defect (i.e. failure to make protein, or altered protein) was not determined.

Relevance

This was an important step in developing the mechanisms of an uncommon genetic disease that will eventually be treatable and preventable with enzyme or gene therapy.

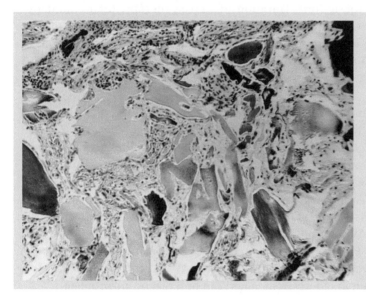

Figure 24.1 Shards of pigmented ochronotic cartilage embedded in synovium.

Paper 4

Corticosteroid therapy associated with ischemic necrosis of bone in systemic lupus erythematosus

Authors

Zizic TM, Marcoux C, Hungerford DS, Dansereau J-V, Stevens MB

Reference

American Journal of Medicine 1985; **79**:596–604

Summary

In this prospective study 52% of 54 patients with systemic lupus erythematosus (SLE) had ischaemic necrosis of bone. Ninety-three sites were involved with hips, knees and shoulders affected most frequently. The dramatic differences between patients with and without ischaemic necrosis were the mean daily doses of prednisone for the month with the highest steroid dose and the highest consecutive 3, 6 and 12 months of therapy with the higher doses favouring the development of the lesions. Duration of steroid therapy, total cumulative steroid dose and mean daily doses in general were not significantly different between the two groups. Patients with ischaemic necrosis were more likely to be cushingoid. A lower mean prednisone dose was required to produce ischaemic necrosis in patients with Raynaud's phenomenon.

Related references

(1) Harrington KD, Murray WR, Koontz SL, Belzer FO. Avascular necrosis after renal transplantation. *Journal of Bone Joint Surgery* 1971; **53**(A):203–X. (One of the early clues to the role of steroids.)

(2) Adarraga DA, Sanchez-Martinez F, Caracuel MA, Escudero A, Collantes E. A case of multiple osteonecrosis in a patient with HIV. *Journal of Clinical Rheumatology* 2000; **6**:41–44. (New causes of AVN continue to be identified.)

(3) Lotke P. Ecker MI. Osteonecrosis of the knee. *Orthopedic Clinics of North America* 1985; **16**:797–808. (AVN at the knee occurs most often in elderly women and can be a diagnostic problem.)

(4) Zizic TM, Hungerford DS, Stevens MB. Ischemic necrosis in systemic lupus erythematosus. I. The early diagnosis of ischemic necrosis of bone. *Medicine* 1980; **59**:134–148. (Increased bone marrow pressure is proposed as a common mechanism for AVN and has led to one approach to early treatment with core decompression.)

Key message

Higher peak steroid doses seem to increase the risk of AVN. This and the other related references have helped make rheumatologists much more aware of AVN as a cause of joint symptoms.

Why it's important

Beginning to understand the relationship to corticosteroid dose in SLE had a variety of impacts. Rheumatologists became better aware of ischaemic necrosis. This is also called AVN, osteonecrosis (ON) or aseptic necrosis (AN). Rheumatologists and orthopaedists began investigating its likely mechanisms in various states in work that continues to this time. Evidence continues to suggest that minimizing peak steroid doses may decrease AVN. The practice of high dosing continues as studies have not evaluated systematically the relative effects of various doses on many manifestations of SLE.

Strength

A prospective study carefully analyzing the role of steroid regimens.

Weakness

1. Limitation of study to SLE making it difficult to isolate the pure role of steroids from an additive effect of steroids and SLE.
2. Very narrow focus on steroids.

Relevance

Ischaemic necrosis remains a frequent complication of therapy of SLE. This and other complications of corticosteroids now account for increasing morbidity in patients with SLE. A diagnosis of ischaemic necrosis should always lead to a search for known underlying diseases and consideration of mechanisms in each situation.

Paper 5

Hemochromatosis and arthritis

Author

Schumacher, HR

Reference

Arthritis and Rheumatism 1964; **7**:41–50

Abstract

Two patients with haemochromatosis and what appears to be a distinctive arthritis are presented. Both showed prominent involvement of the hands, minimal evidence of inflammation, significant x-ray changes and synovial haemosiderin deposition. Five others cases of a similar arthritis were found in a review of 23 cases of idiopathic haemochromatosis. The arthritis is postulated to be the result of iron excess damaging articular tissue in a yet undefined manner.

Summary

Two patients were described in detail and five others reviewed with osteoarthritis-like findings but an unusual distribution that included the PIP and metacarpal phalangeal joints. All were negative for rheumatoid factor. Synovial biopsies did not show inflammation but showed dramatic deposition of haemosiderin primarily localized to the synovial lining cells. Such iron deposition had been previously described but had not been related to any joint symptoms. Two patients without arthritis also had synovial tissue examined and also had iron deposition so that such deposition did not invariably cause arthritis. Possible mechanisms were discussed.

X-rays showed generalized demineralization, irregular articular surfaces, subcortical cysts, periarticular bony proliferation and joint space narrowing. Calcification was described at the lateral meniscus of one knee, which was not commented upon, but turned out to be a finding subsequently seen in many patients.

Related references (1) Schumacher HR. Articular cartilage in the degenerative arthropathy of hemochromatosis. *Arthritis and Rheumatism* 1982; **25**:1460–1468.

(2) Hamilton E, Williams R, Barlow KA, Smith PM. The arthropathy of idiopathic hemochromatosis. *Quarterly Journal of Medicine* 1968; **37**:171–182.

(3) Schumacher HR, Straka PC, Krikker MA, Dudly AT. The arthropathy of hemochromatosis: recent studies. *Annals of the New York Academy of Science* 1988; **526**:224–233.

(4) Hamilton EDD, Domford AB, Laus JW, Williams R. The natural history of arthritis in idiopathic hemachromatosis: progression of the clinical and radiological features over 10 years. *Quarterly Journal of Medicine* 1981; **50**:321–329.

(5) M'Seffar A, Fornaiser VL, Foh IH. Arthropathy as the major clinical indication of occult iron storage disease. *Journal of the American Medical Association* 1977; **238**:1825–1828.

Key message

Hemochromatosis is associated with an arthropathy that previously may have been confused with RA or OA.

Why it's important

This arthropathy has now been identified to be an initial manifestation of haemochromatosis in some cases, and thus it may lead to diagnosis and treatment of this disease before the life-threatening complications of cardiomyopathy, cirrhosis and diabetes. The exact mechanisms of the arthropathy have not been defined. The recent identification of the gene for most familial haemochromatosis sets the stage for renewed investigations into mechanisms.

Strengths

1. An important observation in two cases and expanded with review of additional cases of haemochromatosis for confirmation.
2. Documentation of the synovial deposition of iron predominantly in the lining cells in this disease set the stage for series of observations confirming this important association.

Weaknesses

1. Did not examine implications for treatment of the joints that still remains unsatisfactory.
2. Did not examine bone or cartilage leaving mechanisms unresolved.

Relevance

It identified a new cause of arthropathy. One case and others since have been previously mis-diagnosed as RA leading to inappropriate treatments. This identified an important familial and metabolic disease associated with arthritis.

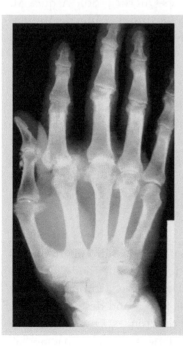
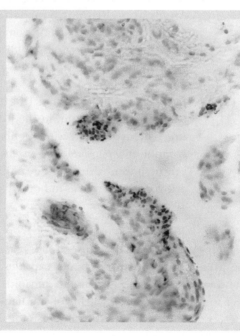

Figure 24.2 (left) X-ray showing classic findings of haemochromatosis.

Figure 24.3 (right) Iron in synovial lining cells in a patient with haemochromatosis.

Paper 6

Synovial amyloidosis in patients undergoing long-term hemodialysis

Authors

Bardin T, Kuntz D, ZingraffJ, Voisin MC, Zeimar A and Lansaman J

Reference

Arthritis and Rheumatism 1985; **28**:1052–1058

Summary

Synovial amyloid deposits were found in 18 patients with end-stage renal failure of various aetiologies who had been treated with long term haemodialysis (mean 116 months). All had carpal tunnel syndrome which was bilateral in 14; four patients also had flexor tenosynovitis and two had destructive arthropathies that required surgical replacement of the hip. Amyloid deposits were confirmed by light microscopy and in 6 by electron microscopy. Nine patients had cystic radiolucencies of bone interpreted as likely due to amyloid.

Related references   **(1)**   Allieu Y, Asencio G, Mailhe D, Baldet P, Mion C. Syndrome du canal carpien chez l'hemodialyse chronique: approche etiopathogenique: apropros de 31 cas operas. *Rev Chir Orthop* 1983; **69**:233–238. (An earlier identification of amyloid in carpal tunnels of dialysis patients.)

               (2)   Munoz-Gomez J, Bergada-Barado E, Gomez-Perez R, Llopart-Buisan E, Subias-Sobrevia E, Rotes-Querol J, Sole-Arques M. Amyloid arthropathy in patients undergoing periodical haemodialysis for chronic renal failure: a new complication. *Annals of Rheumatic Diseases* 1985; **44**:729–733, 1985. (Seven dialysis patients had amyloid arthropathy but no amyloid in subcutaneous fat deposits.)

               (3)   Netter P, Kessler M, Bumel D, Hutin MF, Delones S, Benoit J, Gaucher A. Aluminum in the joint tissues of chronic renal failure patients treated with regular hemodialysis and aluminum compounds. *Journal of Rheumatology* 1984; **11**:66–70. (Aluminum might be another of the many factors involved in dialysis arthropathy as well as in bone disease.)

Key message

Amyloid was convincingly established as the cause of most carpal tunnel syndromes in dialysis patients and was also present in joint synovium and capsules. Juxta articular bone lucencies seemed prominent and were proposed to be due to amyloid. Destructive arthropathies were seen in large joints of four cases, erosive arthritis of the hands in two and destructive spine lesions in seven. These were not explained by any histologic differences. One patient also had the previously recognized apatite deposits. All patients had long durations of haemodialysis with a mean of 116 months and the shortest duration of 74 months.

Why it's important

This and other related studies led to attempts to decrease this complication by examining different dialysis membranes and different regimens. Shorter periods of dialysis before transplantation can decrease the risk of amyloidosis. Recognition of amyloid as the cause of the carpal tunnel syndrome can influence treatment. Local corticosteroids had, at best, transient benefit in these patients. Histopathologic examination of unexplained lesions continues to be important. Later studies confirmed that this amyloid is due to beta 2 microglobulin.

Strengths

1. Large well studied series with confirmation of the role of amyloid in a variety of problems of chronic haemodialysis patients.
2. Extensive x-rays and pathologic studies.

Weaknesses

1. Bone biopsies were not obtained in this report to confirm the presence of amyloid although this has subsequently been confirmed as a factor.
2. The fascinating destructive arthropathy in some patients remained unexplained.

Relevance

Shorter use of dialysis can decrease this complication if transplantation is available. The variety of problems that must be considered in dialysis patients with musculoskeletal problems includes infections, apatite deposition in patients with elevated serum phosphate levels, hyperparathyroidism, or manifestations of the primary disease leading to renal failure.

Section 4

Therapy

CHAPTER 25

Education

Ylva Lindroth

Introduction

Patient education has probably been practised as long as there have been patients and physicians. The reason for the late appearance of patient education in the columns of scientific publications is unclear. Today every practitioner knows that patients will not accept, let alone carry out, a prescribed treatment regime unless it is explained to them. However, as recently as 1976, the importance of patient education was neither acknowledged in medical textbooks nor mentioned in texts on arthritis expressly written for patients. The proper field of medicine was seen to be human biology. We viewed our patients as organisms composed of different parts having different functions. The physician's role was to locate the part that was not fulfilling its function, and then repair that organ by employing external or internal medicine–in short, the reductive model.

In the early 1980s, the reliability of objective, reproducible, numeric 'hard' data were challenged by interest in less confident, subjective 'soft' data. The result was a whole new world of instruments attempting to measure something previously disregarded–the patient's point of view. Using these instruments, it became possible to evaluate the effect of patient education not only on a patient's knowledge and behaviour, but also on the outcome of the disease.

The first classic paper in the field of patient education did not appear until 1982 (Paper 1, Mazzuca). It is a meta-analysis of publications on patient education in cases of chronic disease; arthritis, however, was not mentioned. Although there had been education programmes for patients with rheumatoid arthritis (RA) before, they had never been evaluated and presented in scientific literature. Patients were instructed in the right and wrong way to perform activities of daily living in order to circumvent forces that promoted deformity; but the effect of these programmes was never analysed.

As the afflicted person's role in treatment began to be emphasized, it was vital to assess a patient's perception of RA, and understand how it differed from those of the physicians. This was first done first by Silvers, *et al.* in 1985 (Paper 2). The groundwork for patient education was constructed around the question: what did the patients need to know? Lorig and her collaborators introduced their Arthritis Self-Management Program (ASMP) in 1985 (Paper 3). This study was the first to present an evaluation of arthritis education in an experimental model, namely, a prospective randomized controlled study. A further development of these ideas, modified for another health care system, was presented by Taal, *et al.* in 1993 (Paper 4). Based on experience from a long tradition of patient education programmes in Lund, Sweden and the ASMP from the USA an Australian programme was developed and evaluated (Paper 5). This contained elements of problem-based education further developed. Other means of presenting education cite an approach in which information and support were delivered over the telephone (Paper 6). Looking toward the future, it is hoped that evidence-based medicine will not only include randomized controlled studies, but will also validate the phenomenology of disease. A classic paper of a qualitative method is presented (Paper 7). Donovan, *et al.* tell us in their study what having arthritis means to the patients. A new way of analysing and presenting data has opened our eyes to a broader view of the patient as an important member of a team working to better the outcome of rheumatic disease.

Paper 1

Does patient education for chronic diseases have therapeutic value?

Author

Mazzuca SA

Reference

Journal of Chronic Diseases 1982; **35**:521–529

Summary

This is a review and meta-analysis of publications on patient education from 1970 to 1981. Only such studies were included that were experimental, having a defined allocation of the independent variable (i.e. instruction) to a treatment or control group. Dependent variables were: (a) compliance with therapeutic regimen, (b) physiological progress toward therapeutic goals, and (c) long-term health outcomes. The effect size of each relevant dependent variable was calculated, with a positive result indicating the experimental group being superior to control group. The differential effectiveness of the didactic (increase of knowledge) or behavioural emphasis (promotion of self-management) of the intervention was determined.

Of 320 articles, 63 were viewed as experimental, 32 concerned chronic disease (30 of which allowed the calculation of effect size), and 24 used some kind of randomization (in two cases, altering the experimental conditions). Surprisingly, none of these publications focussed on arthritis.

Related references **(1)** Haynes RB. Strategies for improving compliance. In: *Compliance with Therapeutic Regimens* (Sackett DL, Haynes RB, eds.). Balitmore: Johns Hopkins, 1976: 69–82.

(2) Glass GV. Integrating findings: The meta-analysis of research. In: *Review of Research in Education 5* (Schulman LS, ed.). Itasca, Illinois, 1977: 157–173.

Key message

The literature clearly indicates that patient education has therapeutic value and can improve the course of a chronic disease. Programmes that included behaviour-oriented strategies were more successful in achieving positive change than were didactic interventions which affected knowledge alone.

Why it's important

This article exemplifies the late appearance of publications specifically addressing patient education. During his time of observation (1970–81) Mazzuca found only 320 articles analysing effect of patient education. Twenty-two of these were experimental, randomized, controlled studies dealing with chronic disease. The chronic diseases surveyed were hypertension (10), other heart diseases (5), asthma (3), obesity (3), hyperlipidemia, glaucoma, and renal disease (1 each), and uncategorized diseases (5). There were no evaluative studies of patient education programmes where rheumatic disease was the subject under consideration. At present, there are 4324 references to be found in Med Line during a 2 year period under the key word 'patient education'. These articles focus on many diseases, including arthritis. In comparison with past years, the trend is impressive.

Mazzuca poses the key question, 'Does patient education have therapeutic value?'. He declared that the pattern of diseases appears to have changed over the last 50 years from acute illnesses to such chronic diseases as hypertension, diabetes, lung, and heart ailments. Patient education had advanced the goal of more active participation on the part of the patient in an attempt to maximize therapeutic benefits. However, although some reviews had appeared documenting multidisciplinary patient education efforts and their results, it remained impossible to estimate the degree of efficacy on health status in cases of chronic disease. An earlier review by Haynes (1) had used an *ad hoc* rating system to find statistical and clinical evidence that only providing a patient with information about a particular disease was less effective than interventions that included behavioural strategies. However, Haynes dealt mostly with diseases of short duration and remarked that chronic disease would present a far more challenging problem.

Mazzuca uses meta-analysis (2) to answer his own question. With this method, *each test of a dependent variable yields an estimated effect size, which can be readily interpreted as the change (in standard deviation units) attributable to the experiment's intervention.* He recommends that researchers who want to interpret the clinical importance of their interventions compute the effect size for their dependent variables.

The answer to Mazzuca's leading question can now be seen to be a decisive 'yes'. Patient education does have therapeutic value. After searching in vain for literature on patient education before the appearance of Mazzuca's article, one takes encouragement from his paper and realizes that patient education needs to be evaluated by the same scientific method we employ in other areas of medical research.

Strengths

1. Mazzuca's article provides a good review of publications on patient education.
2. The study's objective methodology, and the author's reasons for excluding many publications are carefully delineated.

Weakness

The interpretation of clinical relevance described in the discussion section appears somewhat tentative.

Relevance

Most authors presenting studies on patient education consider Mazzuca's article a landmark in the field. It poses a fundamental question as to the value of patient education, and goes on to establish the relevance of this approach in the context of other methods of treating chronic rheumatic disease.

Paper 2

Assessing physician/patient perceptions in rheumatoid arthritis. A vital component in patient education

Authors

Silvers IJ, Howell MF, Weisman MH, Mueller MR

Reference

Arthritis and Rheumatism 1985; **28**:300–307

Summary

This study has analysed the needs of patient education regarding the content, provider and delivery methods perceived by 101 patients with RA and 28 rheumatologists. Ninety-two percent of all patients surveyed wanted to learn more about arthritis. All of the physicians conceded that patient education in arthritis management was beneficial, though less than 25% of them had an up-to-date programme to offer their patients. Patients and physicians agreed that certain topics were of importance to them both: medication, patient/physician communication, fraudulent practitioners, and the need to remain ambulatory. Rheumatologists placed great value on psychosocial areas, activities of daily living, sexual concerns, and community resources, while patients rated a knowledge of the disease process, diagnostic procedures, and questions of nutrition most important to them. Both patients and physicians favoured individual over group sessions. There was a difference in opinion over the optimum provider of education, with patients expressing more confidence in pharmacists and nutritionists, whereas doctors preferred programmes that were led by trained volunteers (rather than health professionals).

Key message

Patient education plays an important part of arthritis management by both arthritis patients and physicians. Programmes must be carefully planned, implemented, and evaluated.

Related references **(1)** Green LW, Lewis FM, Levine DM. Balancing statistical data and clinical judgements in the diagnosis of patient educational needs. *Journal of Community Health* 1980; **6**:79–91.

(2) Roter DL. Patient participation in the patient-provider interaction: the effects of patient question asking on the quality of interaction, satisfaction, and compliance. *Health Education Monograph* 1977; **5**:281–315.

Why it's important

When this article appeared in 1985, patient education was practised on the basis of casual clinical observations and individual case studies, often representing a stereotypical attitude toward patients with chronic disease (1). The information given to such patients was what health professionals considered important for them to know. With the exception of studies on heterogeneous groups of patients, there was no empirical data on what the actual needs of patients with RA were.

This study considered the views of patients with defined RA, and those of rheumatologists as well. The active role of patients in the management of their disease had begun to be recognized (2).

The authors found that patient education should be viewed as an important issue for both patients and physicians. Earlier work had indicated that patients did not always understand what their doctors told them; however, no substantial evidence could be found indicating that patient education was considered necessary by the medical profession. Later investigations demonstrated that patients have great misconceptions about the nature of their disease and its treatment, and confirmed the fact that they wanted to know more.

The authors also showed that patients and physicians had different views on the content of a patient education programme (Figures 25.1 and 25.2). While the patients were most interested in achieving more knowledge about the disease process and diagnostic procedures, the physicians found personal, community, and psychosocial areas the most important topics for discussion. This was in agreement with Mazzuka (Paper 1), who stated that programmes including behavioural and psychosocial aspects of the disease were more successful than those dealing with increased knowledge of the disease alone. However, as indicated in the study by Taal and others (Paper 4), answers may change if questions about sensitive topics are phrased differently.

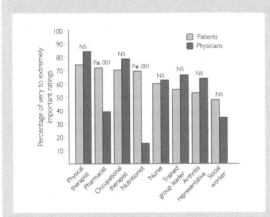

Figure 25.1 Percentages of patients' and physicians' ratings reported as extremely important for non-physician health professionals involved in education.

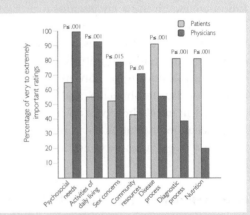

Figure 25.2 Percentages comparing patients' and physicians' ratings reported as extremely important for various topics in arthritis patient education.

Strengths

1. The study focuses on only one disease, RA, and one type of specialist, the rheumatologist.
2. Patients represent a broad range of ages (24–79 years), and the duration of their disease is equally broad (1–49 years).
3. The doctors included came from different health care systems, such as teaching hospitals, private practices, or rheumatology fellows.

Weaknesses

1. The response rate was low for patients (55%), although better for physicians (74%).
2. Only two out of 38 doctors surveyed were women.

Relevance

The importance of this paper lies in questions: what are the self-expressed needs of patients? What do patients want to know, how do they prefer to have this information conveyed, and by whom? What are the attitudes of physicians in this regard?

Paper 3

Outcomes of self-help education for patients with arthritis

Authors

Lorig K, Lubeck D, Kraines RG, Seleznick M, Holman HR

Reference

Arthritis and Rheumatism 1985; **28**:680–685

Summary

A self-help education programme, the Arthritis Self-Management Program (ASMP), was evaluated in a randomized prospective study. The programme is a community-based patient education course given by lay persons over six session. It is conducted for people with arthritis, irrespective of cause. Discussions and exercises in groups were used to improve knowledge, behaviour, and health status. Comparisons were made between the experimental and the control group, and a longitudinal comparison with baseline was made after 20 months. Outcome variables were patient knowledge, exercising, pain, disability, locus of control, number of visits to physician, and participant's satisfaction with physician.

After 4 months, there was an improvement in patient knowledge and a decrease in pain, but no change in disability or number of visits to physician. After 20 months, knowledge and frequency of exercise declined but still remained above base levels. Locus of control did not change.

Related references **(1)** Lorig K, Fries J. *The Arthritis Helpbook*. Reading MA: Addison-Wesley, 1990.

(2) Bandura A. Self-efficacy in human agency. *Annals of Psychology* 1982; **37**:122–147.

Key message

The ASMP, taught by lay-leaders, can lead to increased patient knowledge, changed behaviour, and lessened pain. Improvements seen were still in evidence after 20 months.

Why it's important

When Mazzuca reviewed published articles on patient education, he could find none with rheumatic disease as the target subject. This is the first study of patient education for individuals with arthritis that fulfils his criteria for an experimental study. Since its appearance in 1985, it has become *the* classic paper for those working in the field of patient education. It presents an inexpensive, replicable programme, an evaluation in a randomized, controlled study, and a longitudinal follow-up, measuring changes in patient knowledge, behaviour, and health status.

The Arthritis Helpbook (1) developed for the sessions has been the basis for similar programmes throughout the world, having stimulated health professionals in many countries to institute such a course for patients with arthritis. When the authors later found that changes in health status were not strongly associated with modifications in patient behaviour, they sought reasons for this. They found that those with a documented improvement in their health status also had a feeling of increased personal control over their symptoms. The programme was then redesigned to increase the self-efficacy of the participants, namely, their capability and skill to achieve a desired outcome – something decried by Bandura (2).

The ASMP was originally based on a survey of 100 arthritis patients and 50 practising rheumatologists. The topics of the six sessions were (a) anatomy and physiology, (b) effects and uses of medication, (c) individualized exercise programmes, (d) cognitive pain management, (e) nutrition, (f) patient/physician communication, and (g) problem solving disease-related difficulties.

The programme was designed to be inexpensive and readily available. It is offered to all individuals with arthritis, irrespective of diagnoses; it is community-based and thus given in shopping malls, senior centres, churches, or libraries; and it is conducted by lay-leaders who have been especially trained and are guided by a detailed protocol.

Before the ASMP programme appeared, patient education often took a didactic teaching format: patients were lectured about their arthritis, with the occasional inclusion of slides if medical students were being addressed. This publication introduced strategies for group discussions, the use of contracts, keeping diaries, and weekly feedback sessions. As a result, after this publication, programmes became more interactive, encouraging the participation of group members.

Strengths

1. The outline of the prospective, controlled study to evaluate the impact of the programme on arthritis patients is well-planned and executed.
2. The establishment of patient education programmes for chronic disease sufferers, as a useful part of any therapeutic regime, is a landmark.

Weaknesses

1. The assertion contained in the abstract, claiming that the programme is inexpensive and well-received by patients, physicians, and other health professionals, receives no documentation in the study.
2. Seventy-seven percent of the participants had osteoarthritis, only 10% had RA, and 12% had arthritis of an unspecified kind. There is no report on how the different diagnoses may have influenced the results of the study.

Relevance

A new model for approaching certain aspects of chronic illness, this paper offers thorough documentation of the positive effects of arthritis patient education on patient knowledge, health behaviour, and pain. It has encouraged the further development of other patient education programmes, and pointed out the importance of designing one's evaluation in accordance with scientific method.

Paper 4

Group education for patients with rheumatoid arthritis

Authors

Taal, E, Riemsa RP, Brus HLM, Seydel ER, Rasker JJ, Wiegman O

Reference

Patient Education and Counseling 1993; **20**:177–187

Summary

This Dutch education programme was partly based on the 'Arthritis Self-Management Course' (ASMC) by Lorig and collaborators (1). The task of the programme was to strengthen self-efficacy (2), facilitate the achievement of an individual's expectations, and change patient health behaviours, with the intention of improving health outcomes such as pain, functional ability, and the psychosocial consequences of the disease.

There were some differences, as compared to the Lorig programme: it was taught by health professionals instead of lay-leaders, and the participants all had RA. The programme was evaluated by comparing the effect in an experimental group with a randomly assigned control group. Results after 6 weeks, 4 months, and 14 months showed that patients in the experimental group had increased knowledge of their disease, and had improved physical exercise behaviour and self-efficacy function, as compared with the control group. No effects were found on pain, disease activity, or the psychological and social aspects of the disease.

Related references

(1) Lorig K, Lubeck D, Kraines RG, Seleznick M, Holman HR. Outcomes of self-help education for patients with arthritis. *Arthritis and Rheumatism* 1985; **28**:680–685.

(2) Bandura A. Self-efficacy in human agency. *Annals of Psychology* 1982; **37**:122–147.

Key message

A Dutch educational group programme, which was based on the ASMP by Lorig (1), resulted in improvement with regard to functional disability, joint tenderness, health behaviour, self-efficacy function, and knowledge. After 14 months, positive effects were still visible on self-efficacy function, patient knowledge, and exercise behaviour.

Why it's important

Although a follow-up on the work done by Lorig and collaborators (ASMC), there are some major differences here. The participants in the Dutch study formed a homogenous group and shared a common diagnosis, RA. They were selected from the files of rheumatologists, whereas the participants in Lorig's study were recruited from public service and through the mass media. Moreover, Lorig's group was heterogeneous, most of them suffering from osteoarthritis. Again, the leaders of the Dutch programme were health professionals, as opposed to Lorig's lay-leaders. The topics dealt with were generally the same in both programmes, although Taal's group put greater emphasis on physical exercise and allotted extra time to relaxation techniques. Furthermore, each person in the Dutch study was referred to a physiotherapist for individual instruction, and fewer classroom hours were spent teaching facts. Written material on RA was handed out and information about other resources given. In the discussions, the leaders gave guidelines on how to read and evaluate information about different types of treatment, including alternative therapy. The main emphasis of the programme, the enhancement of self-efficacy, was done by means of patient contracts, goal setting, and feedback (similar to the ASMC). The results of the Dutch programme are compared with those of Lorig and collaborators. The two studies report increased patient knowledge and a change in exercise behaviour. A significant difference is that the Dutch programme did not affect levels of pain or depression, but the principles of pain management are similar. The authors give no explanation for this difference.

Taal and his collaborators found that changes in self-efficacy were only related to function, not to pain or other symptoms. Conversely, Lorig concluded that changes in self-efficacy were associated more with changes in health status than with changes in behaviour.

Strengths

1. The authors aimed at assembling a homogeneous group of including only RA patients between the ages of 21 and 65 years, with a maximum use of second-line anti-rheumatic medication for 8 years.
2. All patients went through a clinical examination which included the assessment of joint tenderness and the taking of blood samples to measure disease activity.

Weaknesses

1. The response rate was low (only 75 of 140 who had been invited agreed to participate). No information is given on the non-respondents.
2. A large number of tests were performed, making it possible that significant changes may have occurred by chance.

Relevance

This paper can be seen as an indication of the further development of patient education. Some ideas from the American programme by Kate Lorig and collaborators have been applied. It does show, however, that each programme has to be adapted to the social structure and health care system of the country where it is introduced.

Paper 5

A controlled evaluation of arthritis education

Authors

Lindroth Y, Bauman A, Barnes C, McCredie M, Brooks PM

Reference

British Journal of Rheumatology 1989; **28**:7–12

Summary

This prospective study evaluated an education programme for people with rheumatoid arthritis (RA) and OA. The intervention group participated in a comprehensively planned six session behaviour-based programme. A questionnaire was given to 100 patients and 95 matched but non-random controls before the programme, 1 month later, and at 3 and 12 months. The intervention group demonstrated improvements in knowledge, self-reported health behaviour and disability scores at 12 months compared to the controls. No difference was reported in symptoms, compliance with therapy, pain perception and locus of control.

Related references	**(1)**	Lorig K, Fries JF. *The Arthritis Helpbook. Reading*: Addison-Wesley, 1980.
	(2)	Althoff B, Nordenskiold U. *Joint Protection. An Alleviating Way of Living*. Uppsala: Pharmacia, 1985.

Key message

Development of a successful patient education programme is facilitated by the involvement of patients at the planning stage. A behavioural-based approach is likely to be most successful, and can lead to improvements in knowledge and behaviour that are long lasting.

Why it's important

Much of the material available to patients for their 'education', as well as many of the packages developed by the professionals, take a didactic, authoritarian approach. One of the most important features of the work described here related to the way in which the intervention was developed. The authors undertook a comprehensive survey of the literature and took note of related work from other centres and disciplines when planning their intervention. They then took the important step of involving both the patients and therapists in a workshop at which the format of the programme was planned.

Another key feature of the programme described in this paper is the the emphasis on changing behaviour of patients as opposed to an emphasis on knowledge, which predominates in many other packages. The outcomes as well as the intervention put major emphasis on activities and behaviour and on the influence of arthritis on these aspects of the participants' lives.

Strengths

1. Careful planning, based on existing literature.
2. Involvement of patients and therapists at the planning stage.
3. Emphasis on health behaviour rather than knowledge.

Weaknesses

1. Neither the planning stage, nor the package of education itself are well described, so that there is very little detail to help others who might want to do a similar study.
2. All outcome measures are self-report based, so that there were no other more 'objective' ways of finding out whether the intervention group's disease status or function improved.
3. The major weakness (acknowledged in the text) is the absence of a randomized controlled trial, the comparative group were different in age and reported problems than the study group.

Relevance

A landmark paper in the development of educational packages for patients with arthritis because of the involvement of patients in planning and the demonstration of long-lasting benefits on health behaviours.

Paper 6

Can the provision of information to patients with osteoarthritis improve functional status?

Authors

Weinberger M, Theriney WM, Booher P, Katz BP

Reference

Arthritis and Rheumatism 1989; **32**:1577–1583

Summary

The aim of this study was to find out whether advising patients over the telephone could affect their functional status in cases of chronic arthritis. Four hundred and thirty-nine patients with osteoarthritis (OA) were randomly assigned to one of four groups receiving information in different ways: (a) by telephone once a month, (b) in person at the clinic, (c) at the clinic and by telephone, and (d) none (i.e. control group). The effect of these interventions was measured by changes in physical health, pain levels, and psychological well-being.

Patients who received telephone intervention only, or who personally visited the clinic *and* had telephone contact, had less pain and disability than the group of patients who only attended the clinic. This may be explained by the fact that the number of contacts were considerably more for those two groups that had ready access to their health care providers by telephone. The authors also propose other explanations: a visit to a clinic may not be the best forum for giving and receiving information, due to the pressure of time and the disturbances one encounters there. Telephone contact, on the other hand, could be made when it suited the patient, and when the patient was feeling relaxed. In addition, it preserves the patient's anonymity. Finally, the telephone is an inexpensive means of giving information, advice, and encouragement.

Key message

Repetitive information, personal advice, and individual encouragement may be conveniently and inexpensively given to patients with OA over the telephone. In practice, this resulted in improved physical health and reduced pain.

Why it's important

This paper presents a new way of conveying information and support to patients, i.e. by use of the telephone. Osteoarthritis, according to the authors, is the most common chronic disease affecting adults. The cost of health care for these individuals is high and, with a view toward the increasing age of the population in the future, the impact of this disease on society is likely to increase. The common symptoms of OA are pain and loss of mobility. This may lead to social isolation and feelings of depression. Traditional treatments have been non-steroidal anti-inflammatory drugs, and exercise programmes. In spite of the fact that earlier studies of patient education have documented the beneficial impact of social support, there continue to be few publications evaluating the effect of this intervention on patients with OA.

According to this study, pain was the main problem for the patients with OA, physical disability caused the least discomfort. Those patients receiving information and support by telephone had less pain and physical disability than other groups did. A surprising result was that clinic intervention only had a detrimental effect on physical functioning! The authors offer four possible explanations: first, these individuals had considerably fewer overall contacts than the others did. Secondly, the competence of the telephone advisors was consistently superior to that of the health care providers in the clinic. Thirdly, patients may have been too ill to pay attention to information given at the clinic. There were also disturbances of other patients seeking care in the clinic, and there was time pressure. This was avoided in the telephone call which could be offered when it suited the patient. Finally a relaxed phone call with some distance between participant and the care giver may have an advantage over a face-to-face contact, which may even be threatening to some individuals. As telephone contacts are an inexpensive means of communication, they can be made with greater frequency. In fact, the mean number of such calls per patient was more than three times the number of clinic visits by the same patient.

Strengths

1. The response rate was high, with 75% of those offered the opportunity agreeing to take part in the study; the follow-up rate was equally so (89.7% of the initial number of participants).
2. The non-respondents and those who failed to follow-up had the same demographic characteristics.
3. An ambitious interviewing programme, involving a great number of subjects, was successfully carried out.

Weaknesses

1. The patients taking part in this study were 70% black, and their level of education was rather low.
2. The authors report in the abstract a 'marginal improvement of psychological health' with a p-value of 0.10. Such a change, so small as to appear almost insignificant, may be a random result.
3. The conclusion that telephone contact is an inexpensive yet effective way of communicating with arthritis patients should be documented by substantial evidence.

Relevance

The authors of this paper raise the issue of providing arthritis patients with social support, information on coping with pain, and instruction on how to perform physical exercise by phone. If this strategy proves to be effective, it would be an inexpensive addition to the total care programme for the management of a very common, disabling disease.

Paper 7

The patient is not a blank sheet: lay beliefs and their relevance to patient education

Authors

Donovan JL, Blake DR, Fleming WG

Reference

British Journal of Rheumatology 1989; **28**:58–61

Summary

This is a qualitative study based on interviews of 32 patients with RA, both before and after their first visit to a rheumatology clinic. It included observations made during these consultations. Interviews were tape-recorded, transcribed, and then analysed using a qualitative method (1). The study describes each patient's perception of arthritis, coping strategies, and expectations in seeking clinical aid. Most of the individuals seen had learned to live with their arthritis, although five of them stated that arthritis had totally disrupted their lives in that they were cut off from the life they had lived before being afflicted. Patients did not talk of symptoms *per se* (i.e. pain and stiffness) but of how pain had affected their lives. Although most had found their own coping strategies, they continued to suffer in their effort to keep going. They expected the doctor to give them information and suggest treatment, which they then would decide whether to heed or not.

Related references	(1)	Glaser B, Strauss A. *Grounded theory*. Chicago: Aldine, 1967.
	(2)	Moll J. Medical communication: recent aspects and relevance to rheumatology. In: *Recent Advances in Rheumatology* (Moll J, Sturrock R, eds.). Bath: Churchill Livingstone, 1986.

Key message

When planning and evaluating patient education, one must bear in mind that any medical advice given to a patient still has to pass through the filter of that person's lay beliefs. Patients are individuals, not blank sheets. The authors suggest a shift from providing didactic information to facilitating more active participation of patients in their own therapy.

Why it's important

This article shows that patient education is more complex than generally assumed. Earlier models of patient education, in which active instruction from rheumatologists and other health professionals was accompanied by passive listening and the absorption of information by patients, may not be enough. In order to be successful, patient education must be viewed as a dialogue between health care provider and patient, i.e. two-way communication.

The method employed in this qualitative study may be new to some medical researchers, although it is familiar in such other fields as sociology and anthropology (1). A small number of individuals are interviewed, and their interviews analysed in detail. A tape recording documents the informal, semi-structured exchange, while the interviewer uses a checklist so that all questions are asked of all subjects.

The article gives the reader a different picture of how patients with arthritis go through life. Great misconceptions can be avoided when one realizes that views on a disease may differ considerably between health professionals and patients. For physicians, illness is commonplace, symptoms are based on biomedical theories, and treatment is self-evident and logical. For patients, on the other hand, illness is abnormal, symptoms are experienced in terms of what one can and cannot do, and medical treatment is only one of several options, including advice from friends, relatives, or alternative cures promoted in the media. Further, the prevalent method of evaluating pain with a visual analogue scale (VAS) tends to reduce a complex feeling to a simple sensation, whereas pain may be influenced by many factors that cannot be accounted for by putting a mark on a 100 mm line. Conflict arising from these different perceptions of illness and treatment may lead to a guilty conscience in some patients for non-compliant behaviour, even though the patient is acting on what subjectively feels like logical reasoning. After the publication of this article, the importance of patients' views on what they wanted or needed to know became clearer. Communication is, by definition, a two-way process (2). Understanding lay-beliefs that individuals bring with them into patient education programme sessions began to be considered seriously.

Strength

The methodology employed results in a lucid presentation in which the tone is conversational and the text, unencumbered by tables or diagrams, is easy to follow.

Weakness

It might have been preferable to outline the new methodology, rather than ask the reader to contact the authors for details.

Relevance

The authors employ a qualitative approach to present information vital to the understanding of disease from a patient's point of view. The knowledge imparted here has been used in planning patient education programmes. After this article appeared, such programmes changed from lecture format, using slides to tell patients about their disease, to interactive formats that often incorporated problem-solving strategies in which patients take an active role in discussing *their own individual problems,* rather than problems which health professionals have selected as common to all patients with arthritis.

CHAPTER 26

Key drug developments

Peter M Brooks

Introduction

This century has seen the development of pharmacological therapy for rheumatic diseases. The century began with the synthesis of salicylic acid, which in some ways spawned the modern pharmaceutical industry and led to many of the treatments we now take for granted in rheumatic diseases. In the early part of the 1900s, salicylates were used extensively for pain relief and as anti-pyretics, although it was not until the 1960s that they were really subjected to clinical trials. Recognition that salicylates were associated with significant side-effects led to the development of indomethacin, phenylbutazone, and other non-steroidal drugs (NSAIDs) which rapidly became the mainstay of pain relief and anti-inflammatory activity. The seminal observations by John Vane in the early 1970s that aspirin and other NSAIDs blocked the production of prostaglandins opened a significant window on inflammation research. Interestingly, in the last decade of this century the discovery that the cyclooxygenase pathway is composed of two enzymes has led to the generation of a new class of specific cyclooxygenase-2 inhibitors which seem to provide the benefits of anti-inflammatory effect with a marked reduction in gastrointestinal adverse events.

The papers I have selected are those that demonstrated, often for the first time in a controlled study, efficacy of a particular drug. Some of the papers, such as the one by Boardman and Hart on the anti-inflammatory effects of salicylates, compare various doses whilst others compare two active agents with a placebo as in the study on sulphasalazine in rheumatoid arthritis (RA), in a double-blind comparison of sulphasalazine with placebo and sodium aurothiomalate. The paper from David Henry's group on gastrointestinal complications of NSAIDs, brought together data from twelve studies of gastro-toxicity and performed a very valuable meta-analysis showing that some NSAIDs were more toxic than others. The group of papers on anti-rheumatic drugs begins with the classic study from Tom Fraser in Glasgow who carried out one of the first controlled clinical trials in medicine comparing gold sodium aurothiomalate with a placebo as part of the Empire Rheumatism Council Multi-centre Trial. This is followed by the classic paper by Phillip Hench and his group at the Mayo Clinic reporting the use of Compound E (hydrocortisone) in severe RA. Controlled studies on penicillamine, sulphasalazine, and methotrexate are also reported. Inclusion of Fred Wolfe's study was important in that it illustrated the strength of large long-term databases in providing us with practical evidence of drug efficacy. This group of studies ends with the paper from Maini's group reporting the first randomized double-blind comparison of monoclonal antibodies versus placebo in RA. This paper heralded a new age for rheumatology, that of biologics, a group of drugs that will lead us into the next millenium, raising significant issues of cost and the potential for long-term side-effects.

After perhaps two decades of activity in the 1960s and 70s when a large range of new NSAIDs were introduced, rheumatology therapeutics went through a relatively quiescent period until the last 5 years. As we enter the next century, Rheumatologists do so surrounded by a range of new anti-rheumatic drugs, specific Cox inhibitors, and biologics. It is an exciting time for Rheumatologists and, more importantly, for patients with rheumatic diseases. Issues of long-term safety and of the cost-effectiveness have, however, to be addressed as never before.

Paper 1

Clinical measurement of the anti-inflammatory effects of salicylates in rheumatoid arthritis

Authors

Boardman PL, Hart FD

Reference

British Medical Journal 1967; **4**:264–268

Summary

Paper demonstrates the anti-inflammatory properties of salicylates as measured by joint size. Comparisons between placebo and prednisolone, paracetamol, and high- and low-dose salicylates were made. Prednisolone and high-dose salicylates were effective in reducing joint size whereas paracetamol and low-dose salicylates were not.

Related references **(1)** Fremont-Smith K, Bayles TB. Salicylate therapy in rheumatoid arthritis. *Journal of the American Medical Association* 1965; **192**:1133–1136.

(2) Calabro JJ, Paulus HE. Anti-inflammatory effects of acetyl salicylic acid in rheumatoid arthritis. *Clinical Orthopaedics and Related Research* 1970; **71**:124–131.

(3) Capell HA, Rennie JAN, Rooney PJ, *et al.* Patients compliance: A novel method of testing non-steroidal anti-inflammatory analgesics in rheumatoid arthritis. *Journal of Rheumatology* 1979; **6**:584–593.

Key message

This was the first paper to demonstrate clearly that high-dose salicylates were effective in the treatment of the inflammation associated with RA. The paper also showed that low doses of salicylate were not anti-inflammatory as was paracetamol.

Why it's important

At the time that the study was carried out there were very few NSAIDs available. Salicylates were widely available and used for the treatment of inflammation and this study was designed to compare placebo with 7.5 mg of prednisolone daily, 6 g of paracetamol, 5.3 g of salicylate and 2.6 g of salicylate. Drug treatment was carried out for a 7 day period and the trial was a cross-over design. In this study, jeweller's rings were used to assess joint size – this methodology was validated against a gauge for measuring joint sizes. Observations were also made regarding the variation of joint size and grip strength, with grip strength increasing and joint size decreasing between morning and evening measurements (Figure 26.1).

Four 2 week cross-over studies were carried out comparing prednisolone with placebo, paracetamol with placebo, high-dose of salicylate with low-dose and low-dose of salicylate with placebo. Treatment periods were for 1 week with a direct cross-over to the alternative treatment. Sequential analysis was used to show that prednisolone and high-dose salicylate were both effective in reducing joint size. Grip strength also improved with prednisolone and high-dose salicylate. Some side-effects were seen on the high-dose salicylate with the major complaint being tinnitus.

This study showed a number of factors: (a) that high-dose salicylate was anti-inflammatory; (b) that low-dose salicylate was not anti-inflammatory; (c) the study validated the use of a simple gauge for measuring joint circumference with the standard jeweller's rings; and (d) the study demonstrated a novel (at the time) clinical trial methodology for assessing anti-inflammatory properties of rapidly acting drugs.

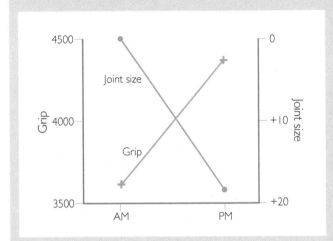

Figure 26.1 Diurnal variation of joint size and grip strength in eight patients with rheumatoid arthritis. Joint size is measured in millimetres (+ indicates improvement). Grip strength is measured in millimetres mercury, the sum for each time being plotted.

Strengths

1. The endpoints were validated in comparison to standard methodology.
2. The paper clearly demonstrated efficacy with prednisolone and with high-dose salicylate.

Weakness

The cross-over design did not allow a wash-out between treatments.

Relevance

This was a pivotal trial in demonstrating the anti-inflammatory effects of aspirin.

Paper 2

Variability in risk of gastrointestinal complications with individual non-steroidal anti-inflammatory drugs: results of a collaborative meta-analysis

Authors

Henry D, L-Y Lim L, Garcia Rodriguez LA, Perez Gutthann S, Carson JL, Griffin M, Savage R, Logan R, Moride Y, Hawkey C, Hill S, Fries JT

Reference

British Medical Journal 1996; **312**:1563–1566

Summary

This paper presents a systematic review of 12 controlled epidemiological studies relating gastrointestinal complications to use of 14 NSAIDs. The relative risks of gastrointestinal complications with individual NSAIDs were ranked in relation to exposure to ibuprofen. Ibuprofen ranked lowest or equal lowest for risk in 10 of the 11 studies reviewed. The low risk of serious gastrointestinal complications of ibuprofen seems to be attributed mainly to lower doses of the drug used in clinical practice.

Table 26.1 Comparison of comparative toxicity of range of drugs with use of ibuprofen as reference for calculating relative risks.

Comparator	No of studies	Pooled relative risk	95% confidence interval for pooled relative risk	P value (heterogeneity)
Ibuprofen	–	1.0*	–*	–*
Fenoprofen	2	1.6	1.0 to 2.5	0.310
Aspirin	6	1.6	1.3 to 2.0	0.685
Diclofenac	8	1.8	1.4 to 2.3	0.778
Sulindac	5	2.1	1.6 to 2.7	0.685
Diflunisal	2	2.2	1.2 to 4.1	0.351
Naproxen	10	2.2	1.7 to 2.9	0.131
Indomethacin	11	2.4	1.9 to 3.1	0.488
Tolmetin	2	3.0	1.8 to 4.9	0.298
Piroxicam	10	3.8	2.7 to 5.2	0.087
Ketoprofen	7	4.2	2.7 to 6.4	0.258
Azapropazone	2	9.2	4.0 to 21.0	0.832

*Reference category for calculating relative risk.

Related references **(1)** Singh, G, Romey DL, Morfeld D, Fries JF. Comparative toxicity of non-steroidal anti-inflammatory agents. *Pharmacology Therapeutics* 1994; **62**:175–191.

(2) Langman MJS, Weil J, Wainwright P, *et al.* Risk of bleeding peptic ulcer associated with individual non-steroidal anti-inflammatory drugs. *The Lancet* 1994; **343**:1075–1078.

Key message

This meta-analysis demonstrates that there are differences in the propensity for NSAIDs to produce serious gastric complications. While some of these differences are related to dose (particularly in relation to ibuprofen) there do seem to be some NSAIDs which cause less gastric toxicity than others.

Why it's important

For many years it has been accepted that all NSAIDs are associated with gastric toxicity and while this remains true, this meta-analysis does demonstrate that there are differences in the potential of gastro-toxicity of NSAIDs. The authors had all produced major individual studies in the gastric toxicity of NSAIDs and were quite rigid in the selection of studies for inclusion in the meta-analysis. The study reported the relative risk with individual drugs and then provided a ranking of the individual NSAIDs to produce the data shown in the table. The importance of dose is emphasized in the paper, particularly in relation to ibuprofen, which tends to be used in low doses.

The paper reaffirms the gastro-toxicity of NSAIDs as a major cause of morbidity and mortality. The meta-analysis of the available epidemiological data does show wide differences between individual drugs and the risk of producing gastrointestinal bleeding or ulcer perforation. Of the drugs in common use, ibuprofen and diclofenac ranked low in toxicity whereas azapropazone, ketoprofen and piroxicam ranked high.

Strength

This study provides a meta-analysis of all the major studies looking at the relationship between NSAID use and gastro-toxicity.

Weakness

Doses used for some of the drugs are not necessarily equipotent from an anti-inflammatory or analgesic point of view.

Relevance

This study emphasizes the differential toxicity of NSAIDs and is important in clinical practice.

Paper 3

N of 1 trials comparing a non-steroidal anti-inflammatory drug with paracetamol in osteoarthritis

Authors

March L, Irwig L, Schwarz J, Simpson J, Chock C, Brooks P

Reference

British Medical Journal 1994; **309**:1041–1046

Summary

This study evaluated the efficacy of paracetamol and a NSAID for symptom relief in osteoarthritis (OA) using n of 1 trial methodology. Patients completed three treatment cycles of 2 weeks each of paracetamol (1 g twice daily) or diclofenac (50 mg twice daily) in identical gelatin capsules. Fifteen patients completed the study and five withdrew early having made a therapeutic decision. Eight of the 20 patients found no clear difference with symptoms being adequately controlled by paracetamol while five preferred the NSAID. After 3 months nine of the 20 patients had adequate symptom control with paracetamol alone. Figure 26.2 shows the pain and stiffness scores in a patient who responded to NSAID.

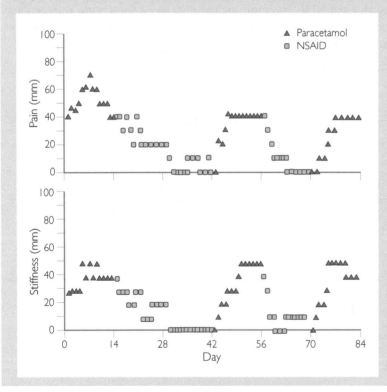

Figure 26.2 Daily visual analogue scores for pain and stiffness in one patient.

Related references **(1)** Williams WJ, Ward JR, Egger MJ, Neuner R, Brooks RH, Clegg DO, *et al.* Comparison of naproxen and acetaminophen in a two year study of the treatment of osteoarthritis of the knee. *Arthritis and Rheumatism* 1993; **36**:1196–1206.

(2) Dieppe E, Cushnagan J, Jasani MK, McRae F, Watt I. A two year placebo-controlled trial of non-steroidal anti-inflammatory therapy in osteoarthritis of the knee joint. *British Journal of Rheumatology* 1993; **32**:595–600.

(3) Dieppe PA Frankel SJ, Toth B. Is research into the treatment of osteoarthritis with non-steroidal anti-inflammatory drugs misdirected? *The Lancet* 1993; **341**:353–354.

Key message

Significant numbers of patients with OA of the knee previously treated with NSAIDs can have their pain adequately controlled with paracetamol for at least up to 3 months. N Of 1 studies are useful for making treatment decisions in OA.

Why it's important

This study demonstrated once again that a significant number of patients with OA of the knee can be controlled, at least in the short-term, with pure analgesics. It also demonstrated that there is a subset of patients with OA of the knee who prefer NSAIDs. This study fits with a number of others suggesting that between a quarter and a third of patients with OA can obtain sufficient pain relief with pure analgesics. This study also demonstrated the usefulness of n of 1 trail methodology in a disease such as OA where symptom control is important. N of 1 trials are particularly applicable to general practice and can be used for therapeutic decision making in an individual patient. The study also demonstrated that patients enjoyed this type of trial in that they felt they gained a better understanding of their arthritis and became more involved in the treatment.

Strength

Simple demonstration of n of 1 trial methodology to assist in treatment decisions.

Weaknesses

1. There were significant drop-outs (10) although five patients only did so after they had made a therapeutic decision.
2. Some of the issues such as use of gelatin capsules to package the active components may detract from the generalizability.

Relevance

The study demonstrates the relevance of simple trial methodology in determining treatment decisions and the ease with which such a trial can be conducted. This trial methodology is particularly relevant to general practice. The study also demonstrates the significant number of patients with OA of the knee who could be treated with paracetamol rather than a NSAID, reducing the potential for adverse drug reactions.

Paper 4

The effect of a hormone of the adrenal cortex (17-hydroxy-11-dehydro-corticosterone-compound E) and of pituitary adreno-corticotropic hormone on rheumatoid arthritis – preliminary report

Authors

Hench PS, Kendall EC, Slocumb CH, Polley HF

Reference

Proceedings of the Staff Meetings of the Mayo Clinic 1949; **24**:181–197

Summary

This study outlines the background to the development of compound E and its use in 14 patients with moderately severe or severe chronic polyarticular arthritis. The patients all had severe disease.

Compound E was given by intramuscular injection. Placebo injections were also given to the patients at irregular intervals. Administration of compound E led to a marked reduction in erythrocyte sedimentation rate (ESR) and resolution of pain and significant disability. Significant side-effects of acne and hirsutism were noted, but these were felt to be mild.

Related references **(1)** Empire Rheumatism Council. Multi-centre controlled trial comparing cortisone acetate and acetyl salicylic acid in the longterm treatment of rheumatoid arthritis. *Annals of Rheumatic Diseases* 1967; **16**:277–289.

(2) Harris ED, Emkey RD, Nicholas JE, *et al.* Low-dose prednisolone therapy in rheumatoid arthritis: a double-blind study. *Journal of Rheumatology* 1988; **24**:125–127.

(3) Kirwan JR and The Arthritis and Rheumatism Council Low-Dose Corticosteroid Study Group. The effect of glucocorticoids on joint destruction in rheumatoid arthritis. *New England Journal of Medicine* 1995; **333**:142–146.

Key message

This was the first study to demonstrate the anti-inflammatory effects of corticosteroids in patients with RA. The responses to treatments were extremely dramatic and few side-effects were reported.

Why it's important

This study heralded a new treatment for RA–corticosteroids, although at the time very small amounts of corticosteroids were available (note the expression of regret from MERCK and Co. Inc. 'because of the exigencies of manufacture, no supplies of compound E are expected for treatment or additional research until some time in 1950 at the earliest, at which time supplies may still be exceedingly small'). The patients treated with compound E all had severe disease with a number being temporarily bedridden or wheelchair bound. These patients all responded dramatically to the treatment with a reduction in pain, swelling and in many cases the return of the ability to walk unaided. Placebo injections were given on occasions to the patients and the effect observed. In some cases (it is reported) even the doctor was unaware that a placebo was being given. Few side-effects were reported during this study, although some patients were noted to have developed hirsutism, a rounding of the face and some transient abdominal pain. Oedema was also reported to occur on occasions. The general feeling however was that the medication was relatively safe. Two female patients were also given small amounts of adrenocorticotropic hormone (ACTH) with dramatic reductions in stiffness, pain on motion and articular tenderness. ESR was also notably reduced in these patients (Figure 26.3). This clinical trial, albeit not well controlled, clearly demonstrated the efficacy of corticosteroids in severe inflammatory RA and this led to the use of corticosteroids which, of course, are still used today.

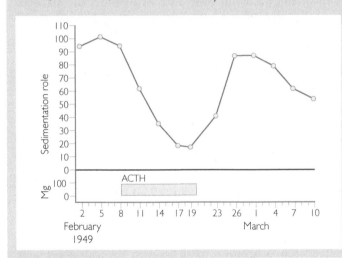

Figure 26.3 Effect of pituitary ACTH on the sedimentation rate of a 45-year-old woman with moderately severe RA of 5 year's duration. The rate decreased markedly during the use of ACTH, then increased rapidly. Note the 'rebound' between 26 February and 10 March; thereafter the rate increased again.

Strengths

1. This is the first time that this medication was used for the treatment of RA.
2. Patients were carefully observed.

Weaknesses

1. There was no real control.
2. Most of the patients were hospitalized and the effect of bed-rest had been significant.
3. In many cases the treatment was short-lived (less than 1 month) and it is perhaps surprising that so many adverse reactions were observed in this short-term trial.

Relevance

This was the first trial of corticosteroids in the management of RA and this heralded a new management strategy for this condition. The report and subsequent research on corticosteroids in RA led to the award of the Nobel Prize to Dr Hench.

Paper 5

Gold treatment in rheumatoid arthritis

Author

Fraser TN

Reference

British Medical Journal 1945; **0**:471–475.

Summary

This study evaluates the effect of intra-muscular gold (gold sodium thiomalate) in comparison to a placebo in patients with RA over a 12 month period. Of 103 patients entered, 57 received gold injections and 46 the inactive control. The intra-muscular (I.M.) injections were given into the buttocks at weekly intervals at doses of 10, 20, and 50 mg followed by nine injections of 100 mg to a total dose of 1 g. A second course in the same dosing schedule was given to 13 patients receiving active drugs and 28 patients on placebo. Clinical improvement occurred in 82% of patients receiving gold but only 45% of patients on placebo. Adverse reactions (mainly skin rashes) were reported in 75% of those on gold but also by 37% of patients receiving placebo.

Related references **(1)** Empire Rheumatism Council: Research Subcommittee. Gold therapy in rheumatoid arthritis. Report of a Multi-Centre Controlled Trial. *Annals of Rheumatic Diseases* 1960; **19**:95–119.

(2) Champion GD, Graham GG, Ziegler JB. The Gold Complexes. *Balliere's Clinical Rheumatology* 1990; **4**:491–534.

(3) Furst DE, Levine S, Srinivasan R, *et al.* A double-blind trial of high versus conventional dosages of gold salts for rheumatoid arthritis. *Arthritis and Rheumatism* 1977; **20**:1473–1480.

Key message

Intra-muscular gold (myocrisin) is effective in a group of patients with RA with acceptable side-effects (primarily skin rashes). A significant proportion of patients with RA also show both objective and subjective improvement over an observation period of 12 months. A relatively high percentage of patients (37%) reported side-effects in the placebo arm.

Why it's important

Although gold therapy had been used in the treatment of polyarthritis since the 1920s, this was probably the first reported controlled trial of gold salts and one of the first controlled trials carried out in rheumatology. This study clearly demonstrates the beneficial effects of gold treatment and also documented the major adverse reactions–skin rashes, mouth ulcers and proteinuria. Interestingly, a significant number of patients receiving placebo also improved and this was put down to the fact that both groups were receiving physiotherapy. Patients were chosen if they had had the condition for 2–5 years, thus eliminating those who might have a spontaneous remission or those long-standing cases where disease activity might be difficult to change.

The author made the point that gold therapy was probably the best form of treatment for RA available at the time but that this should be combined with general physiotherapeutic and orthopaedic measures.

Strength

This was a controlled and blinded study carried out over a significant period of time.

Weakness

The randomization procedure was not described.

Relevance

This study set a benchmark at the time for the assessment of treatments in RA and the results remain relevant to the present day.

Paper 6

Synthetic D-penicillamine in rheumatoid arthritis – double-blind controlled study of a high and low dosage regimen

Authors

Dixon AStJ, Davies J, Dormandy TL, Hamilton EBD, Holt PJL, Mason RM, Thompson M, Webber JCP, Zutschi DW

Reference

Annals of the Rheumatic Diseases 1975; **34**:416–421

Summary

This double-blind controlled multi-centre trail compared the therapeutic and adverse effects of penicillamine in a dosage of either 600 mg or 1200 mg daily in comparison to a group of patients receiving standard treatment and a minimal sub-effective dose of penicillamine (12 mg daily). In this 24 week study doses of both 600 mg and 1200 mg of D-penicillamine daily were superior to standard regimen therapy in RA. The higher dose was not associated with a significantly greater therapeutic benefit but the frequency of adverse reactions (skin rashes, blood dyscrasias and withdrawal from the trial) were higher in the 1200 mg dose group.

Related references (1) Multi-Centre Trial Group. Controlled trial of D-penicillamine in rheumatoid arthritis. *The Lancet* 1973; **1**:275–285.

(2) Situnayake RD, Grindulis KA, McConkey B. Long-term treatment of rheumatoid arthritis with sulphasalazine, gold or D-penicillamine: A comparison using life table methods. *Annals of Rheumatic Diseases* 1987; **46**:177–183.

(3) Ahern MJ, Hall ND, Case K, Maddison PJ. D-penicillamine withdrawal in rheumatoid arthritis. *Annals of Rheumatic Diseases* 1984; **43**:213–217.

Key message

The important finding of this study was that higher doses of D penicillamine (1200 mg daily) were not associated with a superior therapeutic effect than 600 mg doses daily but were associated with an increased frequency of adverse events.

Why it's important

This carefully conducted double-blind multi-centre study addressed the issue of doses of D-penicillamine in patients with RA and its relationship to efficacy and side-effects. Previous studies had demonstrated the efficacy of D-penicillamine in RA and suggested that there was a relationship between dose and adverse events. This study clearly showed differences between the control group and patients treated with both doses of D-penicillamine. However, 67% of patients on the 1200 mg dose noted adverse reactions compared to 50% on the 600 mg dose and 34% of patients on the control (Table 26.2). Serum-copper levels fell significantly and to the same extent on both dosage regimens. This paper stresses the importance of using the lowest dose of penicillamine and that an adequate time (4–8 weeks) should be given for clinical improvement to take place. X-rays of the hands and feet were taken at day 0 and at 24 weeks and were assessed for the number and severity of erosions and an overall impression of change. No trends were seen in either of the treatment groups.

Table 26.2 Responses of patients on D-penicillamine and placebo.

	Control	Daily D-penicillamine dose	
		600 mg	1200 mg
% improved	26	56	70
% patients with adverse effects	34	50	67
% ceasing treatment due to adverse effects	9	20	40

Strength

This was a double-blind study of two dose regimens of D-penicillamine and a placebo which demonstrated a higher incidence of side-effects with a high dose of penicillamine.

Weaknesses

1. This study was of relatively short duration (24 weeks).
2. Mean differences on treatment are reported rather than raw data making clinical significance hard to interpret.

Relevance

This was the first study to address the issue of doses of D penicillamine and its relationship to side-effects and efficacy.

Paper 7

Sulphasalazine in rheumatoid arthritis – a double-blind comparison of sulphasalazine with placebo and sodium aurothiomalate

Authors

Pullar P, Hunter JA, Capell HA

Reference

British Medical Journal 1983; **287**:1102–1104

Summary

Ninety patients with definite or classical RA were randomly allocated to receive sulphasalazine (enteric coated tablets of Salazopyrin), sodium aurothiomalate or sulphasalazine placebo. Sulphasalazine was used in doses of up to 3 g daily. Gold sodium aurothiomalate was administered I.M. at a dose of 50 mg per week after a 10 mg test dose up to a maximum of 1 g or until a clinical response had been obtained, whereafter the frequency of injections was reduced to the minimum necessary to maintain the clinical response. Disease activity was assessed at 6 weekly intervals over a 24 week period. At 24 weeks, 18 patients were still taking sulphasalazine, 18 patients sodium aurothiomalate and 14 placebo. The main reason for stopping treatment were lack of effect (placebo 13, sulphasalazine two, and sodium aurothiomalate one patient) and adverse events (placebo two, sulphasalazine nine, and sodium aurothiomalate 11 patients). The ESR, articular index and index of disease activity demonstrated significant improvement in those patients on active treatment whereas no changes were seen with placebo. The major toxicity for sulphasalazine was gastrointestinal intolerance while rashes were the major cause for stopping the drug in the gold group. Acetylator status was assessed in 28 of the patients treated with sulphasalazine, with 15 being slow acetylators and 13 being fast acetylators. Five of the six patients who stopped taking sulphasalazine because of gastrointestinal intolerance were slow acetylators whereas both patients who stopped because of lack of effect were fast acetylators. The suggestion is made that toxicity and lack of efficacy are related to acetylator phenotype.

Related references (1) Svartz N. Salazopyrin, a new sulfanilamid preparation. *Acta Medica Scandinavica* 1942; **60**:577–598.

(2) Sinclair RJG, Duffy JJR. Salazopyrin in the treatment of rheumatoid arthritis. *Annals of Rheumatic Diseases* 1948; **8**:226–231.

(3) McConkey B, Amos R, Durham S, *et al.* Sulphasalazine in rheumatoid arthritis. *British Medical Journal* 1980; **280**:442–444.

(4) Williams H, Ward J, Dahl S, *et al.* A controlled trial comparing sulphasalazine, gold sodium aurothiomalate, and placebo in rheumatoid arthritis. *Arthritis and Rheumatism* 1988; **31**:702–713.

Key message

Sulphasalazine appears to be an effective second line agent in the management of RA.

Why it's important

This is the first comparative study of sulphasalazine with another disease-modifying anti-rheumatic drug (sodium aurothiomalate). This study clearly showed that the sulphasalazine was effective in patients with active RA although the mean duration of disease was greater than 6 years in all groups, with a range of up 35 years. This may have explained the variable responses noted at the 24 week period (Table 26.3).

Table 26.3 Significance of improvement (p values) in variables at 24 weeks (Wilcoxon (two-tailed) test)

	Placebo	Sulphasalazine	Sodium aurothiomalate
ESR	NS	<0.005	<0.005
Haemoglobin	NS	NS	NS
Platelet count	NS	0.001	NS
Rheumatoid factor	NS	NS	0.05
Articular index	NS	<0.001	0.001
Limbering up time	NS	NS	NS
Pain score	NS	NS	<0.005
Grip strength	NS	<0.005	NS
Index of disease activity	NS	0.005	<0.005

Strengths

1. The study design was well conceived with the outcome measures being assessed by a nurse who was blind to the nature of the therapy.
2. Adverse events were carefully assessed in the study.
3. Acetylator status in those patients receiving sulphasalazine was determined.
4. This study clearly demonstrates the efficacy of Salazopyrin in the treatment of RA with relatively mild side-effects.

Weakness

The raw data for efficacy is not reported in the study and it is therefore hard to assess the importance of the changes.

Relevance

Since the publication of this and other studies of sulphasalazine, the drug has become a standard second-line treatment in RA.

Paper 8

Comparison of low-dose oral pulse methotrexate and placebo in the treatment of rheumatoid arthritis – a controlled clinical trial

Authors

Williams HJ, Willkens RF, Samuelson CO Jr, Alarcon GS, Guttadauria M, Yarboro C, Polisson RP, Weiner SR, Luggen ME, Billingsley LM, Dahl SL, Egger MJ, Reading JC, Ward JR

Reference

Arthritis and Rheumatism 1985; **28**(7):721–730

Summary

This paper describes a prospective, controlled, double-blind, multicentre trial comparing placebo with methotrexate 7.5 mg weekly, taken as three 2.5 mg tablets 12 hours apart. One hundred and ten of 189 patients entered completed 18 weeks of therapy. Methotrexate treatment demonstrated statistically significant improvement over the placebo in the clinical variables of joint pain/tenderness and swelling, rheumatoid nodules, and patient and physician assessments of disease activity (Figure 26.4).

During the trial, one-third of patients receiving methotrexate were withdrawn for adverse drug reactions of which elevated liver enzymes were the most common. All adverse drug effects resolved without sequelae.

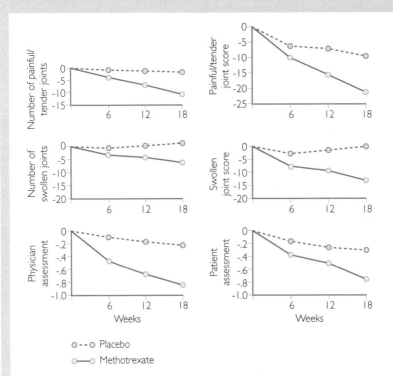

Figure 26.4 Mean change in selected clinical variables by treatment (placebo versus methotrexate) at 6, 12, and 18 weeks of therapy.

Related references **(1)** Andersen EA, West SG, O'Dell JR, *et al.* Weekly pulse methotrexate in rheumatoid arthritis: clinical and immunological effects of a randomized, double-blind study. *Annals of Internal Medicine* 1985; **1–3**:479–486.

(2) Weinblatt ME, Jonathan SC, Fox DA, *et al.* Efficacy of low-dose methotrexate in rheumatoid arthritis. *New England Journal of Medicine* 1985; **312**:818–822.

(3) Kremer JM, Joong KL. The safety and efficacy of the use of methotrexate in long-term therapy for rheumatoid arthritis. *Arthritis and Rheumatism* 1986; **29**:822–831.

Key message

This was the first double-blind trial of low-dose pulse methotrexate in RA to demonstrate efficacy. The size of the study provided sufficient power to detect a difference between the two treatments at the 5% significance level. One hundred and eighty-nine patients fulfilled the entry criteria, but only 110 completed the 18 weeks of therapy, 41 withdrawing from the placebo and 39 from methotrexate. Eighteen patients on methotrexate developed elevated liver enzymes and five developed mucosal ulcers. The study showed that 60% of patients were able to tolerate methotrexate but did identify an incidence of elevated liver function tests. Pancytopenia was also identified in two patients. The conclusion of the study was that methotrexate appeared to be effective in the treatment of RA, but did require close monitoring for toxicity.

Strengths

1. This is a carefully constructed prospective, controlled, double-blind multicentre study.
2. Sufficient power to demonstrates differences between placebo and methotrexate.

Weakness

In terms of a lifetime of RA, it is a relatively short-term study.

Relevance

Methotrexate is still one of the most commonly used anti-rheumatic drugs and its long-term efficacy seems to bear out the initial findings demonstrated by Williams, *et al.*

Paper 9

Termination of slow acting antirheumatic therapy in rheumatoid arthritis: a 14 year prospective evaluation of 1017 consecutive starts

Authors

Wolfe F, Hawley DJ, Cathey MA

Reference

Journal of Rheumatology 1990; **17**(8):994–1002

Summary

This paper provides a very careful review of the treatment outcome with over 1000 new administrations of slow acting anti-rheumatic drugs (SAARDs) in 671 patients followed over a 14 year period. The important observations from this study was the median time for discontinuation of drugs and the reason for that discontinuation. The median time for discontinuation for I.M. gold or auranofin, hydroxychloroquine or penicillamine was 2 years or less, but was over twice that (4.25 years) for methotrexate (Figure 26.5). More patients had to cease their therapy because of an adverse event than for lack of efficacy.

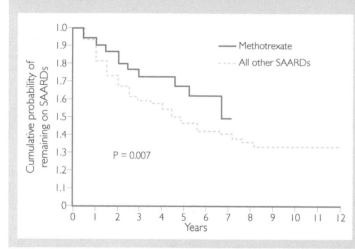

Figure 26.5 Product limit (Kaplan–Meier) cumulative survival analysis of terminations because of lack of efficacy. Cases terminated because of adverse reactions are excluded from this analysis. All other SAARD represent the combined group of I.M. gold, auranofin, hydroxychloroquine, and penicillamine. Difference in cumulative survival is significant at the 0.007 level (Mantel-Cox).

Related references (1) Jessop JD, O'Sullivan MM, Lewis PA, Williams LA, Camilleri JP, Plant MJ, Coles EC. A long-term five year randomized trial of hydroxychloroquine, sodium aurothiomiolate, auranofin and penicillamine in the treatment of patients with rheumatoid arthritis. *British Journal of Rheumatology* 1998; **37**:992–1002.

(2) Van de Putte LBA, Van Gestl AM, Van Riel PLCM. Early treatment of rheumatoid arthritis–rationale, evidence and implications. *Annals of Rheumatic Diseases* 1998; **57**:511–512.

(3) Egmose C, Lund V, Borg G, Petersson H, Berg B, Brodin U, Trang L. Patients with rheumatoid arthritis benefit from second line therapy–five year follow-up of a prospective, double-blind, placebo-controlled study. *Journal of Rheumatology* 1995; **22**:2208–2213.

Key message

Specific antirheumatic drugs are still used widely for the management of RA. Despite their usefulness, there has been growing concern about the side-effects of these agents and the relative efficacy of them. This study was made possible by the establishment and careful follow-up of a cohort of patients with RA who were started on a variety of slow-acting anti-rheumatic drugs over a period of some 14 years. In this study, 671 patients were commenced on 1017 SAARD starts. These patients were all followed at regular intervals and patients were only started once they had already received a second-line agent (this paper reports the history of a second slow-acting anti-rheumatic drug). Over the period of the study (1975–88) the type of drug varied with I.M. gold being commonly used initially, then penicillamine and finally, methotrexate. Those patients commenced on hydroxychloroquine and auranofin seemed to have milder disease while those on methotrexate and penicillamine were more likely to have increased levels of disability and a higher prednisolone dose. The major outcome of this study was the length of time that patients remained on a slow-acting antirheumatic therapy (Figure 26.6). Those patients on methotrexate remained on therapy for significantly longer than those patients on I.M. or oral gold, hydroxychloroquine, or penicillamine. The reasons for discontinuation included both adverse reactions and loss of efficacy. Discontinuation for adverse reactions was more common for all drugs than discontinuation for lack of efficacy, but those patients taking methotrexate remained on the drug for significantly longer periods of time than those on the other medications. Very few (6 of 580) terminations were for remission. The major reasons for drop-out were gastrointestinal and oral ulceration (on methotrexate), proteineuria (on I.M. gold), gastrointestinal (on auranofin) and haematological or renal reasons for penicillamine termination. Nearly a third of patients terminated therapy because of adverse reactions, while 10% of terminations were due to a lack of efficacy.

Strengths

1. The paper presented a significant number of patients followed for a very long time (14 years).
2. Provided practical data to assess and compare individual anti-rheumatic drugs, to assess efficacy and contrast agents.
3. Provided comparative data on side-effects.

Weaknesses

1. The study failed to identify any clear predictors of discontinuation.
2. There were significant differences in the patients treated with different drugs (such as disease duration which was significantly longer in those on methotrexate than those treated with gold), in the level of disability, and the dose of prednisolone. (Although these may have been compensated for somewhat by the large groups involved, they need to be taken into account in interpretation.)

Relevance

This paper demonstrated the importance of the development of long-term databases to investigate therapeutic advances in the management of RA.

Paper 10

Randomized double-blind comparison of chimeric monoclonal antibody to tumour necrosis factor alpha (cA2) versus placebo in rheumatoid arthritis

Authors

Elliott MJ, Maini RN, Feldmann M, Kalden JR, Antoni C, Smolen JS, Leeb B, Breedveld FC, Macfarlane JD, Bijl H, Woody JN

Reference

The Lancet 1994; **344**:1105–1110

Summary

This was the first study of a monoclonal antibody to tumour necrosis factor (TNF) used in a clinical trial. This randomized double-blind trial compared a single infusion of two doses (1 and 10 mg/kg cA2 with placebo) in 73 patients with active RA. At the end of week four using a Paulus 20% response, only four of 24 placebo recipients responded, while 11 of 25 treated with low-dose cA2 and 19 of 24 treated with high-dose cA2 fulfilled these criteria. These results provided the first good human evidence that specific cytokine blockade can be effective in RA.

Related references (1) Wallis WJ, Furst D, Strand V, Keystone E. Biologic agents in immuno-therapy in rheumatoid arthritis–progress and perspective. *Rheumatic Disease Clinics of North America* 1998;**3**:537–565.

(2) Choy EHS, Kingsley GH, Panayi GS. Monoclonal antibody therapy in rheumatoid arthritis. *British Journal of Rheumatology* 1998; **37**:484–490.

(3) Moreland LW, Baumgartner SW, Schiff MH, *et al.* Treatment of rheumatoid arthritis with a recombinant human tumor necrosis factor receptor (p75)–Fc fusion protein. *New England Journal of Medicine* 1997; **337**:141–147.

(4) Elliott MJ, Maini RN, Feldmann M, *et al.* Repeated therapy with monoclonal antibody to tumour necrosis factor (cA2) in patients with rheumatoid arthritis. *The Lancet* 1994; **344**:1125–1127.

Key message

This paper presents compelling clinical evidence that chimeric tumour necrosis alpha plays a significant role in inflammation in RA. The study was extremely carefully conducted, using two doses of TNF antibody and placebo in patients with RA. Significant reductions in clinical features of swollen and tender joint count, pain and overall disease activity were matched with reductions in C-reactive protein and ESR. Both clinical and laboratory parameters fell very rapidly within the first week and remained low (in the high-dose patients) over a period of 4 weeks. The primary endpoint of the study was the achievement in week four of a Paulus 20% response and this was achieved in 19 of 24 patients treated with high-dose. Using the more stringent 50% Paulus criteria, over half of the high-dose patients responded. One of the disappointing features of the study was the relatively short efficacy achieved, particularly with low-dose, with clinical parameters returning towards normal at the end of the 4 week treatment period. In this small study, minor side-effects were noted, although one patient developed pneumonia, which was signified as possibly treatment related.

Why it's important

This study, the first of a series, demonstrated that monoclonal antibodies are useful in suppressing pain and inflammation and defined a new direction for the treatment of RA.

Strength

This is the first study to demonstrate the efficacy of monoclonal antibodies in the treatment of RA.

Weaknesses

1. There were a relatively small number of patients in the study.
2. It was only continued for a 4 week observation period.

Relevance

This study provides one of the benchmarks for the management of RA with monoclonal antibodies.

CHAPTER 27

Exercise and rehabilitation in arthritis

Michael V Hurley

Introduction

This section summarizes important studies that investigated the role of muscle dysfunction and exercise in the management of patients with osteoarthritis (OA) and rheumatoid arthritis (RA). The studies have been placed in the context of the research at the time they were devised and published, and includes later work to show how the fields of research developed from these early studies. It may be surprising how recent most of these 'classic' papers are. The reason for this is that research interest and expertise have only relatively recently been developed in the field of rehabilitation. However, the findings from these studies demonstrate why and how patients with arthritis should exercise to limit the affects of arthritis.

The first two papers highlight why. They show the intimate, but usually disregarded, relationship between peri-articular muscles and intra-articular structures, and emphasize that synovial joints are better viewed as *functional units of movement* composed of bone, cartilage, nerves and muscles. Unfortunately we know very little about the arthritic changes that occur to muscle. Since reversing muscle dysfunction is the main aim of exercise, it is essential to know what changes occur to muscles and understand the implications of these changes, if we are to decide whether patients with arthritis should bother exercising at all. Several papers by Freeman and Wyke in the 1960s showed alteration of joint mechanoreceptors caused muscle sensoriomotor dysfunction (Paper 1), which has subsequently been shown to be associated with disability. The very recent paper by Slemenda, *et al.* (Paper 2) showed quadriceps weakness may precede knee joint damage, and challenges the normal assumption that arthritis causes muscle weakness, suggesting muscle dysfunction may cause arthritic damage.

Whether muscle dysfunction is a cause or a consequence of arthritis and results in disability, muscle is the most 'plastic' component of the functional unit of movement and can be manipulated relatively easily, therefore improving muscle function may ameliorate the effects of arthritis. Three papers demonstrate exercise can improve muscle function, decrease pain and increase function without exacerbating the condition. Minor, *et al.*'s paper (Paper 3) suggests specific, sophisticated exercise regimes may not be essential, but any form of increased physical activity is beneficial. In their paper Nordemar, *et al.* (Paper 5) showed that long-term exercise did not cause long-term damage as has been feared. The final paper by Chamberlain, *et al.* (Paper 4) demonstrates exercising at home is as effective as exercising under supervision in hospital outpatient departments, which improves the cost-effectiveness of exercise. It will also improve patients' adherence, which is important since the size of the patient population with arthritis is large and increasing. This paper also highlights the importance of continuing to exercise to maintain improvements attained during exercise and prevent patients regressing. Strategies need to be developed that will enable patients with arthritis to obtain and maintain benefits from exercise.

These 'classic' papers were not selected because they are definitive studies that are beyond reproach (they have design flaws that may have inflated their results): these papers are 'classics' because they were innovative and initiated new lines of enquiry. Scientifically rigorous studies must confirm their findings, and the regimes refined to enhance their effectiveness and assess their costs, so that effective, affordable, clinically applicable regimes can be implemented that will lead to better management of arthritis. These, however, will be variants of the foundations laid down by the pioneering studies described here.

Paper 1

Articular reflexes at the ankle joint: An electromyographic study of normal and abnormal influences of ankle-joint mechanoreceptors upon reflex activity in the leg muscles

Authors

Freeman MAR, Wyke B

Reference

Journal of Bone and Joint Surgery 1967b; **54**:990–1001

Summary

In up to 17 neurologically intact, lightly anaesthetized cats, passive limb movement and direct stimulation of articular mechanoreceptors and nociceptors altered the EMG activity of the muscles acting across the joint. Variations in discharge from slowly and rapidly adapting mechanoreceptors produced coordinated reflex changes in motor unit activity in limb muscles, increasing activity in some muscle groups and decreasing activity in others. Intra-articular injections of local anaesthetic abolished the articular reflexes by destruction of the articular mechanoreceptors or interruption of the afferent fibres.

Related references **(1)** De Andrade JR, Grant C, Dixon ASJ. Joint distension and reflex muscle inhibition in the knee. *Journal of Bone and Joint Surgery* 1965; **47**(A):313–322.

(2) Ferrell WR, Baxendale RH, Carnachan C, Hart IK. The influence of joint afferent discharge on locomotion, proprioception and activity in conscious cats. *Brain Research* 1985; **347**:41–48.

(3) Hurley M, Scott DL, Rees J, Newham DJ. Sensorimotor changes and functional performance in patients with knee osteoarthritis. *Annals of Rheumatic Diseases* 1997; **56**:641–648.

Key message

Discharge from articular mechanoreceptors contributes to posture and movement by reflex coordination of muscle tone. Alteration to the articular environment may alter discharge from the articular receptors resulting in abnormal posture and movement.

Why it's important

For some time articular receptors had been known to project to spinal and higher centres, and they were considered to be involved in the perception of posture and movement, but the role of articular receptors in the reflex control of muscle tone was unclear. This paper demonstrated articular mechanoreceptors were involved in the coordinated activity and control of muscles across the joint. It established a link between what happens in the articular environment and how this affects motor control via alpha-motor neurones and gamma-motor neurones. The intimate relationship between the joint and muscle activation and control confirmed the findings of other studies from around this time (1). In addition it established the important link between changes in the articular environment and the sensory function of muscle. This relationship suggests a synovial joint should be considered a functional unit comprised of the articular structures, neurones that innervate these structures and the muscles that acts across the joint, effecting movement and protecting the joint via neuromuscular protective mechanisms.

Alteration in motor control affecting posture and movement of conscious cats has been reported in later studies (2). More recently the link between arthritic joint damage and muscle sensorimotor dysfunction has gained increasing interest in terms of its consequences of knee OA on muscle strength, motor control and proprioceptive acuity (3).

Strength

Thorough methodology from experienced research group.

Weaknesses

1. Animal work.
2. Small numbers of animals.
3. Possibility that anaesthesia may be interfering with findings.

Relevance

This study reinforced the intimate physiological relationship between joints and muscles: arthritic damage of intra-articular structures will affect function of the peri-articular muscles, and muscle dysfunction (weakness or proprioceptive deficits) will impair neuromuscular protective mechanisms, exposing the joint to damage.

Paper 2

Quadriceps weakness and osteoarthritis of the knee

Authors

Slemenda C, Brandt KD, Heilman DK, Mazzuca S, Braunstein FM,
Katz BP, Wolinsky FD

Reference

Annals of Internal Medicine 1997; **127**:97–104

Summary

This cross-sectional study investigated the prevalence of muscle weakness, pain, function and
the extent of joint damage in 462 community-based volunteers aged 65 years and over. Joint
damage was assessed from radiographs taken of the knees, the Western Ontario and
MacMaster's University Index for OA knees (a disease-specific questionnaire) was used to
assess pain and function, knee extensor and flexor strength and the lower limb lean tissue
mass were measured. Quadriceps, but not hamstring, weakness was common, and was present in people who had normal lower limb muscle mass. In women with tibiofemoral OA
quadriceps weakness was evident even in the absence of pain. Quadriceps weakness was predictive of radiographic and symptomatic knee OA. Quadriceps weakness may be a risk factor
for knee pain, disability and the progression of joint damage.

Related references **(1)** Hurley M, Scott DL, Kees J, Newham DJ. Sensorimotor changes
and functional performance in patients with knee osteoarthri-
tis. *Annals of Rheumatic Diseases* 1997; **56**:641–648.

(2) McAlindon TE, Cooper C, Kirwan JR, Dieppe PA. Determinants of
disability in osteoarthritis of the knee. *Annals of Rheumatic
Diseases* 1993; **52**:258–262.

(3) Pai Y-C, Rymer, WZ, Chang RW, Sharma L. Effect of age and
osteoarthritis on knee proprioception. *Arthritis and Rheumatism*
1997; **40**:2260–2265.

Key message

Quadriceps weakness is common in patients with and without radiological evidence of knee
OA, and may be a factor in the aetiology of the condition.

Why it's important

Slemenda, *et al.*'s paper took an innovative look at the involvement of quadriceps muscle in knee OA by considering the mechanism through which quadriceps exercise could reduce the pain of knee OA. In their introduction and an accompanying editorial they highlighted how little research had been performed into the changes in muscle that occur in knee OA, and that the link between muscle weakness and knee pain was poorly understood. Using a large community population this paper confirmed other studies demonstrating that quadriceps weakness is a common finding, which is associated with knee OA and disability (1, 2). It also showed that people with weak muscles had normal muscle mass suggesting the cause of the weakness was due to muscle dysfunction rather than atrophy. But the most important aspect of the paper was its proposal that muscle weakness preceded and predicted radiological damage, thus muscle dysfunction might be a factor in the aetiology of knee joint disease. They suggest this may occur by impairment of neuromuscular protective mechanisms that play a vital role in shock absorption during gait. The role of muscle in arthritis is currently gaining much more research attention (1, 3). Improving muscle function may be a strategy for retarding or preventing the progression of joint damage.

Strengths

1. Large representative community population.
2. Well designed, well written report.

Weaknesses

1. Small numbers in some sub-groups limit the inferences that can be drawn from the joint compartments affected.
2. Cross-sectional study, therefore what happens over time cannot be assessed.

Relevance

It was an innovative view of the role of quadriceps weakness in patients with knee OA. There was a lamentable lack of research and understanding of the role muscles might play in the cause and treatment of arthritis. The findings implicated muscle weakness as a factor in the aetiology of knee OA. Since muscle is a very 'plastic' tissue, rehabilitation that improves muscle function may be a strategy in the primary or secondary prevention of joint damage.

Paper 3

Efficacy of physical conditioning exercise in patients with rheumatoid arthritis and osteoarthritis

Authors

Minor M, Hewett J, Webel R, Anderson S, Kay D

Reference

Arthritis and Rheumatism 1989; **32**:1396–1405

Summary

One hundred and twenty patients with symptomatic RA (n = 40) or OA (n = 80) in weight-bearing joints were recruited and baseline assessment of their aerobic capacity, exercise endurance, clinical disease activity, objective tests of functional performance, and the physical and psychological impact of arthritis were performed. The patients were randomized into one of three exercises groups: (a) a land-based walking programme, (b) a pool-based exercises programme, or (c) range of motion exercise. Groups (a) and (b) had an aerobic component to see if the programmes increased aerobic fitness, and group (c) had no aerobic component and acted as a control group. All the participants took part in supervised exercises for 1 hour per week for 12 weeks. After 12 weeks the assessments were repeated, and the patients were recalled for follow-up assessment 6 and 12 months from baseline. Immediately following exercise, aerobic capacity and objective and subjective variables improved in both aerobically exercising groups compared to control group, without exacerbation of disease activity. At 12 month follow-up, 50–60% of the participants of all the groups reported performing more than 60 minutes of physical activity (e.g. formal exercise, household or gardening activities). The improvements of the aerobic exercise groups had been maintained, but in addition the aerobic fitness of the control group had also improved and there were now few differences between the aerobically exercised groups and the control group.

Related references (1) Fisher NM, Gresham GE, Abrams M, Hicks J, Horrigan D, Pendergast DR. Quantitative effects of physical therapy on muscular and functional performance in subjects with osteoarthritis of the knees. *Archives of Physical Medicine and Rehabilitation* 1993; **74**:840–847.

(2) Hurley MV, Scott DL. Improvements in quadriceps sensorimotor function and disability of patients with knee osteoarthritis following a clinically practicable exercise regime. *British Journal of Rheumatology* 1998; **37**:1181–1187.

Key message

Exercise in RA and OA is effective.

Why it's important

This study was instigated because the advantages of regular activity and the dangers of inactivity were well known, but there was concern about advising arthritic patients to exercise because the benefits and risks of exercise for arthritis were contentious. Some studies had shown exercise for arthritis was effective and safe, but these usually involved too few patients and were poorly designed. This relatively large randomized controlled trial showed exercise for arthritis was efficacious and did not exacerbate disease activity in the short/medium-term.

An interesting but unexpected finding was the delayed improvement in aerobic capacity in the control group. The authors hypothesize this may indicate that habitual performance of any form of physical activity is more important than a specific exercise regime. Later reports confirmed that long-term exercise in RA was safe (Paper 4), and studies of OA also showed exercise was beneficial (1). However, although these research regimes were efficacious they were prolonged and labour intensive, making them difficult, very expensive to implement clinically, and have poor patient adherence. Recently exercise regimes have been devised that are shorter but just as effective and safe, and clinically are more practicable (2).

Strengths

1. Randomized controlled trial.
2. Relatively large sample size for the initial intervention part.

Weaknesses

1. Incomplete follow-up due to the drop-out rate, this will decrease the statistical power of the study at 12 month follow-up, and volunteer bias of those that remained in the study will exaggerate these findings.
2. It is unclear how well the self-report exercise habits were verified.
3. From the report the actual method of randomization is unclear, whether an intention-to-treat analysis was used, and whether the evaluators were blind to the interventions, and if the patients were aware of the aim of the study.
4. The alpha-level was set at <0.05, but as no primary outcome variable was stated *a priori* and many variables are reported, the chances of a type II statistical error increases.

Relevance

In spite of the limitations of some aspects of design and omissions in the report this study demonstrated exercise for arthritis is efficacious and safe, and that if patients remained physically active these benefits are maintained. Furthermore these benefits could be attained irrespective of the type of activities that are performed, so patients could benefit from formal exercises or with routine common activities of daily living, which will improve the likelihood of patient adherence.

Paper 4

Physiotherapy in osteoarthritis of the knee.
A controlled trial of hospital versus home exercises

Authors

Chamberlain MA, Care G, Harfield B

Reference

International Journal of Rehabilitation Medicine 1982; **4**:101–106

Summary

Forty-two patients with radiographic and clinical evidence of knee OA had their pain, function, range of movement, ability to lift weights and endurance assessed before and after a rehabilitation regime. They were randomly allocated to receive either: (a) 12 sessions of short wave diathermy and supervised exercise (three times a week for 4 weeks) in an outpatient department and daily home exercises to be performed twice a day; or (b) three supervised sessions of the same exercises in the outpatient department and twice daily home exercises. Both the groups were then discharged with the same advice to perform the exercises daily at home and asked to record their exercise in an 'exercise diary'. Some patients (regardless of whether they were in group (a) or (b)) were told they would be recalled for re-assessment after 12 weeks, while others were not told they would be recalled. Initially pain decreased and function increased by similar amounts in groups (a) and (b). At 12 week re-assessment, 10/14 patients who had been informed in advance they would be re-assessed continued to exercise, and the improvements attained during the initial training phase of the study had been maintained. Only 2/15 patients who were not told they would be re-assessed had continued to exercise, and their improvements in pain and function attained during the initial phase of the study had been lost.

Related references **(1)** Green J, McKenna F, Redfern FJ, Chamberlain MA. Home exercises are as effective as outpatient hydrotherapy for osteoarthritis of the hip. *British Journal of Rheumatology* 1993; **32**:812–815.

(2) O'Reilly S, Muir K, Doherty M. Effectiveness of home exercises on pain and disability from osteoarthritis of the knee: a randomized controlled trial. *Annals of Rheumatic Diseases* 1999; **58**:15–19.

Key message

Simple daily exercises performed at home or in hospital improved pain and function in these patients. These benefits were maintained if the patients continued exercising.

Why it's important

The study was prompted by the length of time physiotherapists spent teaching exercise to large numbers of patients with knee OA, without any good indication that this use of resources was beneficial. A pilot study had suggested with adequate advise home exercises were as effective as supervised hospital treatment. This was borne out in the larger study described above. Several studies were beginning to show the efficacy of exercise in arthritis, but these regimes were prolonged and usually necessitated outpatient treatment. Home exercises are arguably more useful because they avert the need for outpatient treatment which will improve adherence to exercise regimes and cost-effectiveness.

It is also important because the size of the patient population with knee OA is so large, resources are not available to enable them to be treated in outpatient departments. The effectiveness of home exercise has been confirmed in a later study of hydrotherapy for hip OA by the same research group (1), and in a recent larger study of knee OA (2). The study also demonstrated that adherence with a regular home exercise programme can be improved by ensuring patients can perform a simple exercise regime effectively and safely, giving the patients written instructions, and reinforcing the importance of exercise with a diary and follow-up appointment.

Strength

Randomized and blind evaluation.

Weaknesses

1. In some aspects the design and reporting of the study was poor: only one reference cited, the randomization was poorly described, the presentation of the results makes it difficult to assess the size of the changes to enable determining of whether the results were clinically meaningful as well as statistically significant.
2. Some of the objective outcome measures may be inappropriate, invalid and insensitive.
3. Patient numbers were small.

Relevance

Exercise can effectively alleviate the cardinal symptoms of knee OA (pain and disability), but because of limited resources and the size of the patient population long-term hospital outpatient treatment is not feasible. This study demonstrated that home exercise can be just as effective as supervised hospital treatment, cheaper and that relatively simple strategies can be employed to improve adherence so that the exercise and hence the benefits can be maintain in the longer term.

Paper 5

Physical training in rheumatoid arthritis: a controlled long-term study

Authors

Nordemar R, Ekblom B, Zachrisson L, Lundqvist K

Reference

Scandinavian Journal of Rheumatology 1981; **10**:17–30

Summary

In 23 patients with RA the effects of long-term exercising were observed and compared with a control group (n = 23) who did not undergo regular exercise. Initially training consisted of supervised outpatient group exercise, followed by discharge with a static exercise bike for use at home, but over time other recreational exercise activities were encouraged, e.g. swimming, golf, cycling or walking. The patients were followed regularly over 4–8 years, and during this time the training group showed less progress in joint degeneration, better physiological tests, improved clinical variables, reported less sick leave or hospitalized time, and better disease outcomes than the control patients who did not exercise.

Related references (1) Stenstrom C, Lindell B, Swanberg P, Harms-Ringdahl K, Nordemar R. Intensive dynamic training in water for rheumatoid arthritis functional class II: A long term study of effects. *Scandinavian Journal of Rheumatology* 991; **20**:358–365.

(2) Van den Ende CHM, Vliet Vlieland TPM, Munneke M, Hazes JMW. Dynamic exercise therapy in rheumatic arthritis: a systematic review. *British Journal of Rheumatology* 1998, **37**:677–687.

(3) Bearne LM, Scott DL, Hurley MV. Exercise does not increase clinical disease activity measures or plasma pro-inflammatory cytokines in rheumatoid arthritis. *Arthritis and Rheumatism* 1999; **42**(suppl.):530.

Key message

Exercise does not exacerbate disease and may improve some of the effects of the disease. Long-term physical activity is not detrimental to the joints of people affected by RA, inactivity can be.

Why it's important

There had been much controversy as to whether exercise was good or detrimental for patients with inflammatory arthritis. Exercise was considered beneficial for the health of the muscles, articular structures and the patient's general health, but it was argued that exercising inflamed joints might increase pain and cause persistent inflammation and joint damage. In clinical practice exercise of patients with well-controlled RA had shown the benefits of exercise. This paper, and a later study by the group (1) confirmed exercise improved objective and subjective variables affected by the disease, increased function, with possible economic benefits. Although the patients were at risk from injury, this risk was no greater than other populations, and the benefits are likely to outweigh these risks.

A recent systematic review supports the benefits of dynamic exercise in patients with RA (2), and in addition more evidence is accruing showing that neither clinical nor biochemical (plasma concentration of pro-inflammatory cytokines) measures of disease activity are increased by exercise (3). These reports refute the theoretical arguments that exercise in RA is dangerous.

Strength

Longitudinal cohort study.

Weaknesses

1. Methodological deficits (lack of randomization, blinding, probability of strong influence of volunteer bias) will have inflated some of the positive results of the study.
2. Training regime was not well described and varied from 4–8 years, with a mean of 5.4 years.
3. Relatively small patient numbers.

Relevance

If exercise is effective it must be performed regularly or the benefits will be lost. Fears that long-term exercise may accelerate joint damage in inflammatory joint conditions appear to be unfounded. Effective exercise for RA can be performed over a period of time without fear of joint destruction.

INDEX

Classic Papers by chapter

5 Clinical genetics

6 Rheumatoid arthritis

7 Chronic arthritis in children

8 Ankylosing spondylitis

9 Psoriatic arthritis

25 Education

26 Key drug developments

27 Exercise and rehabilitation in arthritis

Classic Papers by title

T - #0055 - 101024 - C464 - 279/191/25 [27] - CB - 9781901865486 - Gloss Lamination